Hemorrhagic Stroke: Pathophysiology and Interventions

Hemorrhagic Stroke: Pathophysiology and Interventions

Edited by Daniella Riggs

hayle
medical

New York

Hayle Medical,
750 Third Avenue, 9ᵗʰ Floor,
New York, NY 10017, USA

Visit us on the World Wide Web at:
www.haylemedical.com

ISBN: 978-1-63241-629-2

Cataloging-in-Publication Data

Hemorrhagic stroke : pathophysiology and interventions / edited by Daniella Riggs.
    p. cm.
Includes bibliographical references and index.
ISBN 978-1-63241-629-2
1. Brain--Hemorrhage. 2. Brain--Pathophysiology. 3. Brain--Diseases. I. Riggs, Daniella.
RC394.H37 H46 2019
616.81--dc23

Table of Contents

Preface...VII

Chapter 1 **Relationship between plasma high mobility group box-1 protein levels and clinical outcomes of aneurysmal subarachnoid hemorrhage**.................................1
Xiang-Dong Zhu, Jing-Sen Chen, Feng Zhou, Qi-Chang Liu, Gao Chen and Jian-Min Zhang

Chapter 2 **Augmented expression of TSPO after intracerebral hemorrhage: a role in inflammation?**...13
Frederick Bonsack IV, Cargill H. Alleyne Jr and Sangeetha Sukumari-Ramesh

Chapter 3 **Nuclear factor-κB activation in perihematomal brain tissue correlates with outcome in patients with intracerebral hemorrhage**.................................27
Ze-Li Zhang, Yu-Guang Liu, Qi-Bing Huang, Hong-Wei Wang, Yan Song, Zhen-Kuan Xu and Feng Li

Chapter 4 **The role of microglia and the TLR4 pathway in neuronal apoptosis and vasospasm after subarachnoid hemorrhage**...34
Khalid A Hanafy

Chapter 5 **The inhibitory effect of mesenchymal stem cell on blood–brain barrier disruption following intracerebral hemorrhage in rats: contribution of TSG-6**.................44
Min Chen, Xifeng Li, Xin Zhang, Xuying He, Lingfeng Lai, Yanchao Liu, Guohui Zhu, Wei Li, Hui Li, Qinrui Fang, Zequn Wang and Chuanzhi Duan

Chapter 6 **Roles of programmed death protein 1/programmed death-ligand 1 in secondary brain injury after intracerebral haemorrhage in rats: selective modulation of microglia polarization to anti-inflammatory phenotype**.................................58
Jie Wu, Liang Sun, Haiying Li, Haitao Shen, Weiwei Zhai, Zhengquan Yu and Gang Chen

Chapter 7 **Dimethylarginines in patients with intracerebral hemorrhage: association with outcome, hematoma enlargement, and edema**...71
Hans Worthmann, Na Li, Jens Martens-Lobenhoffer, Meike Dirks, Ramona Schuppner, Ralf Lichtinghagen, Jan T.Kielstein, Peter Raab, Heinrich Lanfermann, Stefanie M. Bode-Böger and Karin Weissenborn

Chapter 8 **Isoliquiritigenin alleviates early brain injury after experimental intracerebral hemorrhage via suppressing ROS- and/or NF-κB-mediated NLRP3 inflammasome activation by promoting Nrf2 antioxidant pathway**...79
Jun Zeng, Yizhao Chen, Rui Ding, Liang Feng, Zhenghao Fu, Shuo Yang, Xinqing Deng, Zhichong Xie and Shizhong Zheng

Chapter 9 **P2X7R blockade prevents NLRP3 inflammasome activation and brain injury in a rat model of intracerebral hemorrhage: involvement of peroxynitrite**...98
Liang Feng, Yizhao Chen, Rui Ding, Zhenghao Fu, Shuo Yang, Xinqing Deng and Jun Zeng

Chapter 10   **Endogenous hydrogen sulphide attenuates NLRP3 inflammasome-mediated neuroinflammation by suppressing the P2X7 receptor after intracerebral haemorrhage in rats**..115
Hengli Zhao, Pengyu Pan, Yang Yang, Hongfei Ge, Weixiang Chen, Jie Qu, Jiantao Shi, Gaoyu Cui, Xin Liu, Hua Feng and Yujie Chen

Chapter 11   **Deletion of the hemopexin or heme oxygenase-2 gene aggravates brain injury following stroma-free hemoglobin-induced intracerebral hemorrhage**..133
Bo Ma, Jason Patrick Day, Harrison Phillips, Bryan Slootsky, Emanuela Tolosano and Sylvain Doré

Chapter 12   **Neutrophil to lymphocyte ratio predicts intracranial hemorrhage after endovascular thrombectomy in acute ischemic stroke**..145
Slaven Pikija, Laszlo K. Sztriha, Monika Killer-Oberpfalzer, Friedrich Weymayr, Constantin Hecker, Christian Ramesmayer, Larissa Hauer and Johann Sellner

Chapter 13   **Treatment with TO901317, a synthetic liver X receptor agonist, reduces brain damage and attenuates neuroinflammation in experimental intracerebral hemorrhage**...152
Chun-Hu Wu, Chien-Cheng Chen, Chai-You Lai, Tai-Ho Hung, Chao-Chang Lin, Min Chao and Szu-Fu Chen

Chapter 14   **Heme oxygenase-1-mediated neuroprotection in subarachnoid hemorrhage via intracerebroventricular deferoxamine**..169
Robert H. LeBlanc III, Ruiya Chen, Magdy H. Selim and Khalid A. Hanafy

Chapter 15   **Toll-like receptor 4 signaling in intracerebral hemorrhage-induced inflammation and injury**..184
Huang Fang, Peng-Fei Wang, Yu Zhou, Yan-Chun Wang and Qing-Wu Yang

Permissions

List of Contributors

Index

Preface

Hemorrhagic stroke is a medical condition, which results in cell death in the brain due to poor blood flow. The blood flow is affected by some sort of bleeding and can affect the functioning of the brain. Dizziness, inability to move, problems in speaking, inability to feel one side of the body and loss of vision to one side are some of the major symptoms of a stroke. There are two primary categories of hemorrhagic stroke, namely, intracerebral hemorrhage and subarachnoid hemorrhage. Intracerebral hemorrhage refers to the internal bleeding of the brain caused by bleeding within the brain tissue or ventricular system. Subarachnoid hemorrhage refers to the bleeding outside the tissues of the brain but within the skull. This book aims to shed light on some of the unexplored aspects of hemorrhagic stroke. It strives to provide a fair idea about the pathophysiology and interventions related to this medical condition. The case studies included in this book will serve as an excellent guide to develop a comprehensive understanding.

All of the data presented henceforth, was collaborated in the wake of recent advancements in the field. The aim of this book is to present the diversified developments from across the globe in a comprehensible manner. The opinions expressed in each chapter belong solely to the contributing authors. Their interpretations of the topics are the integral part of this book, which I have carefully compiled for a better understanding of the readers.

At the end, I would like to thank all those who dedicated their time and efforts for the successful completion of this book. I also wish to convey my gratitude towards my friends and family who supported me at every step.

Editor

Relationship between plasma high mobility group box-1 protein levels and clinical outcomes of aneurysmal subarachnoid hemorrhage

Xiang-Dong Zhu[*], Jing-Sen Chen, Feng Zhou, Qi-Chang Liu, Gao Chen and Jian-Min Zhang

Abstract

Background: High-mobility group box 1 (HMGB1), originally described as a nuclear protein that binds to and modifies DNA, is now regarded as a central mediator of inflammation by acting as a cytokine. However, the association of HMGB1 in the peripheral blood with disease outcome and cerebrovasospasm has not been examined in patients with aneurysmal subarachnoid hemorrhage.

Methods: In this study, 303 consecutive patients were included. Upon admission, plasma HMGB1 levels were measured by ELISA. The end points were mortality after 1 year, in-hospital mortality, cerebrovasospasm and poor functional outcome (Glasgow Outcome Scale score of 1 to 3) after 1 year.

Results: Upon admission, the plasma HMGB1 level in patients was statistically significantly higher than that in healthy controls. A multivariate analysis showed that the plasma HMGB1 level was an independent predictor of poor functional outcome and mortality after 1 year, in-hospital mortality and cerebrovasospasm. A receiver operating characteristic curve showed that plasma HMGB1 level on admission statistically significantly predicted poor functional outcome and mortality after 1 year, in-hospital mortality and cerebrovasospasm of patients. The area under the curve of the HMGB1 concentration was similar to those of World Federation of Neurological Surgeons (WFNS) score and modified Fisher score for the prediction of poor functional outcome and mortality after 1 year, and in-hospital mortality, but not for the prediction of cerebrovasospasm. In a combined logistic-regression model, HMGB1 improved the area under the curve of WFNS score and modified Fisher score for the prediction of poor functional outcome after 1 year, but not for the prediction of mortality after 1 year, in-hospital mortality, or cerebrovasospasm.

Conclusions: HMGB1 level is a useful, complementary tool to predict functional outcome and mortality after aneurysmal subarachnoid hemorrhage. However, HMGB1 determination does not add to the accuracy of prediction of the clinical outcomes.

Keywords: Aneurysmal subarachnoid hemorrhage, Cerebrovasospasm, Functional outcome, High-mobility group box 1, Mortality

* Correspondence: hzzhuxiangdong@163.com
Department of Neurosurgery, The Second Affiliated Hospital, School of
Medicine, Zhejiang University, 88 Jiefang Road, Hangzhou 310000, PR China

Background

Subarachnoid hemorrhage (SAH) following cerebral aneurysm rupture is associated with high rates of morbidity and mortality [1]. Early prognostication of the risk of death or of a poor long-term outcome would enable optimized care and improved allocation of health-care resources. Several scales of outcome prediction, including the World Federation of Neurological Surgeons (WFNS) score [2] and Fisher score [3], are known to be associated with poor clinical outcomes. However, a readily measurable predictive marker predicting clinical outcomes in patients with SAH would be helpful for early prognostication and risk stratification, and is attracting increasing attention as a potential predictor of outcome in SAH [4].

High-mobility group box 1 (HMGB1) is constitutively expressed in the nuclei of eukaryotic cells. It belongs to a family of high mobility group nuclear proteins that were described in the 1970s as gene regulators that bind to and change the configuration of DNA [5,6]. It later became evident that HMGB1 is actively secreted from cells, has cytokine activities and is a late mediator of endotoxin lethality in mice [7]. Passive release of HMGB1 from necrotic cells also triggers inflammation [8]. Receptors for HMGB1 signaling include receptors for advanced glycation end-products and Toll-like receptors. HMGB1 is a central actor in the inflammatory network because it is induced by a number of cytokines and itself induces a series of inflammatory reactions [9-12].

HMGB1 is widely expressed in various tissues, including the brain [13-15]. The local extracellular accumulation of this cytokine in the brain, as a result of its intracerebroventricular administration or its release from dying neurons during cerebral ischemia, elicits local inflammatory events in mice [16-18]. Moreover, HMGB1 also promotes neuroinflammation in postischemic rat brain [17] and in the neurodegenerative processes associated with Alzheimer's disease [19,20]. Taken together, HMGB1 behaves as a typical immunoregulatory cytokine by promoting astrocyte activation and thus the production of a potent mixture of bioactive protein factors involved in inflammatory/immune responses in the brain [21].

HMGB1 is increased in the cerebrospinal fluid from meningitis patients [22] and in the serum of cerebral ischemia patients [23]. Recent data have identified HMGB1 in the cerebrospinal fluid as a potential biomarker of neurological outcome following SAH in humans [24,25], suggesting HMGB1 may represent a marker of neurological injury. However, no published information exists to date about the association between HMGB1 in the peripheral blood and disease outcome and cerebrovasospasm after SAH. The present study aimed to investigate the ability of plasma HMGB1 to

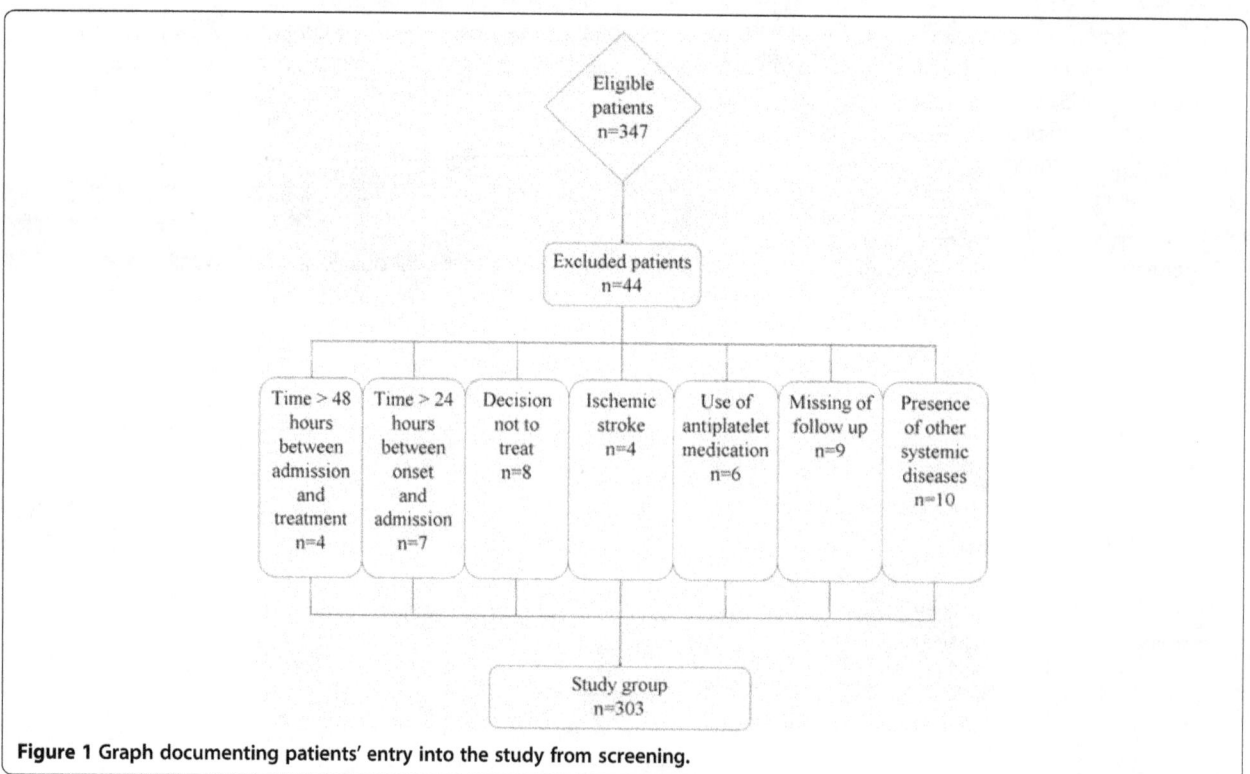

Figure 1 Graph documenting patients' entry into the study from screening.

Table 1 The characteristics for 303 patients

Characteristic	
Sex (male/female)	131/172
Age (years)	43.9 ± 12.4
World Federation of Neurological Surgeons score on admission	2.3 ± 1.2
Modified Fisher score on admission	2.7 ± 1.0
Aneurysmal location	
Posterior communication artery	83 (27.4%)
Internal carotid artery	43 (14.2%)
Anterior communication artery	66 (21.8%)
Middle cerebral artery	45 (14.9%)
Anterior cerebral artery	35 (11.6%)
Posterior cerebral artery	23 (7.6%)
Vertebral artery	8 (2.6%)
Surgery	186 (61.4%)
Aneurysmal size (mm)	7.2 ± 4.9
Rebleeding	16 (5.3%)
Acute hydrocephalus	90 (29.7%)
Intracerebral hemorrhage	39 (12.9%)
Intraventricular hemorrhage	72 (23.8%)
External ventricular drain	109 (36.0%)
Angiographic vasospasm	131 (43.2%)
Computed tomography ischemia	50 (16.5%)
Admission time (hours)	4.7 ± 3.6
Plasma-sampling time (hours)	6.7 ± 4.4
Seizure	44 (14.5%)
Plasma C-reactive protein level (mg/L)	7.1 ± 2.7
plasma D-dimer level (mg/L)	2.1 ± 0.9
Plasma HMGB1 level (ng/mL)	8.5 ± 3.6

Numerical variables were presented as mean ± standard deviation. Categorical variables were expressed as counts (percentage). HMGB1, high mobility group box-1.

predict the disease outcome and cerebrovasospasm in patients with aneurysmal SAH.

Subjects and methods

Study population

Between July 2008 and March 2010, all patients with aneurysmal SAH confirmed by computerized tomography (CT) angiography with or without digital subtraction angiography who were admitted to the Department of Neurosurgery, Second Affiliated Hospital, School of Medicine, Zhejiang University were evaluated in the study. Inclusion criteria were clinical history of SAH within the last 24 hours before admission and the treatment by surgery or coiling within the 48 hours after admission. Exclusion criteria were age less than 18 years, existing previous head trauma, neurological diseases

including ischemic or hemorrhagic stroke, use of antiplatelet or anticoagulant medication, and presence of other prior systemic diseases including uremia, liver cirrhosis, malignancy, chronic heart or lung disease, diabetes mellitus and hypertension.

A control group consisted of 150 healthy subjects without existing previous head trauma, neurological diseases including ischemic or hemorrhagic stroke, use of antiplatelet or anticoagulant medication, and presence of other prior systemic diseases including uremia, liver cirrhosis, malignancy, chronic heart or lung disease, diabetes mellitus and hypertension.

Table 2 The factors associated with 1-year mortality

	Non-survivors	Survivors	P value
	(n = 42)	(n = 261)	
Sex (male/female)	18/24	113/148	0.958
Age (years)	45.4 ± 13.4	43.6 ± 12.2	0.389
WFNS score on admission	4.0 ± 0.7	2.1 ± 1.0	<0.001
Modified Fisher score on admission	4.2 ± 0.6	2.5 ± 0.8	<0.001
Aneurysmal location			0.614
Posterior communication artery	8 (19.0%)	75 (28.7%)	
Internal carotid artery	6 (14.3%)	37 (14.2%)	
Anterior communication artery	9 (21.4%)	57 (21.8%)	
Middle cerebral artery	7 (16.7%)	38 (14.6%)	
Anterior cerebral artery	6 (14.3%)	29 (11.1%)	
Posterior cerebral artery	4 (9.5%)	19 (7.3%)	
Vertebral artery	2 (4.8%)	6 (2.3%)	
Surgery	21 (50.0%)	165 (63.2%)	0.102
Aneurysmal size (mm)	11.1 ± 5.3	6.6 ± 4.5	<0.001
Rebleeding	10 (23.8%)	6 (2.3%)	<0.001
Acute hydrocephalus	25 (59.5%)	65 (24.9%)	0.001
Intracerebral hemorrhage	19 (45.2%)	20 (7.7%)	<0.001
Intraventricular hemorrhage	37 (88.1%)	35 (13.4%)	<0.001
External ventricular drain	38 (90.5%)	71 (27.2%)	<0.001
Angiographic vasospasm	38 (90.5%)	93 (35.6%)	<0.001
Computed tomography ischemia	18 (42.9%)	32 (12.3%)	<0.001
Admission time (hours)	5.5 ± 4.4	4.6 ± 3.5	0.128
Seizure	9 (21.4%)	35 (13.4%)	0.171
Plasma C-reactive protein level (mg/L)	8.7 ± 3.3	6.9 ± 2.6	<0.001
plasma D-dimer level (mg/L)	2.4 ± 1.0	2.0 ± 1.0	0.015
Plasma HMGB1 level (ng/mL)	12.7 ± 3.2	7.9 ± 3.2	<0.001

Numerical variables are presented as mean ± standard deviation. Categorical variables are expressed as counts (percentage). Numerical variables were analyzed by Mann–Whitney U-test or unpaired Student t test. Categorical variables were analyzed by chi-square test or Fisher exact test. HMGB1, high mobility group box-1; n, number of patients; WFNS, World Federation of Neurological Surgeons.

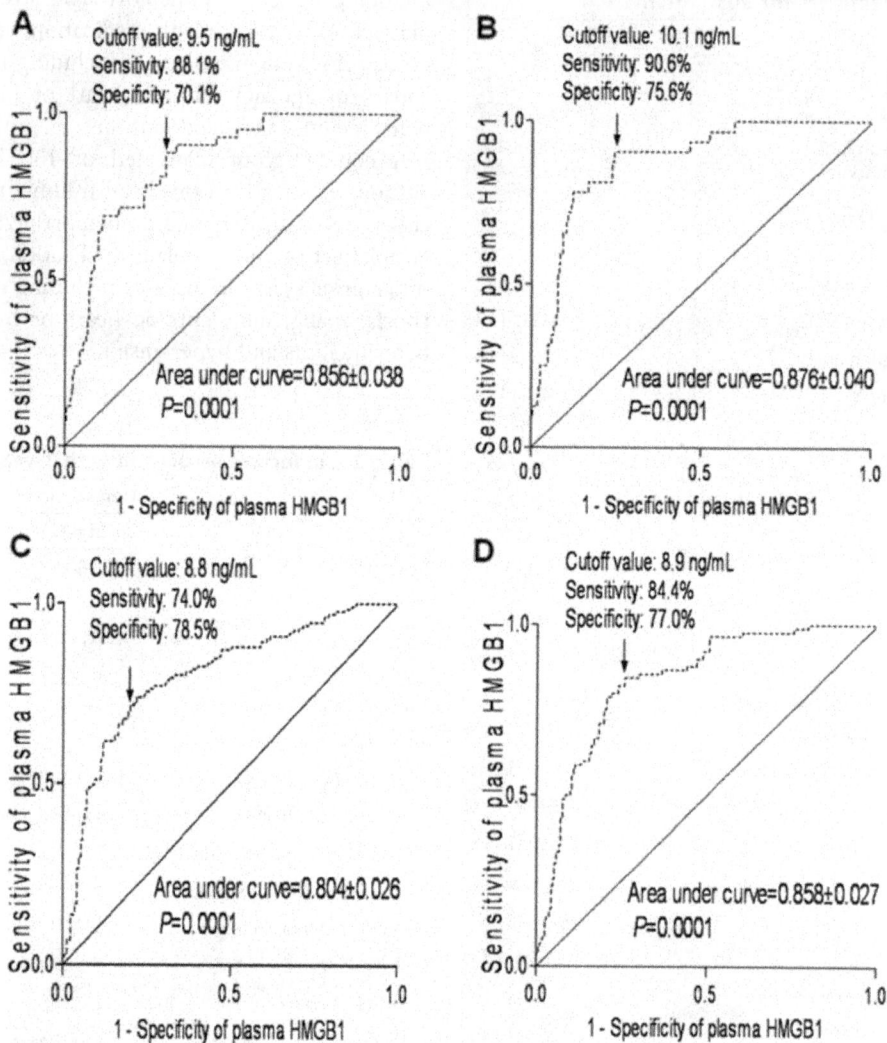

Figure 2 Graph showing receiver operating characteristic curve analysis of plasma high mobility group box-1 (HMGB1) level for (A) 1-year mortality, (B) in-hospital mortality, (C) cerebrovasospasm and (D) 1-year poor functional outcome.

Table 3 Receiver operating characteristic curve analysis of factors predicting the 1-year mortality among 303 patients

	HMGB1	WFNS score	Modified Fisher score
Criterion	>9.5 ng/mL	>3	>3
Area under curve	0.856	0.920	0.927
95% confidence interval	0.812 to 0.894	0.884 to 0.948	0.892 to 0.954
Sensitivity	88.1	78.6	88.1
95% confidence interval	74.4 to 96.0	63.2 to 89.7	74.4 to 96.0
Specificity	70.1	90.4	86.6
95% confidence interval	64.2 to 75.6	86.2 to 93.7	81.8 to 90.5
+ likelihood ratio	2.95	8.20	6.57
95% confidence interval	2.6 to 3.4	7.0 to 9.7	5.8 to 7.4
- likelihood ratio	0.17	0.24	0.14
95% confidence interval	0.07 to 0.4	0.1 to 0.5	0.06 to 0.3
P value	Reference	0.106	0.100

HMGB1, high mobility group box-1; WFNS, World Federation of Neurological Surgeons.

Table 4 The factors associated with in-hospital mortality

	Non-survivors (n = 32)	Survivors (n = 271)	P value
Sex (male/female)	12/20	119/152	0.489
Age (years)	45.4 ± 12.9	43.7 ± 12.3	0.469
WFNS score on admission	3.9 ± 0.7	2.2 ± 1.1	<0.001
Modified Fisher score on admission	4.3 ± 0.6	2.6 ± 0.8	<0.001
Aneurysmal location			0.599
Posterior communication artery	5 (15.6%)	78 (28.8%)	
Internal carotid artery	6 (18.8%)	37 (13.7%)	
Anterior communication artery	8 (25.0%)	58 (21.4%)	
Middle cerebral artery	4 (12.5%)	41 (15.1%)	
Anterior cerebral artery	4 (12.5%)	31 (11.4%)	
Posterior cerebral artery	3 (9.4%)	20 (7.4%)	
Vertebral artery	2 (6.3%)	6 (2.2%)	
Surgery	17 (53.1%)	169 (62.4%)	0.310
Aneurysmal size (mm)	11.9 ± 5.1	6.7 ± 4.5	<0.001
Rebleeding	6 (18.8%)	10 (3.7%)	<0.001
Acute hydrocephalus	19 (59.4%)	71 (26.2%)	<0.001
Intracerebral hemorrhage	15 (46.9%)	24 (8.9%)	<0.001
Intraventricular hemorrhage	31 (96.9%)	41 (15.1%)	<0.001
External ventricular drain	30 (93.8%)	79 (29.2%)	<0.001
Angiographic vasospasm	30 (93.8%)	101 (37.3%)	<0.001
Computed tomography ischemia	16 (50.0%)	34 (12.6%)	<0.001
Admission time (hours)	5.4 ± 4.2	4.6 ± 3.6	0.276
Seizure	7 (21.9%)	37 (13.7%)	0.212
Plasma C-reactive protein level (mg/L)	9.0 ± 3.2	6.9 ± 2.6	<0.001
plasma D-dimer level (mg/L)	2.4 ± 1.1	2.0 ± 1.0	0.045
Plasma HMGB1 level (ng/mL)	13.1 ± 3.1	8.0 ± 3.2	<0.001

Numerical variables are presented as mean ± standard deviation. Categorical variables are expressed as counts (percentage). Numerical variables were analyzed by Mann–Whitney U-test or unpaired Student t test. Categorical variables were analyzed by chi-square test or Fisher exact test. HMGB1, high mobility group box-1; n, number of patients; WFNS, World Federation of Neurological Surgeons.

Written informed consent to participate in the study was obtained from the subjects or their relatives. This protocol was approved by the Ethics Committee of The Second Affiliated Hospital, School of Medicine, Zhejiang University before implementation.

Clinical and radiological assessment

On arrival at the emergency department, a detailed history of vascular risk factors, concomitant medication, Glasgow Coma Scale (GCS) score, body temperature, heart rate, respiratory rate and blood pressure were taken. At admission, clinical severity was assessed using WFNS score [2]. The initial CT was classified according to the modified Fisher score [3]. All CT scans were performed according to the neuroradiology department protocol. Investigators who read them were blinded to clinical information.

Patient management

The type of treatment (surgery or coiling) was decided according to both location and size of the aneurysm by the neurosurgeon and the neuroradiologist. All patients received intravenous nimodipine at a dose of 2 mg/hour from admission until at least day 14, except during periods of uncontrolled increased intracranial pressure during which intravenous nimodipine was discontinued. Seizures were systematically prevented by sodium valproate (200 mg × 3, per os). After surgery or coiling, those patients who had delayed ischemic neurological deficit or cerebrovasospasm were managed with 'triple H' therapy (hypertension with a mean arterial pressure goal greater than 100 mmHg, hypervolemia and hemodilution with a goal hematocrit of 30) through 12 days after hemorrhage. An external ventricular drain was inserted in the case of hydrocephalus on CT and in patients with a high WFNS grade (WFNS score of 3 to 5). Increased intracranial pressure was treated by cerebrospinal fluid drainage, mechanical ventilation, reinforcement of sedation, and, rarely, moderate hypothermia. CT was performed whenever clinical deterioration occurred to search for secondary complications such as hydrocephalus or ischemia.

Clinical onset of cerebral vasospasm was defined as the acute onset of a focal neurologic deficit or a change in the GCS score of 2 or more points. All suspected cases of cerebral vasospasms were confirmed by CT angiography and were then taken to the interventional radiology suite for cerebral angiography. Each vasospasm episode was treated with intra-arterial administration of nimodipine as recently described. This therapy was repeated if necessary. Balloon angioplasty was used as a second-line therapy when nimodipine was judged insufficient. Computed tomography ischemia was referred to as delayed ischemia attributed to vasospasm.

Determination of HMGB1 in plasma

Informed consents were obtained from the study population or family members in all cases before blood was collected. In the control group, venous blood was drawn at study entry. In the SAH patients, venous blood was drawn on admission. The blood samples were immediately placed into sterile EDTA test tubes and centrifuged at 1500 g for 20 minutes at 4°C to collect plasma. Plasma was stored at –70°C until assayed. The concentration of HMGB1 in plasma was analyzed by ELISA using commercial kits (SHINO-TEST Corporations, Kanagawa, Japan) in accordance with the manufacturers'

Table 5 Receiver operating characteristic curve analysis of factors predicting the in-hospital mortality among 303 patients

	HMGB1	WFNS score	Modified Fisher score
Criterion	>10.1 ng/mL	>3	>3
Area under curve	0.876	0.893	0.922
95% confidence interval	0.833 to 0.911	0.853 to 0.926	0.886 to 0.950
Sensitivity	90.6	75.0	90.6
95% confidence interval	75.0 to 97.9	56.6 to 88.5	75.0 to 97.9
Specificity	75.6	87.5	84.1
95% confidence interval	70.1 to 80.6	82.9 to 91.2	79.2 to 88.3
+ likelihood ratio	3.72	5.98	5.71
95% confidence interval	3.3 to 4.2	4.9 to 7.3	5.1 to 6.5
- likelihood ratio	0.12	0.29	0.11
95% confidence interval	0.04 to 0.4	0.1 to 0.6	0.04 to 0.3
P value	Reference	0.707	0.328

HMGB1, high mobility group box-1; WFNS, World Federation of Neurological Surgeons.

instructions. The blood samples were run in duplicate. Researchers running ELISAs were blinded to all patient details.

End point

Participants were followed up until death or completion of 1 year after SAH. Their primary outcome was death (at 1 year or in-hospital) and their secondary outcomes were vasospasm and functional outcome at 1 year. The functional outcome was defined by Glasgow outcome scale (GOS) score. GOS was defined as follows: 1 = death; 2 = persistent vegetative state; 3 = severe disability; 4 = moderate disability; and 5 = good recovery [26]. GOS Scores were dichotomized in good and poor functional outcomes (GOS of 4 to 5 vs. GOS of 1 to 3). For follow-up, we used structure telephone interviews performed by one doctor, blinded to clinical information, and copeptin levels.

Statistical analysis

Statistical analysis was performed with SPSS 10.0 (SPSS Inc., Chicago, IL, USA) and MedCalc 9.6.4.0. (MedCalc Software, Mariakerke, Belgium). The normality of data distribution was assessed by the Kolmogorovor-Smirnov test or Shapiro-Wilk test. All values are expressed as mean ± standard deviation or counts (percentage) unless otherwise specified. Comparisons were made by using (1) chi-square test or Fisher exact test for categorical data, (2) unpaired Student t test for continuous normally distributed variables, and (3) the Mann–Whitney U-test for continuous non-normally distributed variables. The correlations of HMGB1 with WFNS grade and Fisher grade were assessed by Spearman's correlation coefficient. The relations of HMGB1 to the poor functional outcome (GOS 1 to 3), death and cerebrovasospasm

were assessed in a binary logistic-regression model. For multivariate analysis, we included the significantly different outcome predictors as assessed in univariate analysis. A receiver operating characteristic curve was configured to establish the cutoff point of plasma HMGB1 with the optimal sensitivity and specificity for predicting the poor functional outcome (GOS 1 to 3), death and cerebrovasospasm. In a combined logistic-regression model, we estimated the additive benefit of HMGB1 to other predictors (WFNS grade and Fisher grade). A P value of less than 0.05 was considered statistically significant.

Results

Study population characteristics

During the recruitment period 347 patients were admitted with an initial diagnosis of aneurysmal SAH, 312 (89.9%) patients fulfilled the inclusion criteria, and adequate data on admission and follow-up were available for 303 individuals (87.3%) who were finally included in the analysis (Figure 1). Table 1 summarizes the demographic, clinical, laboratory and radiological data of the patients. One hundred and fifty healthy subjects were eligible as controls. The intergroup differences in the age and sex were not statistically significant. After SAH, plasma HMGB1 level on admission in patients was statistically significantly higher than that in healthy controls (8.5 ± 3.6 ng/mL vs. 1.3 ±0.4 ng/mL; $P < 0.001$). Moreover, a significant correlation emerged between plasma HMGB1 level and WFNS score (r = 0.635, $P < 0.001$), as well as between plasma HMGB1 level and modified Fisher score (r = 0.624, $P < 0.001$).

One-year mortality prediction

Forty-two patients (13.9%) died from SAH in 1 year. Higher plasma HMGB1 level was associated with 1-year

Table 6 The factors associated with cerebrovasospasm

	Vasospasm (n = 131)	Non-vasospasm (n = 172)	P value
Sex (male/female)	61/70	70/102	0.307
Age (years)	43.8 ± 12.2	43.9 ± 12.5	0.973
WFNS score on admission	3.2 ± 1.1	1.7 ± 0.9	<0.001
Modified Fisher score on admission	3.5 ± 1.0	2.2 ± 0.6	<0.001
Aneurysmal location			0.813
Posterior communication artery	33 (25.2%)	50 (29.1%)	
Internal carotid artery	20 (15.3%)	23 (13.4%)	
Anterior communication artery	29 (22.1%)	37 (21.5%)	
Middle cerebral artery	22 (16.8%)	23 (13.4%)	
Anterior cerebral artery	16 (12.2%)	19 (11.0%)	
Posterior cerebral artery	7 (5.3%)	16 (9.3%)	
Vertebral artery	4 (3.1%)	4 (2.3%)	
Surgery	86 (65.5%)	100 (58.1%)	0.183
Aneurysmal size (mm)	9.1 ± 5.7	5.8 ± 3.5	<0.001
Rebleeding	10 (7.6%)	6 (3.5%)	0.110
Acute hydrocephalus	71 (54.2%)	19 (11.0%)	<0.001
Intracerebral hemorrhage	26 (19.9%)	13 (7.6%)	0.002
Intraventricular hemorrhage	52 (39.7%)	20 (11.6%)	<0.001
External ventricular drain	90 (68.7%)	19 (11.0%)	<0.001
Admission time (hours)	4.5 ± 3.4	4.9 ± 3.8	0.342
Seizure	17 (13.0%)	27 (15.7%)	0.505
Systolic arterial pressure (mmHg)	134.2 ± 23.6	128.7 ± 21.2	0.033
Diastolic arterial pressure (mmHg)	81.1 ± 15.1	77.5 ± 13.8	0.031
Mean arterial pressure (mmHg)	98.8 ± 16.1	94.6 ± 15.3	0.020
Plasma C-reactive protein level (mg/L)	7.9 ± 3.0	6.6 ± 2.4	<0.001
plasma D-dimer level (mg/L)	2.2 ± 1.1	1.9 ± 0.9	0.011
Plasma HMGB1 level (ng/mL)	10.6 ± 3.4	7.0 ± 2.9	<0.001

Numerical variables are presented as mean ± standard deviation. Categorical variables are expressed as counts (percentage). Numerical variables were analyzed by Mann–Whitney U-test or unpaired Student t test. Categorical variables were analyzed by chi-square test or Fisher exact test. HMGB1, high mobility group box-1; n, number of patients; WFNS, World Federation of Neurological Surgeons.

mortality, as well as other variables shown in Table 2. When the above variables that were found to be significant in the univariate analysis were introduced into the logistic model, a multivariate analysis selected WFNS score (odds ratio, 7.491; 95% confidence interval (CI) 1.361 to 21.351; $P = 0.001$), modified Fisher score (odds ratio, 9.292; 95% CI 2.346 to 23.318; $P = 0.005$) and plasma HMGB1 level (odds ratio, 2.117; 95% CI 1.109 to 7.230; $P = 0.002$) as the independent predictors for 1-year mortality of patients.

A receiver operating characteristic curve showed that plasma HMGB1 level on admission statistically significantly predicted 1-year mortality of patients (Figure 2A). The predictive value of the HMGB1 concentration was similar to those of WFNS score and modified Fisher score (Table 3). In a combined logistic-regression model,

HMGB1 did not statistically significantly improve the area under the curve of WFNS score ($P = 0.107$) or modified Fisher score ($P = 0.160$).

In–hospital mortality prediction

Thirty-two patients (10.6%) died from SAH in the hospital. Higher plasma HMGB1 level was associated with in-hospital mortality, as well as other variables shown in Table 4. When the above variables that were found to be significant in the univariate analysis were introduced into the logistic model, a multivariate analysis selected WFNS score (odds ratio, 4.877; 95% CI 1.448 to 14.301; $P = 0.002$), modified Fisher score (odds ratio, 5.624; 95% CI 2.119 to 16.993; $P = 0.008$) and plasma HMGB1 level (odds ratio, 2.245; 95% CI 1.218 to 8.949; $P = 0.005$) as

Table 7 Receiver operating characteristic curve analysis of factors predicting the cerebrovasospasm among 303 patients

	HMGB1	WFNS score	Modified Fisher score
Criterion	>8.8 ng/mL	>2	>2
Area under curve	0.804	0.879	0.874
95% confidence interval	0.754 to 0.847	0.837 to 0.913	0.831 to 0.909
Sensitivity	74.0	80.9	84.7
95% confidence interval	65.7 to 81.3	73.1 to 87.3	77.4 to 90.4
Specificity	78.5	79.7	76.7
95% confidence interval	71.6 to 84.4	72.9 to 85.4	69.4 to 82.2
+ likelihood ratio	3.44	3.98	3.64
95% confidence interval	3.0 to 3.9	3.6 to 4.4	3.3 to 4.1
- likelihood ratio	0.33	0.24	0.20
95% confidence interval	0.2 to 0.5	0.2 to 0.4	0.1 to 0.3
P value	Reference	0.016	0.017

HMGB1, high mobility group box-1; WFNS, World Federation of Neurological Surgeons.

the independent predictors for in-hospital mortality of patients.

A receiver operating characteristic curve showed that plasma HMGB1 level on admission statistically significantly predicted in-hospital mortality of patients (Figure 2B). The predictive value of the HMGB1 concentration was similar to those of WFNS score and modified Fisher score (Table 5). In a combined logistic-regression model, HMGB1 did not statistically significantly improve the area under the curve of WFNS score ($P = 0.140$) or modified Fisher score ($P = 0.161$).

Cerebrovasospasm prediction

One hundred and thirty-one (43.2%) suffered from cerebrovasospasm in the hospital. Higher plasma HMGB1 level was associated with cerebrovasospasm, as well as other variables shown in Table 6. When the above variables that were found to be significant in the univariate analysis were introduced into the logistic model, a multivariate analysis selected WFNS score (odds ratio, 3.890; 95% CI 1.230 to 8.421; $P = 0.008$), modified Fisher score (odds ratio, 4.713; 95% CI 1.689 to 15.106; $P = 0.001$) and plasma HMGB1 level (odds ratio, 1.249; 95% CI 1.132 to 1.871; $P = 0.011$) as the independent predictors for cerebrovasospasm of patients.

A receiver operating characteristic curve showed that plasma HMGB1 level on admission statistically significantly predicted cerebrovasospasm of patients (Figure 2C). The predictive value of the HMGB1 concentration was lower than those of WFNS score and modified Fisher score (Table 7). In a combined logistic-regression model, HMGB1 did not statistically significantly improve the area under the curve of WFNS score ($P = 0.218$) or modified Fisher score ($P = 0.235$).

Poor neurologic function prediction

Ninety patients (29.7%) suffered from poor neurologic outcome (GOS 1–3) in 1 year. Higher plasma HMGB1 level was associated with 1-year poor neurologic outcome, as well as other variables shown in Table 8. When the above variables that were found to be significant in the univariate analysis were introduced into the logistic model, a multivariate analysis selected WFNS score (odds ratio, 4.872; 95% CI 1.945 to 13.760; $P = 0.004$), modified Fisher score (odds ratio, 5.981; 95% CI 2.519 to 15.379; $P = 0.003$) and plasma HMGB1 level (odds ratio, 1.410; 95% CI 1.112 to 1.914; $P = 0.002$) as the independent predictors for 1-year poor neurologic outcome of patients.

A receiver operating characteristic curve showed that plasma HMGB1 level on admission predicted 1-year poor neurologic outcome of patients statistically significantly (Figure 2D). The predictive value of the HMGB1 concentration was similar to those of WFNS score and modified Fisher score (Table 9). In a combined logistic-regression model, HMGB1 statistically significantly improved the area under curve of WFNS score ($P = 0.007$) and modified Fisher score ($P = 0.014$).

Discussion

This study was conducted to determine if plasma HMGB1 is increased in the circulation of humans with SAH and whether this enhancement correlates with in-hospital mortality, cerebrovasospasm and 1-year poor clinical outcomes in these patients. The admission plasma HMGB1 levels were indeed significantly increased in all patients compared with healthy subjects. Furthermore, an admission plasma HMGB1 level was identified as a reliable and independent marker to predict patients at risk of in-hospital mortality, cerebrovasospasm and 1-year poor

Relationship between plasma high mobility group box-1 protein levels and clinical outcomes of aneurysmal...

9

Table 8 The factors associated with 1-year function outcome

	GOS 1 to 3 (n = 90)	GOS 4 to 5 (n = 213)	P value
Sex (male/female)	42/48	89/124	0.433
Age (years)	44.7 ± 11.3	43.5 ± 12.8	0.422
WFNS score on admission	3.6 ± 0.7	1.8 ± 0.9	<0.001
Modified Fisher score on admission	3.8 ± 0.8	2.3 ± 0.7	<0.001
Aneurysmal location			0.291
Posterior communication artery	24 (26.7%)	59 (27.7%)	
Internal carotid artery	13 (14.4%)	30 (14.1%)	
Anterior communication artery	17 (18.9%)	49 (23.0%)	
Middle cerebral artery	14 (15.6%)	31 (14.6%)	
Anterior cerebral artery	7 (7.8%)	28 (13.1%)	
Posterior cerebral artery	11 (12.2%)	12 (5.6%)	
Vertebral artery	4 (4.4%)	4 (1.9%)	
Surgery	54 (60.0%)	132 (62.0%)	0.747
Aneurysmal size (mm)	10.4 ± 5.8	5.9 ± 3.7	<0.001
Rebleeding	10 (11.1%)	6 (2.8%)	0.003
Acute hydrocephalus	47 (52.2%)	43 (20.2%)	<0.001
Intracerebral hemorrhage	20 (22.2%)	19 (8.9%)	0.002
Intraventricular hemorrhage	59 (65.6%)	12 (5.6%)	<0.001
External ventricular drain	66 (73.3%)	43 (20.2%)	<0.001
Angiographic vasospasm	71 (78.9%)	60 (28.2%)	<0.001
Computed tomography ischemia	28 (31.1%)	22 (10.3%)	<0.001
Admission time (hours)	4.5 ± 3.5	4.8 ± 3.7	0.577
Seizure	19 (21.1%)	25 (11.7%)	0.085
Plasma C-reactive protein level (mg/L)	8.2 ± 3.2	6.7 ± 2.4	<0.001
plasma D-dimer level (mg/L)	2.4 ± 1.2	1.9 ± 0.9	<0.001
Plasma HMGB1 level (ng/mL)	11.5 ± 3.1	7.3 ± 3.0	<0.001

Numerical variables are presented as mean ± standard deviation. Categorical variables are expressed as counts (percentage). Numerical variables were analyzed by Mann–Whitney U-test or unpaired Student t test. Categorical variables were analyzed by chi-square test or Fisher exact test. GOS, Glasgow Outcome Scale; HMGB1, high mobility group box-1; n, number of patients; WFNS, World Federation of Neurological Surgeons.

clinical outcome. Importantly, the prognostic values of HMGB1 were similar to those of WFNS score and modified Fisher score for in-hospital mortality and 1-year poor clinical outcome, substantiating its potential as a new prognostic biomarker.

HMGB1 is a non-histone DNA binding protein that possesses two HMG boxes that are DNA binding domains [27]. As a chromosomal protein, HMGB1 has been implicated in diverse intracellular functions, including the stabilization of nucleosomal structure and the facilitation of gene transcription [28]. Moreover, some evidence identifies HMGB1 as a cytokine-like mediator of delayed endotoxin lethality and acute lung injury [7,29]. HMGB1 is actively secreted by macrophages and monocytes or released by necrotic cells into the extracellular milieu, where it might be involved in the triggering of inflammation [7,8,29,30]. Recombinant HMGB1 has been found to induce acute inflammation in animal models of lung injury and endotoxemia [7,29], and anti-HMGB1 antibody attenuated endotoxin-induced lethality even when administration of antibody was delayed until after early cytokine response [7,31]. In addition, high serum levels of HMGB1 in patients with sepsis or hemorrhagic shock have been reported to be associated with increased mortality and disease severity [7,32].

HMGB1 is widely expressed in various tissues including the brain [13-15]. Moreover, in the brain, HMGB1 has been reported to be released after cytokine stimulation and to be involved in the inflammatory process after it was administered intracerebroventricularly [16,33]. A recent study demonstrates that HMGB1 is massively released into the extracellular milieu during the acute damaging phase and that extracellular HMGB1 might function as a proinflammatory cytokine, activate microglia, and hence stimulate the release of other cytokines and aggravate brain injury in the postischemic brain [17]. Furthermore, HMGB1$^{-/-}$ necrotic cells have a greatly reduced ability to promote inflammation [8]. Although the mechanism by which HMGB1 exerts its proinflammatory cytokine-like effects in the central nervous system is unknown, previous reports have shown that the activations of several mitogen activated protein kinases and nuclear factor kappa B are involved in the proinflammatory effect of HMGB1 [34-36]. These are downstream molecules of receptors for advanced glycation end product or Toll-like receptor family members, which are important receptors in the HMGB1 signaling process [37-40]. Evidence is rapidly accumulating to suggest that HMGB1 may play an important role in brain injury following stroke. Muhammad and colleagues [41] have demonstrated using a mouse middle cerebral artery occlusion model that HMGB1 engagement of receptors for advanced glycation end product triggers inflammation and infarction leading to ischemic brain injury. Recent studies have also reported elevated HMGB1 levels in the cerebrospinal fluid of SAH patients with poor outcome [24,25]. Moreover, another report also found elevated cytosolic HMGB1 in brain parenchyma of SAH animals [15]. To our knowledge, our present study represents the first report of elevated HMGB1 levels in plasma of SAH patients. In our study, a high WFNS score or modified Fisher score upon admission was strongly correlated with the high plasma HMGB1 level. Our data suggest that plasma HMGB1 level in this early period might reflect the initial hemorrhage insult. Connected with the previous studies, our results suggest

Table 9 Receiver operating characteristic curve analysis of factors predicting 1-year poor functional outcome among 303 patients

	HMGB1	WFNS score	Modified Fisher score
Criterion	>8.9 ng/mL	>2	>2
Area under curve	0.858	0.909	0.902
95% confidence interval	0.813 to 0.895	0.871 to 0.939	0.863 to 0.933
Sensitivity	84.4	96.7	95.6
95% confidence interval	75.3 to 91.2	90.6 to 99.3	89.0 to 98.7
Specificity	77.0	74.7	69.5
95% confidence interval	70.8 to 82.5	68.3 to 80.3	62.8 to 75.6
+ likelihood ratio	3.67	3.81	3.13
95% confidence interval	3.3 to 4.1	3.5 to 4.2	2.8 to 3.5
- likelihood ratio	0.2	0.045	0.064
95% confidence interval	0.1 to 0.3	0.01 to 0.1	0.02 to 0.2
P value	Reference	0.104	0.163

HMGB1, high mobility group box-1; WFNS, World Federation of Neurological Surgeons.

HMGB1 may act in concert to promote brain inflammation following SAH.

In this study, a receiver operating characteristic curve showed that plasma HMGB1 level on admission predicted poor functional outcome and mortality after 1 year, and in-hospital mortality of patients obviously. The area under the curve of the HMGB1 concentration was similar to those of WFNS score and modified Fisher score for the prediction of these poor outcomes. In a combined logistic-regression model, HMGB1 improved the area under the curve of WFNS score and modified Fisher score for the prediction of poor functional outcome after 1 year, but not for the prediction of mortality after 1 year or in-hospital mortality. Therefore, the determination of HMGB1 in the plasma of patients on admission provides the ability to distinguish between patients with good and bad outcome. Cerebrovasospasm is regarded as abnormal and prolonged smooth muscle contraction of cerebral arteries; many substances have been involved in the development of cerebral vasospasm following SAH, but the complex mechanism of this arterial narrowing is not yet fully understood [42,43]. The degree of angiographic vasospasm is not always well correlated with the development of neurological deficits in SAH patients, and other influences such as early brain injury due to cortical spreading depression, disruption of the blood–brain barrier, impaired function of the microcirculation, inflammation, and apoptotic cell death may contribute to SAH-induced pathologies [44-48]. This study found that plasma HMGB1 level was an independent predictor for cerebrovasospasm of patients . However, significantly lower accuracy for the prediction of cerebrovasospasm was found for plasma HMGB1 level compared with other clinical grade such as WFNS and modified Fisher score. Hence, plasma levels of HMGB1

on admission are not recommended for the prediction of cerebrovasospasm after SAH. Overall, plasma HMGB1 level has low accuracy for the prediction of cerebrovasospasm and high accuracy for the prediction of 1-year mortality or in-hospital mortality or 1-year poor functional outcome. However, HMGB1 determination does not add to the accuracy of prediction of the clinical outcomes.

In addition, location of the subarachnoid blood can be assessed in the following four anatomical locations: convexity, sylvian fissure, basal cistern, and interhemisphere. However, most of the subarachnoid blood resides in multiple anatomical locations leading to difficulty of classification. Hence, whether HMGB1 levels differ according to SAH location warrants further investigation; maybe this is a limitation in this study. Actually, subarachnoid blood is impossible to gather in just an anatomical location. We need to mention that, in this study, ischemic or hemorrhage stroke referred to stroke in the patients' history. Patients with previous neurological diseases including ischemic or hemorrhagic stroke, or the use of antiplatelet or anticoagulant medication, were excluded because these patients were complicated with vascular risk factors including diabetes mellitus and/or hypertension that were associated with high HMGB1 level [49-52] and became the confounding variables.

Conclusions

In this study, plasma HMGB1 level is a useful, complementary tool to predict functional outcome and mortality after aneurysmal SAH. However, HMGB1 determination does not add to the accuracy of prediction of the clinical outcome.

Abbreviations
CI: confidence interval; CT: computerized tomography; ELISA: enzyme-linked immunosorbent assay; GCS: Glasgow Coma Scale; GOS: Glasgow outcome scale; HMGB1: high mobility group box-1; SAH: subarachnoid hemorrhage; WFNS: World Federation of Neurological Surgeons.

Competing interests
The authors declare that they have no competing interests.

Authors' contributions
XDZ and JSC contributed to the design of the study and drafted the manuscript and participated in the laboratory work. JSC, FZ and QCL enrolled the patients. GC and JMZ contributed to data analysis and interpretation of the results. All authors read and approved the final manuscript.

References
1. Liebenberg WA, Worth R, Firth GB, Olney J, Norris JS: Aneurysmal subarachnoid haemorrhage: guidance in making the correct diagnosis. *Postgrad Med J* 2005, **81**:470–473.
2. Drake C: **Report of world federation of neurological surgeons committee on a universal subarachnoid hemorrhage grading scale.** *J Neurosurg* 1988, **68**:985–986.
3. Fisher CM, Kistler JP, Davis JM: **Relation of cerebral vasospasm to subarachnoid hemorrhage visualized by computerized tomographic scanning.** *Neurosurgery* 1980, **6**:1–9.
4. Turck N, Vutskits L, Sanchez-Pena P, Robin X, Hainard A, Gex-Fabry M, Fouda C, Bassem H, Mueller M, Lisacek F, Puybasset L, Sanchez JC: **A multiparameter panel method for outcome prediction following aneurysmal subarachnoid hemorrhage.** *Intensive Care Med* 2010, **36**:107–115.
5. Goodwin GH, Sanders C, Johns EW: **A new group of chromatin-associated proteins with a high content of acidic and basic amino acids.** *Eur J Biochem* 1973, **38**:14–19.
6. Javaherian K, Liu JF, Wang JC: **Nonhistone proteins HMG1 and HMG2 change the DNA helical structure.** *Science* 1978, **199**:1345–1346.
7. Wang H, Bloom O, Zhang M, Vishnubhakat JM, Ombrellino M, Che J, Frazier A, Yang H, Ivanova S, Borovikova L, Manogue KR, Faist E, Abraham E, Andersson J, Andersson U, Molina PE, Abumrad NN, Sama A, Tracey KJ: **HMG-1 as a late mediator of endotoxin lethality in mice.** *Science* 1999, **285**:248–251.
8. Scaffidi P, Misteli T, Bianchi ME: **Release of chromatin protein HMGB1 by necrotic cells triggers inflammation.** *Nature* 2002, **418**:191–195.
9. Lotze MT, Tracey KJ: **High-mobility group box 1 protein (HMGB1): nuclear weapon in the immune arsenal.** *Nat Rev Immunol* 2005, **5**:331–342.
10. Dumitriu IE, Baruah P, Manfredi AA, Bianchi ME, Rovere-Querini P: **HMGB1: guiding immunity from within.** *Trends Immunol* 2005, **26**:381–387.
11. Bianchi ME, Manfredi AA: **High-mobility group box 1 (HMGB1) protein at the crossroads between innate and adaptive immunity.** *Immunol Rev* 2007, **220**:35–46.
12. Klune JR, Dhupar R, Cardinal J, Billiar TR, Tsung A: **HMGB1: endogenous danger signaling.** *Mol Med* 2008, **14**:476–484.
13. Guazzi S, Strangio A, Franzi AT, Bianchi ME: **HMGB1, an architectural chromatin protein and an extracellular signaling factor, has a spatially and temporally restricted expression pattern in mouse brain.** *Gene Expr Patterns* 2003, **3**:29–33.
14. Watanabe M, Miyajima M, Nakajima M, Arai H, Ogino I, Nakamura S, Kunichika M: **Expression analysis of high mobility group box-1 protein (HMGB-1) in the cerebral cortex, hippocampus, and cerebellum of the congenital hydrocephalus (H-Tx) rat.** *Acta Neurochir Suppl* 2012, **113**:91–96.
15. Murakami K, Koide M, Dumont TM, Russell SR, Tranmer BI, Wellman GC: **Subarachnoid hemorrhage induces gliosis and increased expression of the pro-inflammatory cytokine high mobility group box 1 protein.** *Transl Stroke Res* 2011, **2**:72–79.
16. Agnello D, Wang H, Yang H, Tracey KJ, Ghezzi P: **HMGB-1, a DNA-binding protein with cytokine activity, induces brain TNF and IL-6 production, and mediates anorexia and taste aversion.** *Cytokine* 2002, **18**:231–236.
17. Kim JB, Sig Choi J, Yu YM, Nam K, Piao CS, Kim SW, Lee MH, Han PL, Park JS, Lee JK: **HMGB1, a novel cytokine-like mediator linking acute neuronal death and delayed neuroinflammation in the postischemic brain.** *J Neurosci* 2006, **26**:6413–6421.
18. O'Connor KA, Hansen MK, Rachal Pugh C, Deak MM, Biedenkapp JC, Milligan ED, Johnson JD, Wang H, Maier SF, Tracey KJ, Watkins LR: **Further characterization of high mobility group box 1 (HMGB1) as a proinflammatory cytokine: central nervous system effects.** *Cytokine* 2003, **24**:254–265.
19. Takata K, Kitamura Y, Kakimura J, Shibagaki K, Tsuchiya D, Taniguchi T, Smith MA, Perry G, Shimohama S: **Role of high mobility group protein-1 (HMG1) in amyloid-beta homeostasis.** *Biochem Biophys Res Commun* 2003, **301**:699–703.
20. Takata K, Kitamura Y, Tsuchiya D, Kawasaki T, Taniguchi T, Shimohama S: **High mobility group box protein-1 inhibits microglial Abeta clearance and enhances Abeta neurotoxicity.** *J Neurosci Res* 2004, **78**:880–891.
21. Pedrazzi M, Patrone M, Passalacqua M, Ranzato E, Colamassaro D, Sparatore B, Pontremoli S, Melloni E: **Selective proinflammatory activation of astrocytes by high-mobility group box 1 protein signaling.** *J Immunol* 2007, **179**:8525–8532.
22. Tang D, Kang R, Cao L, Zhang G, Yu Y, Xiao W, Wang H, Xiao X: **A pilot study to detect high mobility group box 1 and heat shock protein 72 in cerebrospinal fluid of pediatric patients with meningitis.** *Crit Care Med* 2008, **36**:291–295.
23. Goldstein RS, Gallowitsch-Puerta M, Yang L, Rosas-Ballina M, Huston JM, Czura CJ, Lee DC, Ward MF, Bruchfeld AN, Wang H, Lesser ML, Church AL, Litroff AH, Sama AE, Tracey KJ: **Elevated high-mobility group box 1 levels in patients with cerebral and myocardial ischemia.** *Shock* 2006, **25**:571–574.
24. Nakahara T, Tsuruta R, Kaneko T, Yamashita S, Fujita M, Kasaoka S, Hashiguchi T, Suzuki M, Maruyama I, Maekawa T: **High-mobility group box 1 protein in CSF of patients with subarachnoid hemorrhage.** *Neurocrit Care* 2009, **11**:362–368.
25. King MD, Laird MD, Ramesh SS, Youssef P, Shakir B, Vender JR, Alleyne CH, Dhandapani KM: **Elucidating novel mechanisms of brain injury following subarachnoid hemorrhage: an emerging role for neuroproteomics.** *Neurosurg Focus* 2010, **28**:E10.
26. Jennett B, Bond M: **Assessment of outcome after severe brain damage.** *Lancet* 1975, **1**:480–484.
27. Landsman D, Bustin MA: **Signature for the HMG-1 box DNA-binding proteins.** *Bioessays* 1993, **15**:539–546.
28. Bustin M: **Regulation of DNA-dependent activities by the functional motifs of the high-mobility-group chromosomal proteins.** *Mol Cell Biol* 1999, **19**:5237–5246.
29. Abraham E, Arcaroli J, Carmody A, Wang H, Tracey KJ: **HMG-1 as a mediator of acute lung inflammation.** *J Immunol* 2000, **165**:2950–2954.
30. Bonaldi T, Talamo F, Scaffidi P, Ferrera D, Porto A, Bachi A, Rubartelli A, Agresti A, Bianchi ME: **Monocytic cells hyperacetylate chromatin protein HMGB1 to redirect it towards secretion.** *EMBO J* 2003, **22**:5551–5560.
31. Yang H, Ochani M, Li J, Qiang X, Tanovic M, Harris HE, Susarla SM, Ulloa L, Wang H, DiRaimo R, Czura CJ, Wang H, Roth J, Warren HS, Fink MP, Fenton MJ, Andersson U, Tracey KJ: **Reversing established sepsis with antagonists of endogenous high-mobility group box 1.** *Proc Natl Acad Sci USA* 2004, **101**:296–301.
32. Ombrellino M, Wang H, Ajemian MS, Talhouk A, Scher LA, Friedman SG, Tracey KJ: **Increased serum concentrations of high-mobility group protein 1 in haemorrhagic shock.** *Lancet* 1999, **354**:1446–1447.
33. Wang H, Vishnubhakat JM, Bloom O, Zhang M, Ombrellino M, Sama A, Tracey KJ: **Proinflammatory cytokines (tumor necrosis factor and interleukin 1) stimulate release of high mobility group protein-1 by pituicytes.** *Surgery* 1999, **126**:389–392.
34. Huttunen HJ, Fages C, Rauvala H: **Receptor for advanced glycation end products (RAGE)-mediated neurite outgrowth and activation of NF-kB require the cytoplasmic domain of the receptor but different downstream signaling pathways.** *J Biol Chem* 1999, **274**:19919–19924.
35. Taguchi A, Blood DC, del Toro G, Canet A, Lee DC, Qu W, Tanji N, Lu Y, Lalla E, Fu C, Hofmann MA, Kislinger T, Ingram M, Lu A, Tanaka H, Hori O, Ogawa S, Stern DM, Schmidt AM: **Blockade of RAGE amphoterin signalling suppresses tumour growth and metastases.** *Nature* 2000, **405**:354–360.

36. Park JS, Arcaroli J, Yum HK, Yang H, Wang H, Yang KY, Choe KH, Strassheim D, Pitts TM, Tracey KJ, Abraham E: **Activation of gene expression in human neutrophils by high mobility group box 1 protein.** *Am J Physiol Cell Physiol* 2003, **284**:C870–C879.

37. Schmidt AM, Yan SD, Yan SF, Stern DM: **The biology of the receptor for advanced glycation end products and its ligands.** *Biochim Biophys Acta* 2000, **1498**:99–111.

38. Huttunen HJ, Rauvala H: **Amphoterin as an extracellular regulator of cell motility: from discovery to disease.** *J Int Med* 2004, **255**:351–366.

39. Park JS, Svetkauskaite D, He Q, Kim JY, Strassheim D, Ishizaka A, Abraham E: **Involvement of Toll-like receptors 2 and 4 in cellular activation by high mobility group box 1 protein.** *J Biol Chem* 2004, **279**:7370–7377.

40. Tsung A, Sahai R, Tanaka H, Nakao A, Fink MP, Lotze MT, Yang H, Li J, Tracey KJ, Geller DA, Billiar TR: **The nuclear factor HMGB1 mediates hepatic injury after murine liver ischemia-reperfusion.** *J Exp Med* 2005, **201**:1135–1143.

41. Muhammad S, Barakat W, Stoyanov S, Murikinati S, Yang H, Tracey KJ, Bendszus M, Rossetti G, Nawroth PP, Bierhaus A, Schwaninger M: **The HMGB1 receptor RAGE mediates ischemic brain damage.** *J Neurosci* 2008, **28**:12023–12031.

42. Sobey CG, Faraci FM: **Subarachnoid haemorrhage: what happens to the cerebral arteries?** *Clin Exp Pharmacol Physiol* 1998, **25**:867–876.

43. Cook DA: **Mechanisms of cerebral vasospasm in subarachnoid haemorrhage.** *Pharmacol Ther* 1995, **66**:259–284.

44. Hansen-Schwartz J, Vajkoczy P, Macdonald RL, Pluta RM, Zhang JH: **Cerebral vasospasm: looking beyond vasoconstriction.** *Trends Pharmacol Sci* 2007, **28**:252–256.

45. Pluta RM, Hansen-Schwartz J, Dreier J, Vajkoczy P, Macdonald RL, Nishizawa S, Kasuya H, Wellman G, Keller E, Zauner A, Dorsch N, Clark J, Ono S, Kiris T, Leroux P, Zhang JH: **Cerebral vasospasm following subarachnoid hemorrhage: time for a new world of thought.** *Neurol Res* 2009, **31**:151–158.

46. Sabri M, Kawashima A, Ai J, Macdonald RL: **Neuronal and astrocytic apoptosis after subarachnoid hemorrhage: a possible cause for poor prognosis.** *Brain Res* 2008, **1238**:163–171.

47. Vergouwen MD, Vermeulen M, Coert BA, Stroes ES, Roos YB: **Microthrombosis after aneurysmal subarachnoid hemorrhage: an additional explanation for delayed cerebral ischemia.** *J Cereb Blood Flow Metab* 2008, **28**:1761–1770.

48. Wellman GC: **Ion channels and calcium signaling in cerebral arteries following subarachnoid hemorrhage.** *Neurol Res* 2006, **28**:690–702.

49. Skrha J Jr, Kalousová M, Svarcová J, Muravská A, Kvasnička J, Landová L, Zima T, Skrha J: **Relationship of soluble RAGE and RAGE ligands HMGB1 and EN-RAGE to endothelial dysfunction in Type 1 and Type 2 diabetes mellitus.** *Exp Clin Endocrinol Diabetes* 2012, **120**:277–281.

50. Haraba R, Uyy E, Suica VI, Ivan L, Antohe F: **Fluvastatin reduces the high mobility group box 1 protein expression in hyperlipidemia.** *Int J Cardiol* 2011, **150**:105–107.

51. Tang D, Kang R, Zeh HJ 3rd, Lotze MT: **High-mobility group box 1, oxidative stress, and disease.** *Antioxid Redox Signal* 2011, **14**:1315–1335.

52. Ding HS, Yang J: **High mobility group box-1 and cardiovascular diseases.** *Saudi Med J* 2010, **31**:486–489.

2

Augmented expression of TSPO after intracerebral hemorrhage: a role in inflammation?

Frederick Bonsack IV, Cargill H. Alleyne Jr and Sangeetha Sukumari-Ramesh[*]

Abstract

Background: Intracerebral hemorrhage (ICH) is a potentially fatal stroke subtype accounting for 10–15 % of all strokes. Despite neurosurgical intervention and supportive care, the 30-day mortality rate remains 30–50 % with ICH survivors frequently displaying neurological impairment and requiring long-term assisted care. Although accumulating evidence demonstrates the role of neuroinflammation in secondary brain injury and delayed fatality after ICH, the molecular regulators of neuroinflammation remain poorly defined after ICH.

Methods: In the present study, ICH was induced in CD1 male mice by collagenase injection method and given the emerging role of TSPO (18-kDa translocator protein) in neuroinflammation, immunofluorescence staining of brain sections was performed to characterize the temporal expression pattern and cellular and subcellular localization of TSPO after ICH. Further, both genetic and pharmacological studies were employed to assess the functional role of TSPO in neuroinflammation.

Results: The expression of TSPO was found to be increased in the peri-hematomal brain region 1 to 7 days post-injury, peaking on day 3 to day 5 in comparison to sham. Further, the TSPO expression was mostly observed in microglia/macrophages, the inflammatory cells of the central nervous system, suggesting an unexplored role of TSPO in neuroinflammatory responses after ICH. Further, the subcellular localization studies revealed prominent perinuclear expression of TSPO after ICH. Moreover, both genetic and pharmacological studies revealed a regulatory role of TSPO in the release of pro-inflammatory cytokines in a macrophage cell line, RAW 264.7.

Conclusions: Altogether, the data suggest that TSPO induction after ICH could be an intrinsic mechanism to prevent an exacerbated inflammatory response and raise the possibility of targeting TSPO for the attenuation of secondary brain injury after ICH.

Keywords: Microglial activation, ICH, TSPO

Background

Intracerebral hemorrhage (ICH) is a common and often a fatal stroke subtype that accounts for 10–15 % of all stroke events [1]. In-hospital rates of mortality and patient disability following ICH are 40 and 80 % respectively [2] and the 1-month mortality rate is 30–50 % [3, 4]. In addition, a vast majority of ICH survivors do not regain their independence within 6 months of symptom onset and at 6 months only 20 % achieve independence in their daily lives [4, 5]. Despite recent advances in preclinical research,

* Correspondence: sramesh@gru.edu
Department of Neurosurgery, Medical College of Georgia, Augusta University, 1120 15th Street, CA1010, Augusta, GA 30912, USA

there is no effective treatment for ICH. Notably, the current treatment options are largely limited to providing mechanical ventilation and supportive care. The need for new therapeutic approaches for ICH has prompted a search for the molecular and cellular mechanisms that underlie brain damage after ICH.

TSPO is an 18-kDa trans-membrane protein of 169 amino acids, found primarily in the mitochondrial outer membrane [6]. TSPO was first identified as a diazepam-binding protein found in peripheral tissues; hence the previous denomination as peripheral-type benzodiazepine receptor [7, 8]. It is found in most species from bacteria to humans and the cDNA encoding TSPO has been cloned from various species such as rodents, bovines, and humans [9–13] among which there is an 80 % sequence homology [6]. TSPO has been implicated in many cellular processes including cell proliferation and differentiation, apoptosis, immunomodulation, tetrapyrrole biosynthesis, oxidative stress, steroid biosynthesis, and mitochondrial physiology [14–17]. In particular, TSPO was thought to be required and essential for the translocation of cholesterol from the outer mitochondrial membrane to the inner mitochondrial membrane, a limiting step for steroidogenesis [15, 18–20]. However, recent studies demonstrate that knockdown of TSPO in different cell types had no effect on viability and more importantly, that global TSPO knockout mice were viable and exhibited unaltered steroidogenesis [21–23], suggesting an elusive and conflicting role of TSPO in mammalian cells.

In the normal brain, TSPO expression is low, and it is found mainly in glia and at very low levels in neurons [8, 24–26]. However upon brain injury, augmented expression of TSPO is observed in activated glial cells [27–31] and serves as a biomarker for disease activity in Alzheimer's and Parkinson's disease [32, 33]. Synthetic ligands to TSPO are also investigated as therapeutic agents for various CNS disorders [34]. ICH results in both primary and secondary brain insults, and neuroinflammation characterized by glial activation is regarded as a major component of secondary brain injury mechanisms after ICH. However, the molecular expression and the functional role of TSPO after hemorrhagic brain injury have not been studied previously. The purpose of this study was to explore the temporal expression pattern and characterize the cellular localization of TSPO after ICH.

Methods

ICH

Animal studies were reviewed and approved by the Committee on Animal Use for Research and Education at Augusta University, in compliance with NIH and USDA guidelines. Male CD-1 mice (8–10 weeks old; Charles River) were anesthetized with an intraperitoneal injection of ketamine and xylazine and positioned prone in a stereotaxic head frame (Stoelting, WI, USA). A small animal temperature controller (David Kopf Instruments, USA) was used to maintain the body temperature at 37 ± 0.5 °C throughout surgery. With a high-speed dental drill (Dremel, USA), a 0.5-mm burr hole was made 2.2 mm lateral to the bregma, taking care not to damage the underlying dura. A 26-G Hamilton syringe containing 0.04 U of bacterial type IV collagenase (Sigma, St. Louis, MO, USA) in 0.5-μl saline was inserted with stereotaxic guidance 3.0 mm into the left striatum to induce spontaneous ICH [35, 36]. After removal of the needle, the burr hole was sealed with bone wax and the

incision was surgically stapled. Sham animals underwent the same surgical procedure, but only a saline injection (0.5 μl) was performed. Mice were maintained at 37 °C until recovery.

Immunohistochemistry

Deeply anesthetized mice were transcardially perfused with 0.1-M phosphate-buffered saline (pH 7.4; PBS), followed by 4 % paraformaldehyde in PBS. The brains were post-fixed overnight in 4 % paraformaldehyde and cryoprotected in 30 % sucrose at 4 °C until the brains were permeated. They were snap-frozen and sectioned at 25 μm using a cryostat. The coronal sections mounted on glass slides were incubated at 20 °C with 10 % normal donkey serum in PBS containing 0.4 % Triton X-100 for 1 h, followed by incubation with primary antibodies [Iba1 (ionized calcium binding adaptor molecule; 1:100; goat polyclonal; Abcam, MA, USA), TSPO (1:250; rabbit monoclonal; Abcam, MA, USA), glial fibrillary acidic protein (GFAP, 1:1000; goat polyclonal; Abcam, MA, USA), NeuN (1:100; mouse monoclonal; EMD Millipore, MA, USA), CD16/32 (1:100; rat monoclonal; BD Biosciences, CA, USA), CD206 (1:100; mouse monoclonal; BD Biosciences, CA, USA), and proliferating cell nuclear antigen (PCNA, 1:100; mouse monoclonal ; Cell Signaling, MA, USA)] at 4 °C for 24 h in 0.2 % Triton X-100 containing PBS. Sections were washed and incubated with appropriate Alexa Fluor-tagged secondary antibody (1:1000; Invitrogen/Life Technologies, USA; Alexa Fluor 594 conjugated donkey anti-Rat IgG, Alexa Fluor 594 or Alexa Fluor 488 conjugated donkey anti-Rabbit IgG, Alexa Fluor 594 or Alexa Fluor 488 conjugated donkey anti-Mouse IgG, and Alexa Fluor 488 conjugated donkey anti-Goat IgG) at room temperature for 1 h in 0.2 % Triton X-100 containing PBS. After washing, the sections were cover slipped with a mounting media containing DAPI (DAPI-Fluoromount-G; SouthernBiotech, AL, USA), a nuclear stain. Immunofluorescence was determined using a Zeiss LSM510 Meta confocal laser microscope and cellular colocalization was determined, as described earlier [37]. We analyzed 3 non-consecutive sections per animal and a minimum of 3–5 random fields around the hematoma. The fluorescence intensity of immunoreactivity and the number of immunopositive cells were estimated using ImageJ software (NIH, USA). The number of immunoreactive cells per mouse were quantified (3–5 fields per section and 3 sections per mouse, $n = 3$ mice/group) and averaged as positive cells per 0.1 mm^2 in the peri-hematomal brain region. Quantitative assessment of colocalization between TSPO and CD16/32 or CD206 fluorescent signals was performed by calculating the overlap coefficient (ranging from 0 %; minimum colocalization to 100 %; maximum colocalization) using the Zeiss Zen2009 (NY, USA) software. An average of 10–15 cells were analyzed per section (3 sections per mouse; $n = 3$ mice/group) and overlap co-efficient was calculated.

Cell culture and enzyme-linked immunoassay (ELISA)

The mouse macrophage cell line, RAW 264.7 purchased from ATCC (American Type Culture Collection), was maintained in Dulbecco's modified Eagle's medium supplemented with 5 % fetal bovine serum and 5 % bovine growth serum, 5 % CO_2, and 100 % humidity. Cells were added to tissue culture plates, allowed to adhere overnight, and then stimulated with hemin (30 μM). TSPO agonist or antagonist was added 1 h prior to hemin addition, and the hemin treatment was conducted for 18 h in the presence of TSPO agonist or antagonist and the supernatant was collected. The release of pro-inflammatory cytokines such as (tumor necrosis factor-α) TNF-α and (interleukin-6) IL-6 into the supernatant was estimated using ELISA as per manufacturer's instructions. (RayBiotech, Inc., Norcross, GA, USA). Briefly, pre-coated 96-well ELISA plates for different captured antibodies were incubated overnight at 4 °C with cell culture supernatant and different concentrations of standard protein, 100 μl per well. Unbound materials were washed out, and biotinylated respective anti-cytokine detection antibody was added to each well. The plates were incubated for 1 h at room temperature. After washing, 100 μl of streptavidin-HRP conjugate was added to the wells and incubation was continued for another 45 min at room temperature. After washing, color development was performed by incubation with substrate solution. After adding stop solution, the optical density at 450 nm was determined for each well using a microtiter plate reader (Bio-TeK, Epoch) and the concentrations of

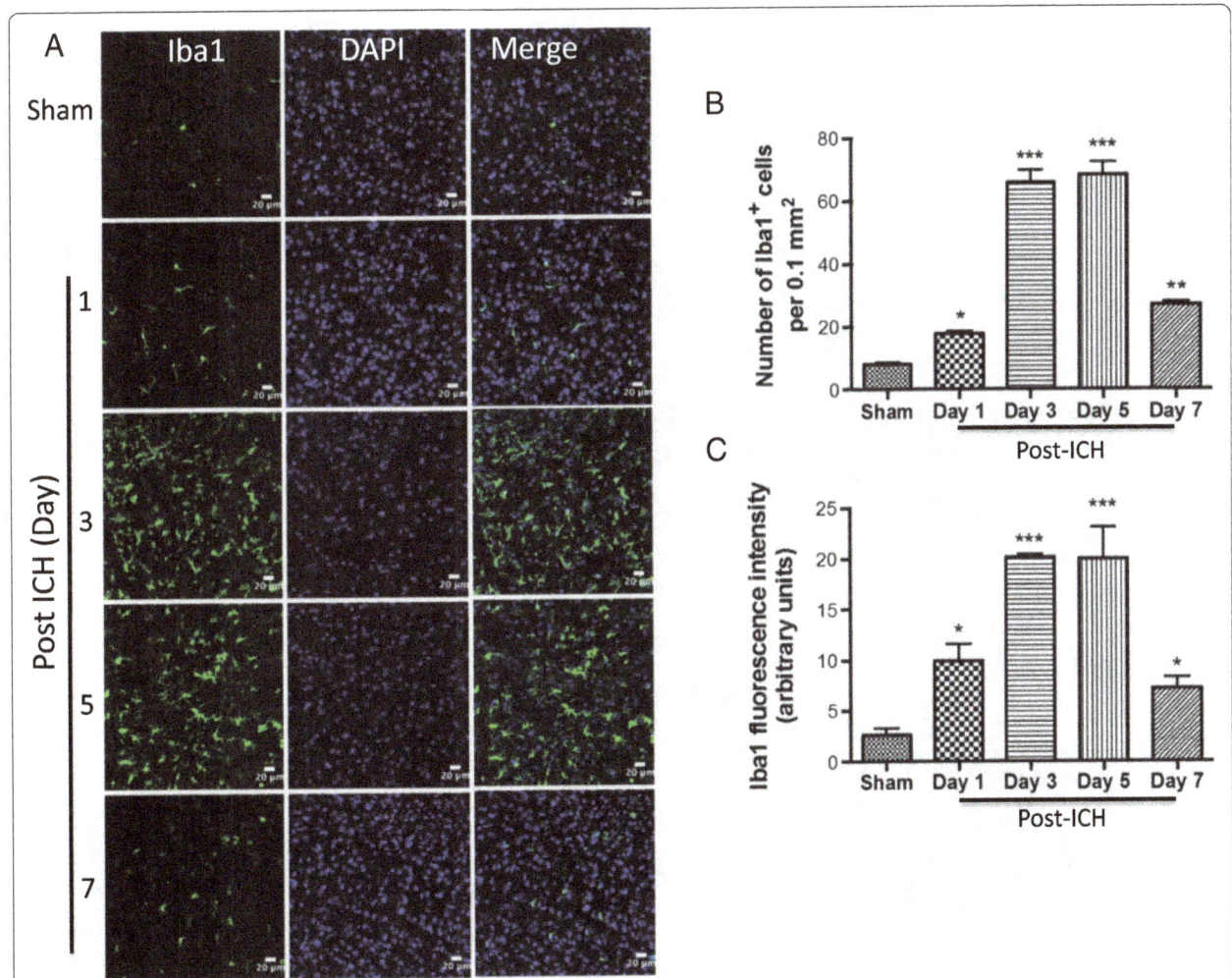

Fig. 1 Microglial/macrophage activation and ICH. Brain sections were immunostained for Iba1 (**a**) as described in the "Methods" section. After counter staining the sections with DAPI, the staining was analyzed using confocal microscopy. ICH remarkably induced microglial/macrophage activation as evidenced by cellular hypertrophy with enhanced Iba1 staining. Scale bar = 20 μm $n = 3$–6/group. **b** The average number of Iba1-positive cells per 0.1 mm^2 in the ipsilateral striatum. **c** The fluorescence intensity quantification of Iba1 immunoreactivity using ImageJ (NIH, USA). *$p < 0.05$, **$p < 0.01$, ***$p < 0.001$ vs. sham

the samples were determined in comparison to the respective standard concentration curve.

Genetic knockdown of TSPO

RAW 264.7 cells were transfected with either control siRNA (ON-TARGETplus Non-targeting Pool; GE Dharmacon) or TSPO siRNA (SMARTpool: ON-TARGETplus TSPO siRNA; GE Dharmacon). Briefly, the cells were plated overnight and transfected with control or TSPO siRNA using HiPerFect Transfection Reagent (QIAGEN) according to manufacturer's instructions. Target gene knockdown was verified 48-h post-transfection by qRT-PCR. To accomplish this, total RNA was isolated (SV RNA Isolation System, Promega), and quantitative RT-PCR was performed on a Cepheid SmartCycler II using a SuperScript III Platinum SYBR Green One-Step RT-

PCR kit (Invitrogen, Carlsbad, CA, USA). Primers were as follows: TSPO (5′AGAAACCCTCTTGGCATCCG3′(F), 5′ GCCATACCCCATGGCTGAATA 3′(R) and RPS3: (FP 5′-AATGAACCGAAGCACACCATA-3′; RP 5′-ATCAG AGAGTTGACCGCAGTT-3′). Product specificity was confirmed by melting curve analysis and gene expression levels were quantified using a cDNA standard curve. Data were normalized to *RPS3*, a housekeeping gene that was unaffected by the experimental conditions.

Statistical analysis

The data were analyzed using one-way analysis of variance followed by Student-Newman-Keuls post hoc test and were expressed as mean ± SE. A *p* value of <0.05 was considered to be significant.

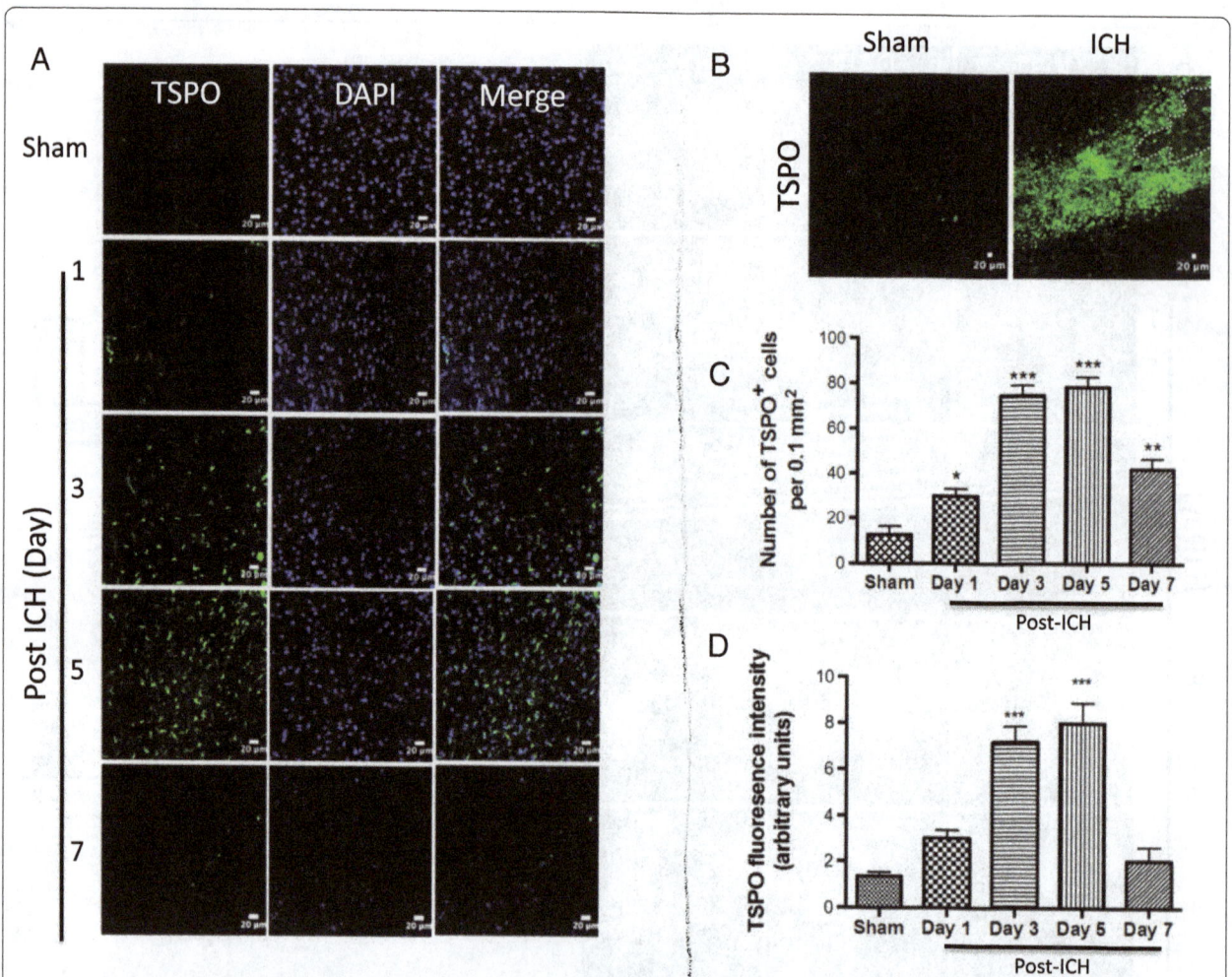

Fig. 2 TSPO expression and ICH. **a** Representative confocal images demonstrating the temporal expression pattern of TSPO immunostaining in the brain tissue of ICH or sham. The confocal images were obtained from the peri-hematomal brain area of ICH 1–7 days post-injury or from the comparable brain region of sham. ICH remarkably augmented TSPO expression. Scale bar = 20 μm; n = 4–6/group. **b** The low magnification image depicting the profound induction of TSPO in the peri-hematomal brain region 5 days post-ICH or sham. **c** The average number of TSPO-positive cells per 0.1 mm^2 in the ipsilateral striatum. **d** The fluorescence intensity quantification of TSPO immunoreactivity using ImageJ (NIH, USA). *$p < 0.05$, **$p < 0.01$, ***$p < 0.001$ vs. sham

Results

Temporal expression pattern of TSPO after ICH

Microglia are believed to be the first non-neuronal cells to react to a brain injury and are regarded as the major source of expression of pro-inflammatory cytokines after ICH [38]. Given the emerging role of TSPO in neuroinflammation, our goal was to characterize the immune response 1 to 7 days post-hemorrhagic injury because the kinetics of cytokine expression within the first week after experimental ICH is quite dynamic. In addition, important clinical sequelae begin to appear within the first 7-day post-ICH [39]. We found a very prominent microglia/macrophage activation at day 1 and it peaked at 3 to 5 days post-ICH as evidenced by a significant induction in both Iba1 (microglia/macrophage marker) immunofluorescence intensity and the number of Iba1-immunoreactive cells around the hematoma in comparison to sham (Fig. 1a–c). Notably, consistent with the previous reports [40, 41], Iba1-positive cells in the peri-hematomal area after ICH predominantly exhibited activated/reactive morphology with hypertrophic cell body and short processes in comparison to the ramified morphology observed in sham-injured mice (Fig. 1a). Notably, there was approximately

an 8-fold increase ($p < 0.001$) in the number of Iba1-positive cells and Iba1 immunofluorescence intensity ($p < 0.001$) on day 3 and day 5, post-ICH in comparison to sham (Fig. 1b, c). However, it is known that Iba1 recognizes both microglia and macrophages, therefore the prominent induction in Iba1-positive cells after ICH could be either due to the proliferation and/or migration of microglia or due to the infiltration of macrophages after a brain injury. Furthermore, a week after ICH, microglia/macrophage activation tended to reduce; however, it did not reach sham levels (Fig 1a–c), suggesting a prolonged activation of microglia/macrophage after ICH. To evaluate TSPO expression after ICH, we performed immunofluorescence staining of brain sections acquired at different time points after surgery. TSPO was expressed at low levels in sham-operated mice as assessed by immunohistochemistry (Fig. 2) and no TSPO immunoreactivity was observed in the contralateral hemisphere (data not shown). In contrast, TSPO induction was observed in the peri-hematomal brain region 1 to 7 days post-injury with a remarkable up regulation observed on day 3 and day 5 post-injury (Fig. 2a, c, d). The quantification of the number of TSPO-immunoreactive cells and immunofluorescence

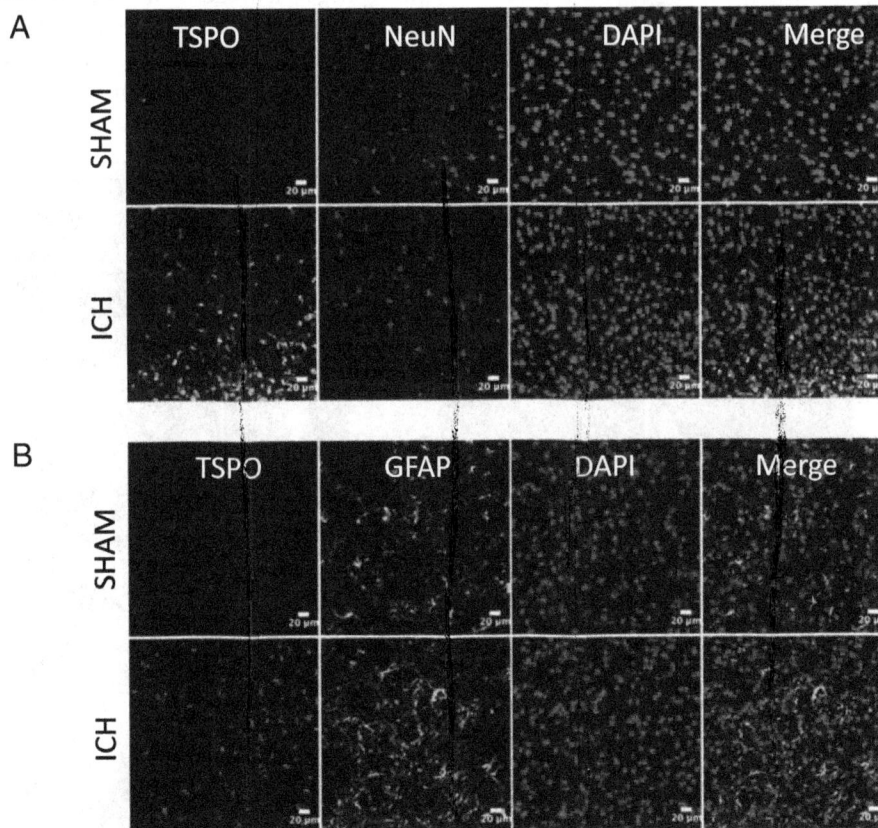

Fig. 3 Cellular localization of TSPO. Double immunolabeling of brain sections from sham/ICH mice were performed for **a** TSPO and NeuN and **b** TSPO and GFAP 5 days post-surgery. TSPO expression was absent in both NeuN-positive and GFAP-positive cells after ICH. Scale bar = 20 μm; n = 3/group

intensity analysis together confirmed a significant induction of TSPO expression on day 3 and day 5 in comparison to sham (Fig. 2c, d). Along these lines, there was approximately a 6-fold increase ($p < 0.001$) in TSPO immunoreactivity on day 3 and day 5 post-ICH in comparison to sham (Fig. 2c, d).

Cellular and subcellular localization of TSPO expression after ICH

To establish the cellular localization of TSPO after ICH, we employed double immunohistochemical labeling. TSPO expression was not found in GFAP- and NeuN-positive cells suggesting the absence of TSPO expression in astrocytes and neurons, respectively, after ICH (Fig. 3). In contrast, a remarkable colocalization of TSPO was observed in Iba1-positive cells, suggesting that TSPO-expressing cells after ICH are mostly microglia/macrophages, the inflammatory cells of CNS (Fig. 4). Notably, microglia/macrophages exhibited polarization after ICH and the analysis of immunopositive cell number and fluorescence intensity together revealed a significant induction of pro-inflammatory M1 microglia/macrophage marker, CD16/32 expression in the peri-hematomal brain region at 3 to 7 days post-injury, peaking on day 5, in comparison to sham (Fig. 5a–c). Further, CD16/32 expression was mostly confined to Iba1-positive cells after ICH (Fig. 5d) and the number of CD16/32-positive cells increased 6- and 10-fold ($p < 0.001$) on day 3 and day 5 post-ICH, respectively, in comparison

to sham (Fig. 5b). Of note, the expression of anti-inflammatory M2 microglia/macrophage marker, CD206, was observed mostly on day 1 and day 3 post-ICH, with a peak expression observed on day 3 (Fig. 6a–c). There was a 6-fold increase ($p < 0.001$) in CD206-positive cells on day 3 post-ICH in comparison to sham (Fig. 6b) and the expression of CD206 colocalized with Iba1 (Fig. 6d). Moreover, both CD16/32 - and CD206-positive cells co-expressed TSPO further emphasizing the role of TSPO in neuroinflammatory responses after ICH (Fig. 7a, b). Quantitative colocalization analysis of images revealed a percentage of colocalization of 58.06 ± 2.3 and 46.97 ± 1.7 % between TSPO and CD16/32 or CD206, respectively, post-ICH (Fig. 7c, d). Though there was a difference in overlap of 11.09 % between the two, it was not statistically significant (data not shown). Furthermore, the subcellular localization of TSPO revealed prominent perinuclear expression of TSPO upon colocalization with PCNA, a nuclear marker of proliferating cells (Fig. 8).

Pharmacological and genetic modulation of TSPO signaling significantly alters the release of pro-inflammatory cytokines

To establish the functional role of TSPO in microglial/macrophage activation, we studied whether a TSPO agonist, Ro5-4864, is able to modulate hemin-mediated inflammatory reaction. Hemin is a metabolite, which accumulates at high concentration in intracranial hematomas

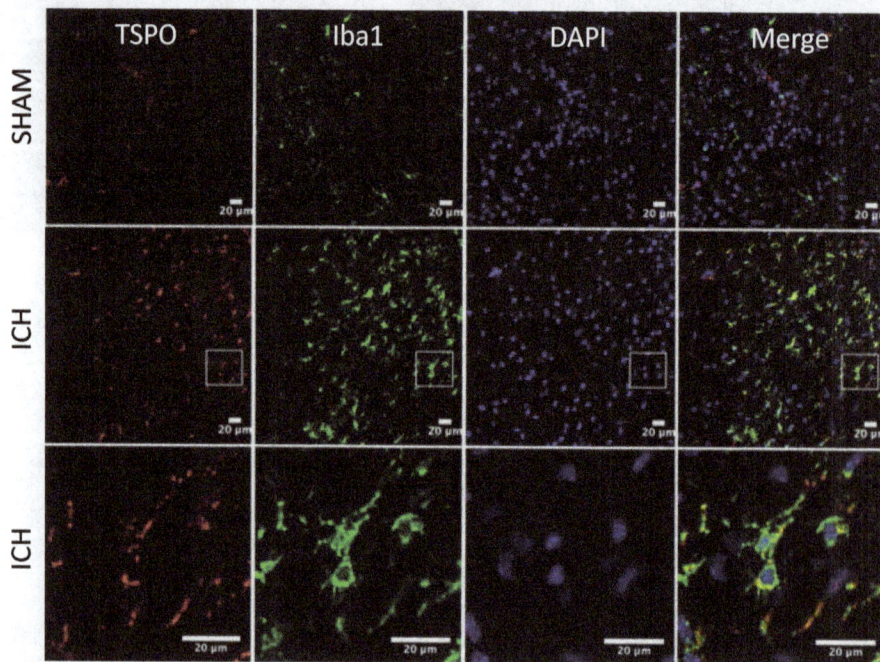

Fig. 4 TSPO expression in microglia/macrophage. Double immunolabeling of brain sections were performed for TSPO and Iba1 5 days post-injury. A very prominent expression of TSPO was observed in Iba1-positive cells and the lowest panel depicts high magnification image. Scale bar = 20 μm; n = 3/group

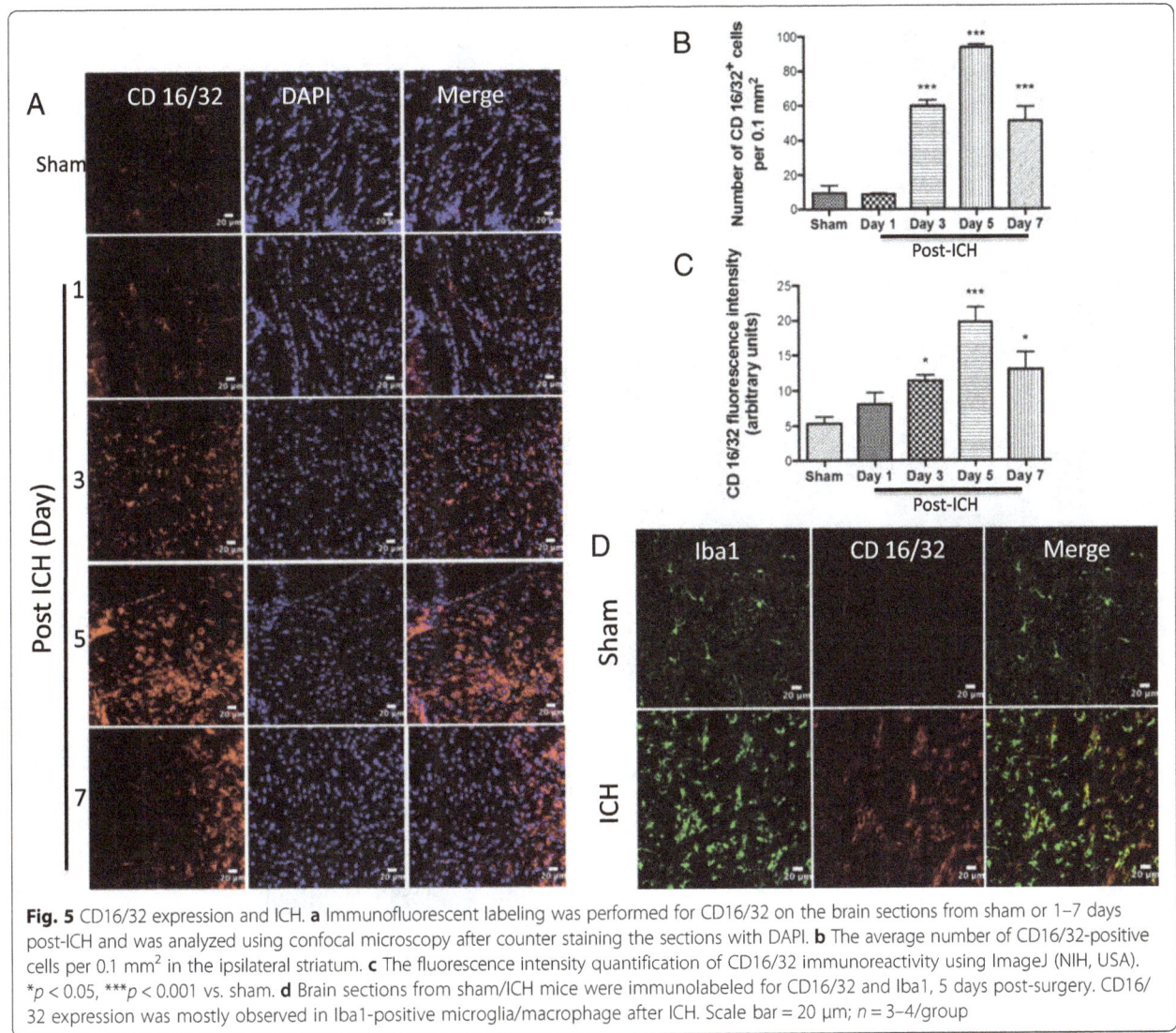

Fig. 5 CD16/32 expression and ICH. **a** Immunofluorescent labeling was performed for CD16/32 on the brain sections from sham or 1–7 days post-ICH and was analyzed using confocal microscopy after counter staining the sections with DAPI. **b** The average number of CD16/32-positive cells per 0.1 mm^2 in the ipsilateral striatum. **c** The fluorescence intensity quantification of CD16/32 immunoreactivity using ImageJ (NIH, USA). *$p < 0.05$, ***$p < 0.001$ vs. sham. **d** Brain sections from sham/ICH mice were immunolabeled for CD16/32 and Iba1, 5 days post-surgery. CD16/32 expression was mostly observed in Iba1-positive microglia/macrophage after ICH. Scale bar = 20 μm; $n = 3$–4/group

and is known to induce microglial activation via TLR-4 (Toll-like receptor-4) signaling mechanism [42]. Hemin treatment significantly augmented the release of pro-inflammatory cytokines TNF-α and IL-6 from murine macrophage cell line, RAW 264.7 cells, as evidenced by ELISA, whereas the incubation of cells with TSPO agonist, Ro5-4864, attenuated hemin-induced release of both TNF-α and IL-6 (Fig. 9). Along these lines, Ro5-4864 (5 and 10 μM) significantly reduced hemin-induced release of TNF-α by 87 and 97 %, respectively (Fig. 9a; $p < 0.05$ vs. hemin alone), and IL-6 by 52 and 79 %, respectively (Fig. 9b; $p < 0.001$ vs. hemin alone). Further, TSPO antagonist (PK11195) did not reduce hemin-induced TNF-α secretion (data not shown). To validate this further, we performed siRNA-mediated genetic knockdown of TSPO expression in RAW 264.7 cells and examined the inflammatory response. Notably, silencing of TSPO expression in RAW 264.7 cells by siRNA significantly reduced the TSPO expression by 52.6 % (Fig. 10a; $p < 0.001$ vs. control) and augmented hemin-induced release of TNF-α and IL-6 by 2-fold in comparison to controls (Fig. 10b, c; $p < 0.01$ vs. hemin-treated control). Altogether, the data derived from both pharmacological and genetic studies suggest that TSPO may serve as a negative regulator of inflammation after ICH.

Discussion

Intracerebral hemorrhage (ICH) is a stroke subtype resulting from the spontaneous extravasation of blood into the brain parenchyma. Though chronic hypertension, amyloid angiopathy, and advanced age are recognized as the prominent risk factors of ICH, the risk factors also include but not limited to ethnic differences and lifestyle factors such as smoking and alcohol intake [43]. Currently, the

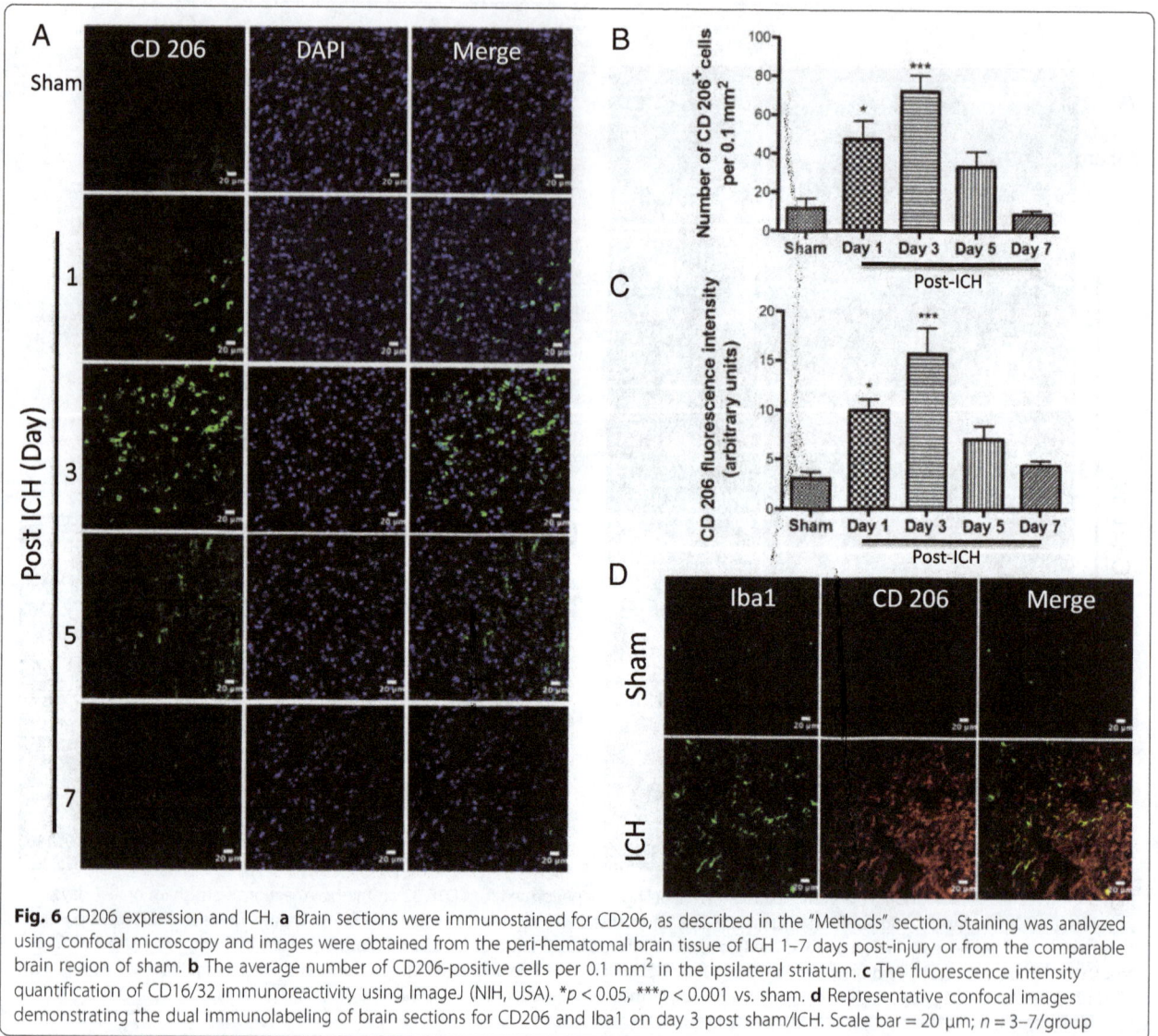

Fig. 6 CD206 expression and ICH. **a** Brain sections were immunostained for CD206, as described in the "Methods" section. Staining was analyzed using confocal microscopy and images were obtained from the peri-hematomal brain tissue of ICH 1–7 days post-injury or from the comparable brain region of sham. **b** The average number of CD206-positive cells per 0.1 mm² in the ipsilateral striatum. **c** The fluorescence intensity quantification of CD16/32 immunoreactivity using ImageJ (NIH, USA). *p < 0.05, ***p < 0.001 vs. sham. **d** Representative confocal images demonstrating the dual immunolabeling of brain sections for CD206 and Iba1 on day 3 post sham/ICH. Scale bar = 20 µm; n = 3–7/group

worldwide incidence of ICH is 2 million cases per year [2], with approximately 120,000 cases per year in the USA [44–46]. However, the incidence is expected to have doubled by 2050 [39] due to aging and the spreading use of anticoagulants [47]. Though ICH is a major public health problem, no effective medical or surgical therapy has been firmly established. Given the critical role of microglia/macrophage-mediated inflammation in ICH-induced secondary brain injury, a thorough understanding of the molecular regulators of inflammation in hemorrhagic brain injury is critical. This study identifies for the first time the microglia/macrophage expression of TSPO and the existence of M1 and M2 microglia/macrophage phenotypes in a preclinical model of ICH.

Secondary inflammatory damage to brain tissue has emerged as a common link between different types of central nervous system disorders [48–51]. ICH results in both primary and secondary brain insults, and several clinical and preclinical studies have suggested a significant contribution of neuroinflammation to the pathophysiology of ICH [47, 52, 53]. Notably, activated microglia and newly recruited peripheral macrophages are regarded as the key cellular regulators of neuroinflammation after ICH based on their local release of cytokines, chemokines, prostaglandins, proteases, ferrous iron, and other immunoactive molecules [52, 54, 55]. Under normal conditions, microglia retain a relative quiescent phenotype for constant monitoring of the brain parenchyma [56]. As influenced by their environment, both resident microglia and peripheral macrophages assume pro-inflammatory M1 and anti-inflammatory M2 phenotypes. M1 polarized microglia/macrophages produce largely deleterious

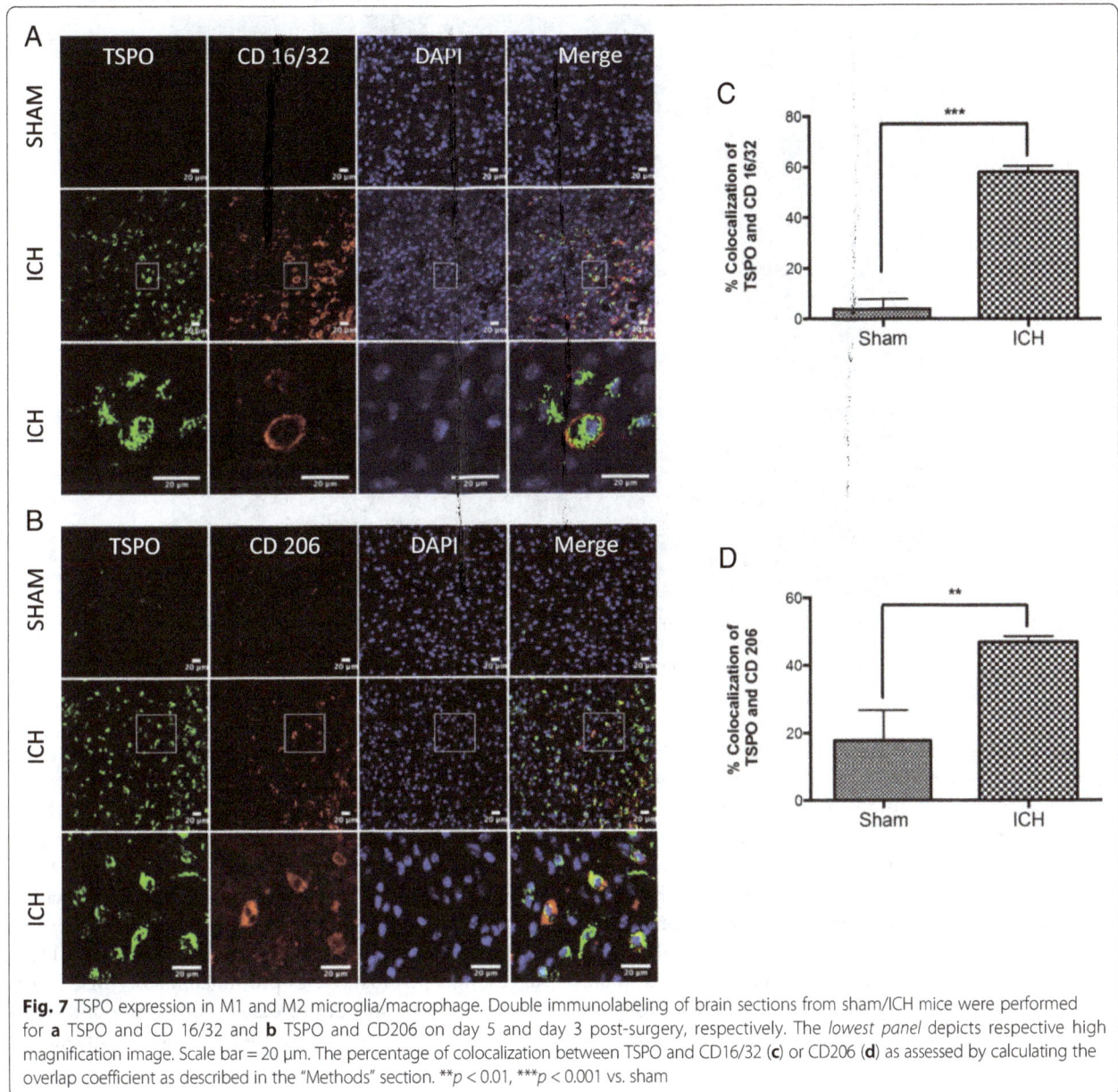

Fig. 7 TSPO expression in M1 and M2 microglia/macrophage. Double immunolabeling of brain sections from sham/ICH mice were performed for **a** TSPO and CD 16/32 and **b** TSPO and CD206 on day 5 and day 3 post-surgery, respectively. The *lowest panel* depicts respective high magnification image. Scale bar = 20 μm. The percentage of colocalization between TSPO and CD16/32 (**c**) or CD206 (**d**) as assessed by calculating the overlap coefficient as described in the "Methods" section. **$p < 0.01$, ***$p < 0.001$ vs. sham

pro-inflammatory cytokines such as TNF-α, IL-1β, and pro-oxidant enzymes such as inducible nitric oxide synthase [57, 58]. In contrast, M2-polarized microglia/macrophages produce neurotrophic factors and have been associated with regenerative effects after brain injury [59]. However, the microglia/macrophage polarization after ICH is largely uncharacterized and herein we demonstrate for the first time the temporal pattern of microglia/macrophage polarization after ICH.

The inflammatory response to ICH is characterized by a rapid activation of resident microglia within minutes after the onset of ICH and the activated microglia/macrophage are found in and around the hematoma [52, 54, 60]. The early response of microglia/macrophage to ICH suggests that components of the hematoma may trigger microglial activation. Consistently, the hematoma components such as erythrocytes and its lysed products (Hb, heme, and iron), thrombin (blood coagulation factor), and complements are capable of activating microglia/macrophages [61–64]. However, the precise molecular mechanism of microglia/macrophage activation after ICH remains unclear. Further, hemin, a hemoglobin metabolite which accumulates at high concentration in intracranial hematomas [65], can induce inflammatory brain injury after ICH [64]. Altogether, inflammatory signaling triggered by hematoma components leads to microglial

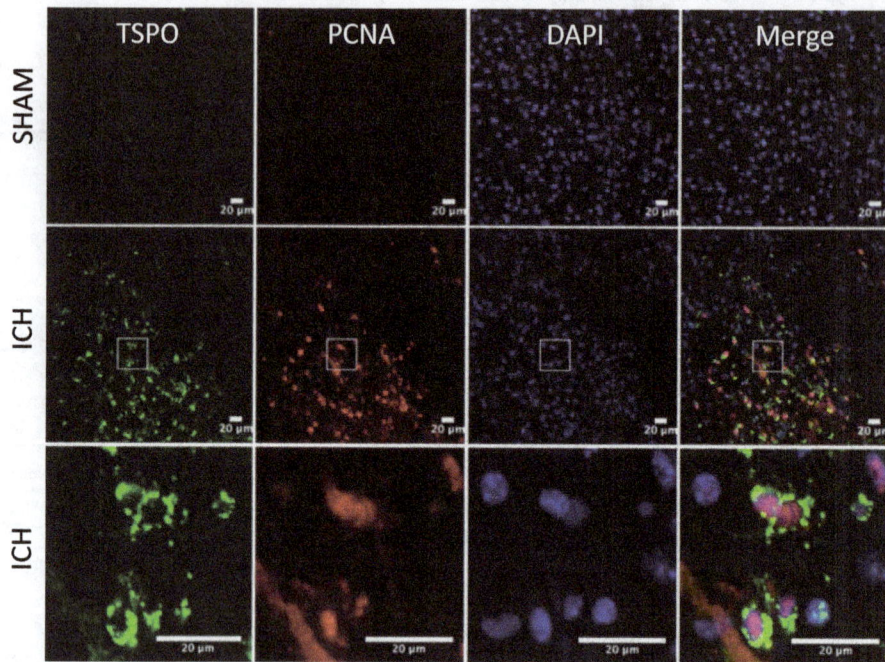

Fig. 8 Subcellular localization of TSPO. Dual-label fluorescence immunohistochemistry was performed for proliferating cell nuclear antigen (PCNA), a cellular proliferation marker, and TSPO, in sham-operated mice or at 5 days post-ICH and prominent perinuclear expression of TSPO was observed after ICH and the *lowest panel* depicts high magnification image. Scale bar = 20 μm

activation, peripheral inflammatory cell infiltration, and release of pro-inflammatory mediators, eventually resulting in massive brain cell death and neurological deficits. However, intrinsic regulators of microglia/macrophage activation after ICH remain largely uncharacterized.

Herein, we demonstrate for the first time that the TSPO expression is elevated after ICH and the peak expression is observed on day 3 to day 5 post-ICH, the time point that exhibits very prominent microglia/macrophage activation. Furthermore, TSPO expression was observed mostly in the Iba1-positive microglia or macrophage whereas TSPO

expression was not observed in either GFAP- or NeuN-positive cells, making TSPO a suitable molecular target to modulate microglia/macrophage functions after ICH. Furthermore, microglia/macrophage exhibited both pro-inflammatory M1 and anti-inflammatory M2 phenotypes after ICH. The expression of M1 cell surface marker CD16/32 is found to be prolonged after ICH in contrast to an early occurrence of M2, cell surface marker, CD206 suggesting a possible role of pro-inflammatory M1 microglia/macrophage in ICH-mediated both acute and long-term neurological deficits. Further, the early occurrence of

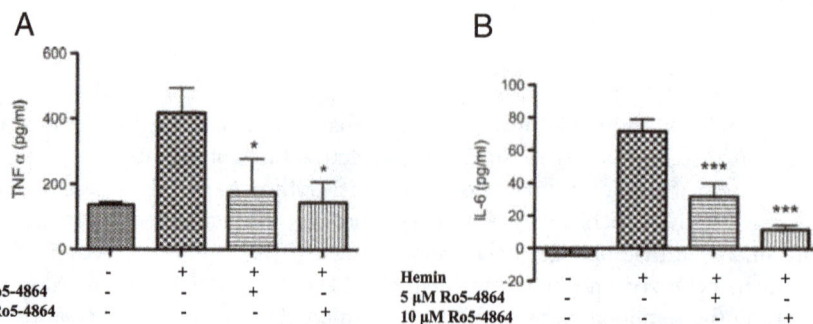

Fig. 9 Ro5-4864-attenuated hemin-induced release of TNF-α and IL-6. RAW 264.7 cells were plated overnight and TSPO agonist, Ro5-4864, was added 1 h prior to hemin (30 μM) addition and the hemin treatment was conducted in the presence of Ro5-4864 and the supernatant was collected. The release of TNF-α (**a**) and IL-6 (**b**) into the supernatant was estimated using ELISA as per manufacturer's instructions. (RayBiotech, Inc., Norcross, GA, USA). Ro5-4864 treatment significantly attenuated the hemin-induced release of TNF-α and IL-6. $n = 4$–9; $^*p < 0.05$, $^{***}p < 0.001$ vs. hemin alone

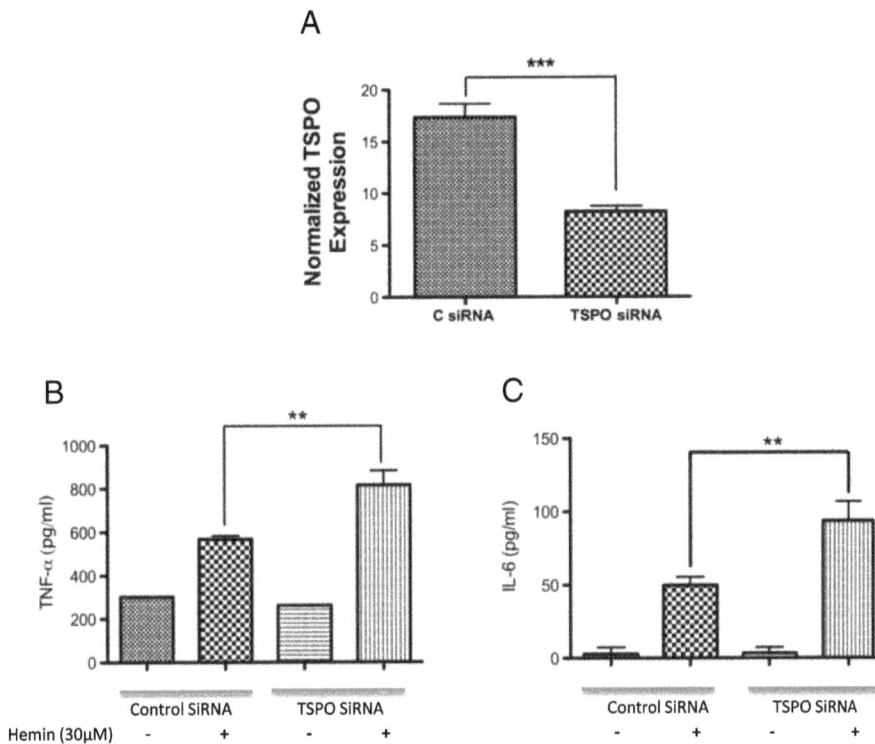

Fig. 10 Genetic knockdown of TSPO augmented hemin-induced release of TNF-α and IL-6. **a** Genetic knockdown of TSPO in RAW. 264.7 cells were achieved employing TSPO siRNA as described in the "Methods" section. Genetic knockdown of TSPO significantly augmented the hemin-induced release of both TNF-α (**b**) and IL-6 (**c**) in RAW 264.7 cells. $n = 3$–4; **$p < 0.01$ vs. hemin-treated control, ***$p < 0.001$ vs. control

CD206-positive M2 microglia/macrophage after ICH could be an intrinsic mechanism to remove cellular debris derived from hematoma or to restore brain homeostasis. More importantly, the expression of TSPO in both M1 and M2 microglia/macrophage as demonstrated herein suggests an unexplored role of TSPO in neuroinflammatory responses after ICH. In addition, a TSPO agonist attenuated hemin-mediated release of TNF-α and IL-6 from RAW 264.7 cells, suggesting that TSPO can be therapeutically targeted to attenuate neuroinflammatory response after ICH and this was further supported by the genetic knockdown studies. However, further studies are required to characterize the cell-specific role of TSPO expression in M1 and M2 microglia/macrophage after ICH. Though, CD16/32 and CD 206 are widely used and regarded as signature markers of M1 and M2 microglia/macrophage phenotypes, respectively, the use of a single molecular marker in characterizing either M1 or M2 microglia/macrophage remains as a limitation of the study. Further, given the occurrence of differential microglia/macrophage phenotypes after a brain injury, the possibility of expression of TSPO in other microglia/macrophage phenotypes apart from M1 and M2 cannot be completely ruled out. Notably, LPS (lipopolysaccharide), a potent ligand of TLR-4 augmented TSPO expression in BV2 microglial cells

[66]. Moreover, in actively proliferating cells and in LPS-induced cultured retinal microglia, the expression of TSPO has been observed in the perinuclear and nuclear area [66, 67]. Consistently, the subcellular localization of TSPO revealed prominent perinuclear expression after ICH suggesting a role of TSPO in microglial proliferation which is often associated with neurodegenerative conditions [68] further emphasizing the therapeutic potential of TSPO. It has been previously reported that IL-1β and TNF-α can stimulate microglial proliferation [69–71]. However, the mechanism by which TSPO regulates neuroinflammation after ICH needs further investigation.

Further, emerging evidences suggest that the administration of TSPO-selective ligands may be useful in the treatment of neuroinflammatory conditions [72–74] and may exert neuroprotection after seizures and brain injury by suppressing microglial activation [72, 75–78]. Moreover, minocycline-mediated attenuation of retinal degeneration was associated with reduction in microglial reactivity and the expression of TSPO [79]. Notably, the primary endogenous ligands of TSPO include a polypeptide called diazepam-binding inhibitor (DBI) and its shorter peptide cleavage products called endozepines [80]. These molecules are expressed and secreted by glial populations in the CNS [81]. It is postulated that the ligand-mediated TSPO signaling in microglia can increase mitochondrial cholesterol flux, facilitating the production of modulatory neurosteroids that in turn repress inflammatory genes in a cell-autonomous manner [66]. Endogenous TSPO signaling may also result in other physiological changes in microglia including regulation of calcium influx [82], mitochondrial function [6], and apoptosis [83], all of which may modulate microglial activation. However, neither the precise role of TSPO nor the exact mechanism by which TSPO-specific ligands confer neuroprotection is known. Though TSPO ligands have been widely used for brain imaging of neuroinflammation, in several neuropathological conditions such as Alzheimer's disease (AD), Parkinson's disease, and Huntington's disease, no such imaging technique is currently available to monitor microglial activation after ICH. The low level of expression in uninjured brain regions coupled with the injury-induced remarkable induction makes TSPO a suitable candidate to monitor inflammation after ICH. Altogether, the data derived from this study suggest a therapeutic and diagnostic potential of TSPO after ICH.

Conclusions

The present study reports for the first time that TSPO expression is found to be increased in the peri-hematomal brain region 1 to 7 days post-ICH, peaking on day 3 to day 5 in comparison to sham. Further, the expression of TSPO is mostly observed in microglia/macrophages suggesting a possible role of TSPO in neuroinflammatory response after ICH and this is further supported by its occurrence in M1 and M2 microglia/macrophage phenotypes after ICH. Notably, the subcellular localization studies revealed prominent perinuclear expression of TSPO after ICH. Though this observation is consistent with the in vitro studies with cultured microglia [66], the precise functional significance of TSPO expression in this subcellular area requires further investigation. Moreover, both genetic and pharmacological studies revealed a regulatory role of TSPO in the release of pro-inflammatory cytokines in a macrophage cell line, RAW 264.7. Altogether, the data suggest that TSPO induction after ICH could be an intrinsic mechanism to prevent an exacerbated inflammatory response and raise the possibility of targeting TSPO for the attenuation of secondary brain injury after ICH.

Abbreviations
CD 16/32, cluster of differentiation 16/32; CD 206, cluster of differentiation 206; cDNA, complementary DNA; CNS, central nervous system; DAPI, 4′,6-diamidino-2-phenylindole; ELISA, enzyme-linked immunosorbent assay; GFAP, glial fibrillary acidic protein; Hb, hemoglobin; Iba1, ionized calcium binding adaptor molecule 1; ICH, intracerebral hemorrhage; IL-6, interleukin 6; LPS, lipopolysaccharide; NeuN, neuronal nuclei; PBS, phosphate-buffered saline; PCNA, proliferating cell nuclear antigen; RPS3, ribosomal protein S3; RT-PCR, reverse transcription polymerase chain reaction; SE, standard error; siRNA, small interfering ribonucleic acid; TLR-4, Toll-like receptor 4; TNF-α, tumor necrosis factor alpha; TSPO, 18-kDa translocator protein

Acknowledgements
Not applicable.

Funding
This work was supported by a grant from the American Heart Association (14SDG18730034) to SSR. None of the funding bodies had a role in the study design, data collection, data analysis, data interpretation, or writing of the manuscript.

Authors' contributions
FB carried out the immunohistochemical and cell culture studies and participated in the data analysis. CA participated in timely project discussions. SSR conceived and designed the experiments. SSR also conducted the animal surgeries, genetic studies, and data analysis and drafted the manuscript. All authors read and approved the final manuscript.

Competing interests
The authors declare that they have no competing interests.

References
1. Qureshi AI, Ling GS, Khan J, Suri MF, Miskolczi L, et al. Quantitative analysis of injured, necrotic, and apoptotic cells in a new experimental model of intracerebral hemorrhage. Crit Care Med. 2001;29:152–7.
2. van Asch CJ, Luitse MJ, Rinkel GJ, van der Tweel I, Algra A, et al. Incidence, case fatality, and functional outcome of intracerebral haemorrhage over time, according to age, sex, and ethnic origin: a systematic review and meta-analysis. Lancet Neurol. 2010;9:167–76.
3. Nilsson OG, Lindgren A, Brandt L, Saveland H. Prediction of death in patients with primary intracerebral hemorrhage: a prospective study of a defined population. J Neurosurg. 2002;97:531–6.
4. Broderick JP, Adams Jr HP, Barsan W, Feinberg W, Feldmann E, et al. Guidelines for the management of spontaneous intracerebral hemorrhage: a statement for healthcare professionals from a special writing group of the Stroke Council, American Heart Association. Stroke. 1999;30:905–15.
5. Broderick J, Connolly S, Feldmann E, Hanley D, Kase C, et al. Guidelines for the management of spontaneous intracerebral hemorrhage in adults: 2007 update: a guideline from the American Heart Association/American Stroke Association Stroke Council, High Blood Pressure Research Council, and the Quality of Care and Outcomes in Research Interdisciplinary Working Group. Stroke. 2007;38:2001–23.
6. Casellas P, Galiegue S, Basile AS. Peripheral benzodiazepine receptors and mitochondrial function. Neurochem Int. 2002;40:475–86.
7. Braestrup C, Albrechtsen R, Squires RF. High densities of benzodiazepine receptors in human cortical areas. Nature. 1977;269:702–4.
8. Papadopoulos V, Baraldi M, Guilarte TR, Knudsen TB, Lacapere JJ, et al. Translocator protein (18 kDa): new nomenclature for the peripheral-type benzodiazepine receptor based on its structure and molecular function. Trends Pharmacol Sci. 2006;27:402–9.
9. Sprengel R, Werner P, Seeburg PH, Mukhin AG, Santi MR, et al. Molecular cloning and expression of cDNA encoding a peripheral-type benzodiazepine receptor. J Biol Chem. 1989;264:20415–21.
10. Parola AL, Stump DG, Pepperl DJ, Krueger KE, Regan JW, et al. Cloning and expression of a pharmacologically unique bovine peripheral-type benzodiazepine receptor isoquinoline binding protein. J Biol Chem. 1991;266:14082–7.

11. Riond J, Mattei MG, Kaghad M, Dumont X, Guillemot JC, et al. Molecular cloning and chromosomal localization of a human peripheral-type benzodiazepine receptor. Eur J Biochem. 1991;195:305–11.

12. Chang YJ, McCabe RT, Rennert H, Budarf ML, Sayegh R, et al. The human "peripheral-type" benzodiazepine receptor: regional mapping of the gene and characterization of the receptor expressed from cDNA. DNA Cell Biol. 1992;11:471–80.

13. Garnier M, Dimchev AB, Boujrad N, Price JM, Musto NA, et al. In vitro reconstitution of a functional peripheral-type benzodiazepine receptor from mouse Leydig tumor cells. Mol Pharmacol. 1994;45:201–11.

14. Anholt RR, Pedersen PL, De Souza EB, Snyder SH. The peripheral-type benzodiazepine receptor. Localization to the mitochondrial outer membrane. J Biol Chem. 1986;261:576–83.

15. Mukhin AG, Papadopoulos V, Costa E, Krueger KE. Mitochondrial benzodiazepine receptors regulate steroid biosynthesis. Proc Natl Acad Sci U S A. 1989;86:9813–6.

16. Krueger KE, Papadopoulos V. Peripheral-type benzodiazepine receptors mediate translocation of cholesterol from outer to inner mitochondrial membranes in adrenocortical cells. J Biol Chem. 1990;265:15015–22.

17. Rupprecht R, Papadopoulos V, Rammes G, Baghai TC, Fan J, et al. Translocator protein (18 kDa) (TSPO) as a therapeutic target for neurological and psychiatric disorders. Nat Rev Drug Discov. 2010;9:971–88.

18. Costa E, Auta J, Guidotti A, Korneyev A, Romeo E. The pharmacology of neurosteroidogenesis. J Steroid Biochem Mol Biol. 1994;49:385–9.

19. Lacapere JJ, Papadopoulos V. Peripheral-type benzodiazepine receptor: structure and function of a cholesterol-binding protein in steroid and bile acid biosynthesis. Steroids. 2003;68:569–85.

20. Romeo E, Cavallaro S, Korneyev A, Kozikowski AP, Ma D, et al. Stimulation of brain steroidogenesis by 2-aryl-indole-3-acetamide derivatives acting at the mitochondrial diazepam-binding inhibitor receptor complex. J Pharmacol Exp Ther. 1993;267:462–71.

21. Morohaku K, Pelton SH, Daugherty DJ, Butler WR, Deng W, et al. Translocator protein/peripheral benzodiazepine receptor is not required for steroid hormone biosynthesis. Endocrinology. 2014;155:89–97.

22. Banati RB, Middleton RJ, Chan R, Hatty CR, Kam WW, et al. Positron emission tomography and functional characterization of a complete PBR/TSPO knockout. Nat Commun. 2014;5:5452.

23. Tu LN, Morohaku K, Manna PR, Pelton SH, Butler WR, et al. Peripheral benzodiazepine receptor/translocator protein global knock-out mice are viable with no effects on steroid hormone biosynthesis. J Biol Chem. 2014;289:27444–54.

24. Chen MK, Guilarte TR. Translocator protein 18 kDa (TSPO): molecular sensor of brain injury and repair. Pharmacol Ther. 2008;118:1–17.

25. Cosenza-Nashat M, Zhao ML, Suh HS, Morgan J, Natividad R, et al. Expression of the translocator protein of 18 kDa by microglia, macrophages and astrocytes based on immunohistochemical localization in abnormal human brain. Neuropathol Appl Neurobiol. 2009;35:306–28.

26. Veenman L, Papadopoulos V, Gavish M. Channel-like functions of the 18-kDa translocator protein (TSPO): regulation of apoptosis and steroidogenesis as part of the host-defense response. Curr Pharm Des. 2007;13:2385–405.

27. Liu J, Rone MB, Papadopoulos V. Protein-protein interactions mediate mitochondrial cholesterol transport and steroid biosynthesis. J Biol Chem. 2006;281:38879–93.

28. Maeda J, Higuchi M, Inaji M, Ji B, Haneda E, et al. Phase-dependent roles of reactive microglia and astrocytes in nervous system injury as delineated by imaging of peripheral benzodiazepine receptor. Brain Res. 2007;1157: 100–11.

29. Zurcher NR, Loggia ML, Lawson R, Chonde DB, Izquierdo-Garcia D, et al. Increased in vivo glial activation in patients with amyotrophic lateral sclerosis: assessed with [(11)C]-PBR28. Neuroimage Clin. 2015;7:409–14.

30. Karlstetter M, Nothdurfter C, Aslanidis A, Moeller K, Horn F, et al. Translocator protein (18 kDa) (TSPO) is expressed in reactive retinal microglia and modulates microglial inflammation and phagocytosis. J Neuroinflammation. 2014;11:3.

31. Liu GJ, Middleton RJ, Hatty CR, Kam WW, Chan R, et al. The 18 kDa translocator protein, microglia and neuroinflammation. Brain Pathol. 2014;24:631–53.

32. Politis M, Su P, Piccini P. Imaging of microglia in patients with neurodegenerative disorders. Front Pharmacol. 2012;3:96.

33. Venneti S, Lopresti BJ, Wiley CA. Molecular imaging of microglia/macrophages in the brain. Glia. 2013;61:10–23.

34. Nothdurfter C, Baghai TC, Schule C, Rupprecht R. Translocator protein (18 kDa) (TSPO) as a therapeutic target for anxiety and neurologic disorders. Eur Arch Psychiatry Clin Neurosci. 2012;262 Suppl 2:S107–12.

35. Sukumari-Ramesh S, Alleyne Jr CH, Dhandapani KM. Astrocyte-specific expression of survivin after intracerebral hemorrhage in mice: a possible role in reactive gliosis? J Neurotrauma. 2012;29:2798–804.

36. Sukumari-Ramesh S, Alleyne Jr CH, Dhandapani KM. Astrogliosis: a target for intervention in intracerebral hemorrhage? Transl Stroke Res. 2012;3:80–7.

37. Laird MD, Sukumari-Ramesh S, Swift AE, Meiler SE, Vender JR, et al. Curcumin attenuates cerebral edema following traumatic brain injury in mice: a possible role for aquaporin-4? J Neurochem. 2010;113:637–48.

38. Emsley HC, Tyrrell PJ. Inflammation and infection in clinical stroke. J Cereb Blood Flow Metab. 2002;22:1399–419.

39. Qureshi AI, Tuhrim S, Broderick JP, Batjer HH, Hondo H, et al. Spontaneous intracerebral hemorrhage. N Engl J Med. 2001;344:1450–60.

40. Sukumari-Ramesh S, Alleyne Jr CH, Dhandapani KM. The histone deacetylase inhibitor suberoylanilide hydroxamic acid (SAHA) confers acute neuroprotection after intracerebral hemorrhage in mice. Transl Stroke Res. 2016;7:141–8.

41. Sukumari-Ramesh S, Alleyne Jr CH. Post-injury administration of tert-butylhydroquinone attenuates acute neurological injury after intracerebral hemorrhage in mice. J Mol Neurosci. 2016;58:525–31.

42. Lin S, Yin Q, Zhong Q, Lv FL, Zhou Y, et al. Heme activates TLR4-mediated inflammatory injury via MyD88/TRIF signaling pathway in intracerebral hemorrhage. J Neuroinflammation. 2012;9:46.

43. O'Donnell MJ, Xavier D, Liu L, Zhang H, Chin SL, et al. Risk factors for ischaemic and intracerebral haemorrhagic stroke in 22 countries (the INTERSTROKE study): a case-control study. Lancet. 2010;376:112–23.

44. Aguilar MI, Freeman WD. Spontaneous intracerebral hemorrhage. Semin Neurol. 2010;30:555–64.

45. Broderick J, Connolly S, Feldmann E, Hanley D, Kase C, et al. Guidelines for the management of spontaneous intracerebral hemorrhage in adults: 2007 update: a guideline from the American Heart Association/American Stroke Association Stroke Council, High Blood Pressure Research Council, and the Quality of Care and Outcomes in Research Interdisciplinary Working Group. Circulation. 2007;116:e391–413.

46. Ribo M, Grotta JC. Latest advances in intracerebral hemorrhage. Curr Neurol Neurosci Rep. 2006;6:17–22.

47. Wang J. Preclinical and clinical research on inflammation after intracerebral hemorrhage. Prog Neurobiol. 2010;92:463–77.

48. Xi G, Keep RF, Hoff JT. Mechanisms of brain injury after intracerebral haemorrhage. Lancet Neurol. 2006;5:53–63.

49. Diringer MN. Intracerebral hemorrhage: pathophysiology and management. Crit Care Med. 1993;21:1591–603.

50. Greve MW, Zink BJ. Pathophysiology of traumatic brain injury. Mt Sinai J Med. 2009;76:97–104.

51. Dirnagl U, Iadecola C, Moskowitz MA. Pathobiology of ischaemic stroke: an integrated view. Trends Neurosci. 1999;22:391–7.

52. Wang J, Dore S. Inflammation after intracerebral hemorrhage. J Cereb Blood Flow Metab. 2007;27:894–908.

53. Carmichael ST, Vespa PM, Saver JL, Coppola G, Geschwind DH, et al. Genomic profiles of damage and protection in human intracerebral hemorrhage. J Cereb Blood Flow Metab. 2008;28:1860–75.

54. Aronowski J, Hall CE. New horizons for primary intracerebral hemorrhage treatment: experience from preclinical studies. Neurol Res. 2005;27:268–79.

55. Zhang D, Hu X, Qian L, Wilson B, Lee C, et al. Prostaglandin E2 released from activated microglia enhances astrocyte proliferation in vitro. Toxicol Appl Pharmacol. 2009;238:64–70.

56. Nimmerjahn A, Kirchhoff F, Helmchen F. Resting microglial cells are highly dynamic surveillants of brain parenchyma in vivo. Science. 2005;308:1314–8.

57. Liao B, Zhao W, Beers DR, Henkel JS, Appel SH. Transformation from a neuroprotective to a neurotoxic microglial phenotype in a mouse model of ALS. Exp Neurol. 2012;237:147–52.

58. Kobayashi K, Imagama S, Ohgomori T, Hirano K, Uchimura K, et al. Minocycline selectively inhibits M1 polarization of microglia. Cell Death Dis. 2013;4, e525.

59. Ponomarev ED, Maresz K, Tan Y, Dittel BN. CNS-derived interleukin-4 is essential for the regulation of autoimmune inflammation and induces a state of alternative activation in microglial cells. J Neurosci. 2007;27:10714–21.

60. Wang J, Rogove AD, Tsirka AE, Tsirka SE. Protective role of tuftsin fragment 1-3 in an animal model of intracerebral hemorrhage. Ann Neurol. 2003;54:655–64.

61. Moller T, Hanisch UK, Ransom BR. Thrombin-induced activation of cultured rodent microglia. J Neurochem. 2000;75:1539–47.
62. van Rossum D, Hanisch UK. Microglia. Metab Brain Dis. 2004;19:393–411.
63. Aronowski J, Zhao X. Molecular pathophysiology of cerebral hemorrhage: secondary brain injury. Stroke. 2011;42:1781–6.
64. Babu R, Bagley JH, Di C, Friedman AH, Adamson C. Thrombin and hemin as central factors in the mechanisms of intracerebral hemorrhage-induced secondary brain injury and as potential targets for intervention. Neurosurg Focus. 2012;32, E8.
65. Letarte PB, Lieberman K, Nagatani K, Haworth RA, Odell GB, et al. Hemin: levels in experimental subarachnoid hematoma and effects on dissociated vascular smooth-muscle cells. J Neurosurg. 1993;79:252–5.
66. Wang M, Wang X, Zhao L, Ma W, Rodriguez IR, et al. Macroglia-microglia interactions via TSPO signaling regulates microglial activation in the mouse retina. J Neurosci. 2014;34:3793–806.
67. Kuhlmann AC, Guilarte TR. Cellular and subcellular localization of peripheral benzodiazepine receptors after trimethyltin neurotoxicity. J Neurochem. 2000;74:1694–704.
68. Gomez-Nicola D, Fransen NL, Suzzi S, Perry VH. Regulation of microglial proliferation during chronic neurodegeneration. J Neurosci. 2013;33:2481–93.
69. Ganter S, Northoff H, Mannel D, Gebicke-Harter PJ. Growth control of cultured microglia. J Neurosci Res. 1992;33:218–30.
70. Kloss CU, Kreutzberg GW, Raivich G. Proliferation of ramified microglia on an astrocyte monolayer: characterization of stimulatory and inhibitory cytokines. J Neurosci Res. 1997;49:248–54.
71. Mander PK, Jekabsone A, Brown GC. Microglia proliferation is regulated by hydrogen peroxide from NADPH oxidase. J Immunol. 2006;176:1046–52.
72. Veiga S, Carrero P, Pernia O, Azcoitia I, Garcia-Segura LM. Translocator protein 18 kDa is involved in the regulation of reactive gliosis. Glia. 2007;55:1426–36.
73. Ma L, Zhang H, Liu N, Wang PQ, Guo WZ, et al. TSPO ligand PK11195 alleviates neuroinflammation and beta-amyloid generation induced by systemic LPS administration. Brain Res Bull. 2016;121:192–200.
74. Zhao YY, Yu JZ, Li QY, Ma CG, Lu CZ, et al. TSPO-specific ligand vinpocetine exerts a neuroprotective effect by suppressing microglial inflammation. Neuron Glia Biol. 2011;7:187–97.
75. Ferzaz B, Brault E, Bourliaud G, Robert JP, Poughon G, et al. SSR180575 (7-chloro-N, N,5-trimethyl-4-oxo-3-phenyl-3,5-dihydro-4H-pyridazino[4,5-b]indole-1 -acetamide), a peripheral benzodiazepine receptor ligand, promotes neuronal survival and repair. J Pharmacol Exp Ther. 2002;301: 1067–78.
76. Ryu JK, Choi HB, McLarnon JG. Peripheral benzodiazepine receptor ligand PK11195 reduces microglial activation and neuronal death in quinolinic acid-injected rat striatum. Neurobiol Dis. 2005;20:550–61.
77. Veenman L, Leschiner S, Spanier I, Weisinger G, Weizman A, et al. PK 11195 attenuates kainic acid-induced seizures and alterations in peripheral-type benzodiazepine receptor (PBR) protein components in the rat brain. J Neurochem. 2002;80:917–27.
78. Veiga S, Azcoitia I, Garcia-Segura LM. Ro5-4864, a peripheral benzodiazepine receptor ligand, reduces reactive gliosis and protects hippocampal hilar neurons from kainic acid excitotoxicity. J Neurosci Res. 2005;80:129–37.
79. Scholz R, Sobotka M, Caramoy A, Stempfl T, Moehle C, et al. Minocycline counter-regulates pro-inflammatory microglia responses in the retina and protects from degeneration. J Neuroinflammation. 2015;12:209.
80. Ferrero P, Santi MR, Conti-Tronconi B, Costa E, Guidotti A. Study of an octadecaneuropeptide derived from diazepam binding inhibitor (DBI): biological activity and presence in rat brain. Proc Natl Acad Sci U S A. 1986;83:827–31.
81. Yanase H, Shimizu H, Yamada K, Iwanaga T. Cellular localization of the diazepam binding inhibitor in glial cells with special reference to its coexistence with brain-type fatty acid binding protein. Arch Histol Cytol. 2002;65:27–36.
82. Hong SH, Choi HB, Kim SU, McLarnon JG. Mitochondrial ligand inhibits store-operated calcium influx and COX-2 production in human microglia. J Neurosci Res. 2006;83:1293–8.
83. Hirsch T, Decaudin D, Susin SA, Marchetti P, Larochette N, et al. PK11195, a ligand of the mitochondrial benzodiazepine receptor, facilitates the induction of apoptosis and reverses Bcl-2-mediated cytoprotection. Exp Cell Res. 1998;241:426–34.

3

Nuclear factor-κB activation in perihematomal brain tissue correlates with outcome in patients with intracerebral hemorrhage

Ze-Li Zhang[1], Yu-Guang Liu[2*], Qi-Bing Huang[1], Hong-Wei Wang[2], Yan Song[2], Zhen-Kuan Xu[2] and Feng Li[2*]

Abstract

Background: Nuclear factor-κB (NF-κB) plays an important role in the inflammatory response after intracerebral hemorrhage (ICH). We therefore proposed that NF-κB activation in perihematomal brain tissue might correlate with clinical outcome in patients with ICH. To confirm this, we studied clinical data of 45 patients with ICH and NF-κB activation in perihematomal brain tissue and analyzed predictors of clinical outcome as well as the predictive value of NF-κB activation.

Methods: Forty-five patients with spontaneous basal ganglia hemorrhage were prospectively investigated. The clinical data were collected, which include demographics, alcohol and tobacco abuse, stroke risk factors, neuroimaging variables at presentation, Glasgow Coma Scale (GCS) at admission, number of days in hospital, mechanical ventilation, pneumonia, and outcome. Clinical outcome was assessed by the modified Rankin Scale at 6 months after ICH. Perihematomal brain tissue was collected, and NF-κB activation was detected using immunohistochemistry. Univariate analysis and multivariate logistic regression analysis were performed to determine predictors of the poor outcome.

Results: Immunohistochemical detection showed that NF-κB p65 was expressed in the nuclei of neurons and glial cells in all patients. The number of nuclear NF-κB p65-positive cells was 54 ± 21. Six months after ICH, 18 (40%) patients achieved a favorable functional outcome (mRS ≤ 3) while 27 (60%) had a poor functional outcome (mRS 4 to 6). In univariate analysis, predictors of poor functional outcome were lower GCS score on admission ($P = 0.004$), larger hematoma volume ($P = 0.004$), intraventricular extension ($P = 0.047$), midline shift ($P = 0.005$), NF-κB activation ($P < 0.0001$), mechanical ventilation ($P = 0.018$), and co-morbidity with pneumonia ($P = 0.002$). In multivariate logistic regression analysis, NF-κB activation was the only independent predictor of poor outcome at 6 months after ICH.

Conclusions: NF-κB activation is closely related to clinical outcome 6 months after ICH in humans. Therefore, it could be useful to predict prognosis of ICH accurately and should be further evaluated as a target for therapeutic strategies of ICH in the future.

Keywords: NF-κB, Intracerebral hemorrhage, Outcome, Predictor, Patient

* Correspondence: NS3000@126.com; tylor1216@163.com
[2]Department of Neurosurgery, Qilu Hospital of Shandong University and
Brain Science Research Institute of Shandong University, No. 107 Wenhuaxi
Road, 250012 Jinan, Shandong Province, People's Republic of China
Full list of author information is available at the end of the article

Introduction

Primary intracerebral hemorrhage (ICH) is still a frequent form of cerebrovascular diseases despite improved control of hypertension. It accounts for 30% of all cases of stroke in China, approximately twice higher than that in the West, and is one of the leading causes of stroke-related mortality and morbidity worldwide [1-3]. Functional outcome in survivors is also poor with fewer than 20% being independent at 6 months [4]. Previous studies have shown that the prognosis of patients with ICH is affected by series of factors, such as age, high blood pressure, hematoma volume, Glasgow Coma Scale (GCS) score on admission, stroke risk factors, underlying disease, leukocyte counts, neuroimaging, operation, complications, and so on [5-11], so it is always difficult for us to predict the outcome accurately.

A series of pathophysiological changes in brain tissue arises after ICH [12]. Previous studies revealed that a large number of inflammatory cells surround the hematoma in the rat model of ICH and that the inflammatory response is an important mechanism of secondary brain damage after ICH [13,14]. Nuclear factor-κB (NF-κB) has been recognized as a critical regulator of inflammatory responses since its discovery [15]. In unstimulated cells, inactive NF-κB is sequestered in the cytoplasm by inhibitory protein IκB. NF-κB can be activated by a wide array of factors such as thrombin, tumor necrosis factor-α (TNF-α), interleukin-1 (IL-1), oxidative stress, and growth factors [16]. Then, the free NF-κB rapidly migrates into the nucleus, binds to DNA, and promotes the transcription of genes for the release of inflammatory substances. So NF-κB plays an important role in the inflammatory response after ICH [17].

Given the important role played by NF-κB in the secondary brain damage after ICH, we imagine that NF-κB activation in perihematomal brain tissue was closely related to the clinical outcome of patients with ICH. In other words, NF-κB could be used to predict the clinical outcome. In order to confirm this, we collected 45 patients with basal ganglia hemorrhage, studied the clinical data and perihematomal brain tissue, and analyzed the predictors of the clinical outcome as well as the predicting value of NF-κB activation.

Materials and methods

Study population

All patients with spontaneous basal ganglia hemorrhage admitted to the Emergency Neurosurgery Department of Shandong University Qilu Hospital from October 2011 to August 2013 were screened for this study. Inclusion criteria were time from symptom onset to specimen collection 6 to 12 h, hematoma volume 30 to 90 ml, and hematoma evacuation operation conducted along the nonfunctional cortex. The intracerebral hemorrhage volume

was measured using the ABC/2 method according to the CT scanning [18]. Exclusion criteria were rebleeding, secondary ICH (such as head trauma, aneurysm, vascular malformation, hemorrhagic infarction, cerebral vein and sinus thrombosis, tumor, anticoagulant, blood thinners, or coagulopathy-related hemorrhage), history that may affect the study (such as bleeding, inflammation, trauma, surgery), use of drugs that affect the immune system (ibuprofen, hormones, illicit drug, cocaine or other stimulants, and so on), presence of underlying diseases within the previous month, or refusal of participation.

Ethics approval

The study protocol was approved by the Ethics Committee of Qilu Hospital. All patients' families received a comprehensive description of the study and gave written informed consent for their relatives' participation. The specimen for the study was waste brain tissue discarded during surgery, and the collection process did not cause any additional damage to the patient.

Clinical data and specimen collection

Clinical data of patients were collected on admission or during hospitalization. The variables include demographics (age and gender), alcohol and tobacco abuse, a detailed history of stroke risk factors (hypertension, diabetes mellitus, coronary heart disease, and chronic obstructive pulmonary diseases (COPD)), neuroimaging variables at presentation (hematoma volume, intraventricular extension, midline shift, hydrocephalus, brain edema), GCS on admission, number of days in hospital, mechanical ventilation, pneumonia, and outcome. The midline shift was determined by the distance between midline and septum pellucidum according to the CT scanning.

The proximity to the ICH is a key factor in the inflammatory response. Therefore, the specimen (no less than $0.5 \ cm^3$ per patient) was collected according to the standard that the distance between specimen and hematoma was 1 cm. In order to reduce the traction injury to the adjacent brain tissue, cortical fistula was made according to the ICH location during operation. Specimen was collected in this process by the same surgeon, and the distance between specimen and hematoma can be measured directly. So the samples were collected in the same way each time. The brain tissue was quickly fixed with 10% formalin and embedded in wax for immunohistochemistry (IHC) detection of NF-κB activation.

Detection of NF-κB activation

The activation of NF-κB was detected by IHC. The tissue sections (4 μm thick) were dewaxed, rehydrated, rinsed with distilled water and phosphate-buffered saline (PBS), repaired with EDTA, quenched with 3% H_2O_2, exposed to primary antibody (anti-NF-κB p65 antibody, B7162 rabbit polyclonal, ANBO, USA), and incubated at 4°C overnight. Sections were then washed with PBS, incubated in polymer helper for 25 min at room temperature, washed again, and incubated with non-biotin rabbit hypersensitivity two-step secondary antibody (PV-9001, GBI, USA) for 25 min at room temperature. Finally, the sections were stained with diaminobenzidine-H$_2$O$_2$ solution, washed, dehydrated in graded ethanol, immersed in xylene, and covered with a coverslip. In order to identify the cell type of nucleus NF-κB positive cells (neurons or glial cells), double-labeled IHC was performed on all of the 45 specimens, using the primary antibody (anti-NF-κB p65 antibody, B7162 rabbit polyclonal, ANBO, USA; anti-GFAP antibody, TA500336 mouse monoclonal, ZSGB-BIO, CHN; anti-NSE antibody, ZM-0203 mouse monoclonal, ZSGB-BIO, CHN) and double staining kit (DS-0005, ZSGB-BIO, CHN). The double-labeled IHC was performed according to the instructions of the double staining kit.

The slices were observed under the multi-head microscope by five professors of pathology in a blinded fashion. A total of five no-repeat fields (×400 high magnification) were randomly selected, the nucleus NF-κB positive cells were identified, and the numbers of positive cells in the five fields were added up as the result. The numbers of positive cells recorded by the five pathologists were consistent.

Functional outcome assessment

Clinical outcome was assessed by modified Rankin Scale (mRS) at 6 months after ICH. The follow-up was made by telephone interview or face-to-face assessment. In this study, the patients were relatively serious due to the hematoma volume, and three points can be considered as a good prognosis. Therefore, poor clinical outcome was defined as mRS ≥ 4 assessed at the 6-month follow-up.

Statistical analysis

The normally and non-normally distributed continuous variables were expressed as mean ± standard derivation and median (IQR), respectively. In univariate analysis, normally distributed continuous variables were analyzed with Student's t-test, non-normally distributed continuous variables were analyzed with Mann–Whitney U test, and categorical variables were analyzed with chi-square test. Stepwise forward logistic regression was used to determine independent predictors for poor functional outcome at 6 months after ICH. All tests were two-tailed, and statistical significance was determined at α level of 0.05. Statistical analysis and charting were performed using SPSS 19.0 and Excel 2003.

Results

Clinical data and NF-κB activation

The clinical data and NF-κB activation are listed in Table 1. The number of patients with 30 to 90 ml basal

ganglia ICH was 419 in total, and 92 (22.0%) refused surgery because of serious underlying disease or some other personal reasons (such as economic reasons and so on). All of the others (327, 78.0%) were treated with surgery in our department. Among patients with an ICH size of 30 to 90 ml that underwent surgical decompression, a total of 45 patients met our study's inclusion criteria, with an age of 53.87 ± 10.78 years (range 35 to 77 years), 29 males and 16 females. Thirty-seven (82.2%) had one or more underlying diseases: 26 (57.8%) had hypertension, 11 (24.4%) diabetes mellitus, 5 (11.1%) COPD, and 11 (24.4%) coronary artery diseases. Fourteen (31.1%) were smokers, and 11 (24.4%) were drinkers. The GCS score on admission was 5 to 13.

CT scan was performed on all of the 45 patients. The intracerebral hematoma volume was 59.44 ± 14.26 ml. Eighteen (40.0%) had intraventricular extension, 10 (22.2%) had acute hydrocephalus, 13 (28.9%) had perihematoma brain edema, and 24 (53.3%) had midline shift ≥1 cm.

Hematoma evacuation operation was performed on all patients along the non-functional cortex, while ventricular drainage was performed on 16 (35.6%) and craniectomy on 12 (26.7%). Mechanical ventilation was required in 14 (31.1%) patients, and pneumonia was diagnosed in 20 (44.4%) patients. The body temperature was controlled between 36.0°C and 37.0°C with the help of drugs or physical cooling. Osmotherapy (mannitol or hypertonic saline) was used pre- or post-operation. Mannitol was used according to the clinical manifestations and imaging. Serum sodium was maintained at 145 mmol/l or higher if necessary. The numbers of days in hospital were 18.29 ± 6.89. Do-not-attempt resuscitation or withdrawal-of-care did not exist in all of the 45 patients.

Immunohistochemical detection showed that NF-κB p65 was expressed in the nucleus of cells in all of the 45 patients (Figure 1), suggesting that NF-κB was activated and migrated into the nucleus. Double-labeled IHC showed that NF-κB p65 was expressed in the nucleus of both neurons and glial cells (Figure 1). The numbers of nucleus NF-κB p65-positive cells ranged from 9 to 95, and the total number was 54.38 ± 20.97.

The numbers of patients mRS scored 0 to 6 at 6 months after ICH were 0, 3 (6.5%), 8 (17.4%), 7 (15.2%), 9 (19.6%), 16 (34.8%), and 2 (4.3%); thus, 18 (40.0%) patients achieved a favorable functional outcome (mRS ≤ 3) while 27 (60.0%) had a poor functional outcome (mRS 4 to 6).

Predictors of poor outcome at 6 months after ICH

In univariate analysis of the 6-month outcome, predictors of poor functional outcome were lower GCS score on admission ($P = 0.004$), larger hematoma volume ($P = 0.004$), intraventricular extension ($P = 0.047$), midline shift ($P = 0.005$), and NF-κB activation ($P < 0.0001$). In addition, significantly more patients with poor outcome needed

Table 1 Predictive value of the characteristics on univariate analysis

Characteristics	Total ($n = 45$)	Good outcome ($n = 18$)	Poor outcome ($n = 27$)	Odds ratio (95% CI)	P value
Demographics					
Male sex	29 (64.4)	10 (55.6)	19 (70.4)	1.900 (0.548 to 6.590)	0.309[a]
Age, years	53.87 ± 10.78	51.50 ± 10.40	55.44 ± 10.93		0.233[b]
GCS score on admission	9 (4)	11 (3.5)	9 (2)		0.004[c]
Risk factors					
Smoking	14 (31.1)	5 (27.8)	9 (33.3)	1.300 (0.352 to 4.796)	0.693[a]
Alcohol abuse	11 (24.4)	5 (27.8)	6 (22.2)	0.743 (0.188 to 2.934)	0.671[a]
Hypertension	26 (57.8)	10 (55.6)	16 (59.3)	1.164 (0.348 to 3.885)	0.805[a]
Diabetes mellitus	11 (24.4)	4 (22.2)	8 (29.6)	1.474 (0.369 to 5.885)	0.582[a]
Coronary heart disease	11 (24.4)	3 (16.7)	8 (29.6)	2.105 (0.475 to 9.338)	0.322[a]
COPD	5 (11.1)	1 (5.6)	4 (14.8)	2.957 (0.303 to 28.882)	0.333[a]
Radiologic variables					
Hematoma volume, ml	59.44 ± 14.26	52.17 ± 13.10	64.30 ± 13.06		0.004[b]
Intraventricular extension	18 (40.0)	4 (22.2)	14 (51.9)	3.769 (0.984 to 14.443)	0.047[a]
Hydrocephalus	10 (22.2)	2 (11.1)	8 (29.6)	3.368 (0.624 to 18.185)	0.143[a]
Midline shift ≥1 cm	24 (53.3)	5 (27.8)	19 (70.4)	6.175 (1.647 to 23.148)	0.005[a]
Brain edema	13 (28.9)	3 (16.7)	10 (37.0)	2.941 (0.680 to 12.730)	0.140[a]
Hospitalizations					
Mechanical ventilation	14 (31.1)	2 (11.1)	12 (44.4)	6.400 (1.224 to 33.482)	0.018[a]
Pneumonia	20 (44.4)	3 (16.7)	17 (63.0)	8.500 (1.964 to 36.790)	0.002[a]
NF-κB activation	54.38 ± 20.97	37.11 ± 16.51	65.89 ± 14.91	2.929 (1.616 to 5.311)[d]	0[b]

[a]Chi-square test for categorical variables, data was expressed as n (%); [b]Student's t-test for normally distributed continuous variables, data was expressed as mean ± SD; [c]Mann-Whitney U test for non-normally distributed continuous variables, data was expressed as median (IQR); [d]The numbers of nucleus NF-κB p65-positive cells were stratified by 10, and OR (95% CI) was calculated according to the binary logistic regression analysis.

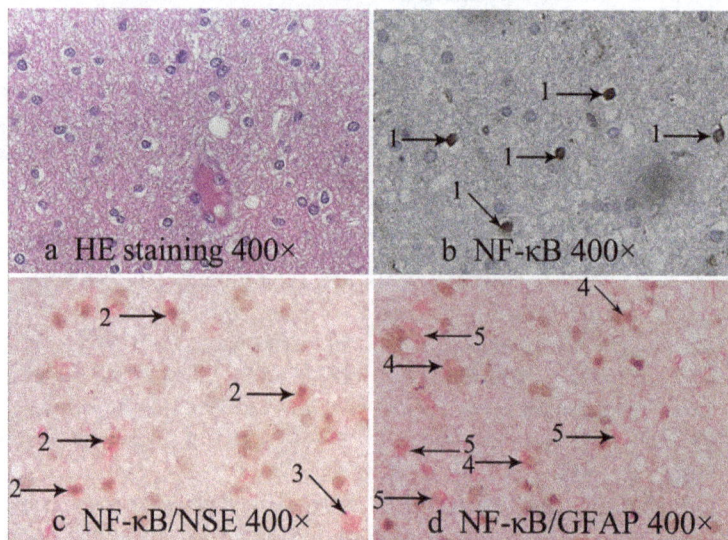

Figure 1 The microscopic images of NF-κB p65 detected with IHC. Microscopic images (400×) showed that NF-κB p65 expressed in nucleus of neurons and glial cells. **(a)** HE staining. **(b)** NF-κB p65 detected with IHC. **(c)** NF-κB p65/NSE double-labeled IHC. **(d)** NF-κB p65/GFAP double-labeled IHC. 1 → indicates nucleus NF-κB p65-positive neurons or glial cells, 2 → indicates nucleus NF-κB p65-positive neurons, 3 → indicates nucleus NF-κB p65-negative neurons, 4 → indicates nucleus NF-κB p65-positive glial cells, and 5 → indicates nucleus NF-κB p65-negative glial cells. HE, hematoxylin and eosin; NF-κB, nuclear factor-κB; NSE, neuron-specific enolase; GFAP, glial fibrillary acidic protein.

mechanical ventilation ($P = 0.018$) and suffered from pneumonia ($P = 0.002$). There was no significant difference in sex, age, all of the researched risk factors, brain edema, or hydrocephalus on admission. Then, the numbers of nucleus NF-κB p65-positive cells were stratified by 10, and the result was 1 case for 0~, 2 for 10 ~ and 20~, 8 for 30~, 5 for 40~, 6 for 50~, 8 for 60 ~ and 70~, 3 for 80~, and 2 for 90~. According to the binary logistic regression analysis, β value was 1.075, OR was 2.929, and the 95% CI was 1.616 to 5.311 (Table 1).

In the multivariate analysis, the variable entrance cut-off was set as 0.10 according to the results of univariate analysis. Therefore, GCS score on admission, hematoma volume, intraventricular extension, midline shift, and NF-κB activation were selected for multivariate analysis using logistic regression. With stepwise logistic regression, NF-κB activation was the only independent predictor of the 6-month outcome. The prognostic accuracy of NF-κB activation was assessed with ROC curve analysis. The area under curve (AUC) of NF-κB activation was 0.893 (95% CI 0.787 to 0.999), which was higher than that of GCS score on admission (0.748, 95% CI 0.590 to 0.906), hematoma volume (0.744, 95% CI 0.598 to 0.890), and midline shift (0.713, 95% CI 0.556 to 0.870) (Figure 2).

Relationship between baseline data and NF-κB activation

The relationship between every baseline data and NF-κB activation was analyzed. Continuous variables were analyzed with binary linear regression, and categorical variables were analyzed with one-way ANOVA. The results showed that NF-κB activation was significantly related

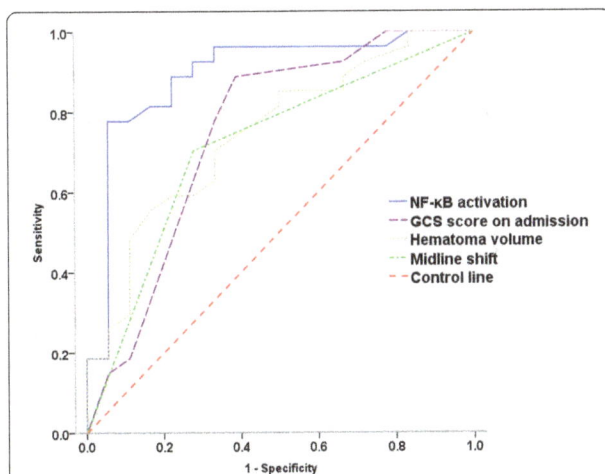

Figure 2 The ROC curve of predictors to predict the poor clinical outcome. The AUC of NF-κB activation, GCS score on admission, hematoma volume, and midline shift were 0.893 (95% CI 0.787 to 0.999), 0.748 (95% CI 0.590 to 0.906), 0.744 (95% CI 0.598 to 0.890), and 0.713 (95% CI 0.556 to 0.870), respectively. NF-κB, nuclear factor-κB; GCS, Glasgow Coma Scale.

to GCS score on admission ($P < 0.0001$), hematoma volume ($P < 0.0001$), and midline shift ($P = 0.006$) and not significantly related to sex, age, risk factors, or radiologic variables except midline shift.

Discussion

The present study examines the relationships among clinical data, NF-κB activation, and the 6-month outcome following primary ICH and produces the following major findings. First, in univariate analysis, GCS score on admission, hematoma volume, intraventricular extension, midline shift, mechanical ventilation, pneumonia, and NF-κB activation were predictors of the 6-month functional outcome. Second, in multivariate analysis, only NF-κB activation was independently associated with the 6-month outcome. Third, on the linear regression analysis, NF-κB activation was closely related to GCS score on admission, hematoma volume, and midline shift.

In this study, GCS score on admission, hematoma volume, intraventricular extension, and midline shift were predictors of the 6-month outcome, and this was consistent with the literature [5-11]. But one thing should be noted is that preoperative brain edema was not related to the 6-month outcome according to the univariate analysis. The reason for this may be that the CT scanning was performed within 10 h after onset of ICH, when the edema just begun and had not reached the peak.

It is interesting that this study first newly identified NF-κB activation as the only independent factor to predict the poor clinical outcome after ICH according to the multivariate analysis. This is mainly because that NF-κB activation is affected by many baseline factors. In the linear regression analysis, NF-κB activation was closed related to GCS score on admission, hematoma volume, and midline shift. Therefore, NF-κB activation might be affected by the combined effect of the three factors and then became the only independent factor.

The close relationship between NF-κB activation and the 6-month outcome is probably due to the function of NF-κB's downstream factors. NF-κB is a ubiquitous transcription factor and a member of a family of proteins which are critical regulators of a variety of responses, including inflammation [19]. In unstimulated cells, inactive NF-κB is sequestered in the cytoplasm by inhibitory protein IκB, which prevents its translocation to the nucleus. In response to various external pathogenic stimuli, including thrombin, TNF-α, IL-1β, oxidative stress, growth factors, and so on [16,20,21], specific kinases phosphorylate IκB, leading to its proteolysis and dissociation from NF-κB. The free, newly activated NF-κB migrates into the cell nucleus, where it binds to specific NF-κB response elements in the promoters of target genes. This promotes the transcription of genes for the release of series of inflammatory substances, such as TNF-α, IL-1β, induced nitric oxide synthase (iNOS), intercellular adhesion molecule-1 (ICAM-1), and so on. These substances are closely related to the secondary neuronal injuries after ICH, including blood–brain barrier disruption, brain edema, and neuronal cell death [22-29], which lead to poor functional outcome.

The results of this study have two major significances for the treatment of ICH in the future. First, based on these results, NF-κB activation in the perihematomal tissue is closely related to the outcome of ICH patients, so it can be detected to predict the prognosis of ICH accurately. Second and more importantly, these findings offer a potential therapeutic target for patients with ICH. It might be possible to improve the outcome of ICH patients by interfering NF-κB activation. Studies on animal ICH model have confirmed that some measures, such as application of 6-O-acetyl shanzhiside methyl ester, tauroursodeoxycholic acid in 2 h after ICH, and neural stem cell transplantation, could reduce the NF-κB activation [30-32]. Therefore, these measures might be taken to treat human ICH after clinical trials in the future.

There are several limitations in the current study that should be addressed. On one hand, the sample size of this study was relatively small and the patients enrolled were relatively serious, because the brain tissue could only be collected from patients with poor grades, who needed surgery to evacuate the hematoma. The result of this study may not be representative for all ICH patients. Therefore, we will continue collecting more cases in order to obtain a more convincible result. On the other hand, although NF-κB activation in the perihematomal tissue is closely related to the outcome of ICH patients, it is still questionable whether NF-κB activation directly leads to poor functional outcome or NF-κB activation is just a compensatory mechanism to protect the brain tissue from damage. In other words, promoting or inhibiting NF-κB activation to improve the outcome of ICH patients is still unclear. To clarify this issue, we will study the ICH rat model, using gene overexpression, RNA interference, and specific inhibition technology to interfere NF-κB activation at the different stages after ICH, detect the cell death, observe the behavioral changes of rats, and finally clarify the effect of NF-κB activation to the cell death and outcome in different stages. Then, different measures can be performed in different stages to improve the outcome of ICH.

Conclusion

In summary, in the current study, we found that NF-κB activation was closely related to the 6-month clinical outcome after primary ICH in humans. Therefore, it can be detected to predict the prognosis of ICH accurately. Furthermore, these findings offer a potential therapeutic target for patients with ICH. It might be possible to improve the outcome of ICH patients by interfering NF-κB activation in the future.

Abbreviations
AUC: area under curve; COPD: chronic obstructive pulmonary diseases; GCS: Glasgow Coma Scale; ICAM-1: intercellular adhesion molecule-1; ICH: intracerebral hemorrhage; IHC: immunohistochemistry; IL-1β: interleukin-1β; iNOS: induced nitric oxide synthase; NF-κB: nuclear factor-κB; NIK: NF-κB-inducing kinase; ROC curve: receiver operating characteristic curve; TNF-α: tumor necrosis factor-α.

Competing interests
The authors declare that they have no competing interests.

Authors' contributions
ZZ collected the specimen and the clinical data, participated in the experiments, performed the statistical analysis, and prepared the manuscript. YL and FL supervised all aspects of the project and revised the manuscript for important intellectual content. QH, HW, YS, and ZX collected the specimen and the clinical data. All authors read and approved the final manuscript.

Acknowledgements
This study is supported by the Youth Found of Shandong University Qilu Hospital (The relationship between NF-κB activation and outcome in patients with intracerebral hemorrhage), China Postdoctoral Science Foundation (2014 T70661, 2014 M560562), and National Natural Science Foundation of China (81301127).

Author details
[1]Department of Emergency Surgery, Qilu Hospital of Shandong University, No. 107 Wenhuaxi Road, 250012 Jinan, Shandong Province, People's Republic of China. [2]Department of Neurosurgery, Qilu Hospital of Shandong University and Brain Science Research Institute of Shandong University, No. 107 Wenhuaxi Road, 250012 Jinan, Shandong Province, People's Republic of China.

References
1. Narayan SK, Sivaprasad P, Sushma S, Sahoo RK, Dutta TK. Etiology and outcome determinants of intracerebral hemorrhage in a south Indian population, a hospital-based study. Ann Indian Acad Neurol. 2012;15(4):263–6.
2. Al Q, Tuhrim ST, Broderick JP, Batjer HH, Hondo H, Hanley DF. Spontaneous intracerebral hemorrhage. N Engl J Med. 2001;344:1450–60.
3. Zhang LF, Yang J, Hong Z, Yuan GG, Zhou BF, Zhao LC, et al. Proportion of different types of subtypes of stroke in China. Stroke. 2003;34(9):2091–6.
4. Counsell C, Boonyakarnkul S, Dennis M, Sandercock P, Bamford J, Burn J, et al. Primary intracerebral haemorrhage in the Oxfordshire Community Stroke Project, 2: prognosis. Cerebrovasc Dis. 1995;5:26–34.
5. Hardemark HG, Wesslen N, Persson L. Influence of clinical factors, CT findings and early management on outcome in supratentorial intracerebral hemorrhage. Cerebrovasc Dis. 1999;9(1):10–21.
6. Rathor MY, Rani MF, Jamalludin AR, Amran M, Shahrin TC, Shah A. Prediction of functional outcome in patients with primary intracerebral hemorrhage by clinical-computed tomographic correlations. J Res Med Sci. 2012;17(11):1056–62.
7. Diedler J, Sykora M, Hahn P, Heerlein K, Schölzke MN, Kellert L, et al. Low hemoglobin is associated with poor functional outcome after non-traumatic, supratentorial intracerebral hemorrhage. Crit Care. 2010;14(2):R63.
8. Ganti L, Jain A, Yerragondu N, Jain M, Bellolio MF, Gilmore RM, et al. Female gender remains an independent risk factor for poor outcome after acute nontraumatic intracerebral hemorrhage. Neurol Res Int. 2013;2013:219097.
9. Li N, Liu YF, Ma L, Worthmann H, Wang YL, Wang YJ, et al. Association of molecular markers with perihematomal edema and clinical outcome in intracerebral hemorrhage. Stroke. 2013;44(3):658–63.
10. Sakamoto Y, Koga M, Yamagami H, Okuda S, Okada Y, Kimura K, et al. Systolic blood pressure after intravenous antihypertensive treatment and clinical outcomes in hyperacute intracerebral hemorrhage: the

stroke acute management with urgent risk-factor assessment and improvement-intracerebral hemorrhage study. Stroke. 2013;44(7):1846–51.

11. Agnihotri S, Czap A, Staff I, Fortunato G, McCullough LD. Peripheral leukocyte counts and outcomes after intracerebral hemorrhage. J Neuroinflammation. 2011;8:160.

12. Hwang BY, Appelboom G, Ayer A, Kellner CP, Kotchetkov IS, Gigante PR, et al. Advances in neuroprotective strategies: potential therapies for intracerebral hemorrhage. Cerebrovasc Dis. 2011;31(3):211–22.

13. Xi G, Keep RF, Hoff JT. Mechanisms of brain injury after intracerebral haemorrhage. Lancet Neurol. 2006;5:53–63.

14. Gong C, Hoff JT, Keep RF. A cute inflammatory reaction following experimental intracerebral hemorrhage in rat. Brain Res. 2000;871(1):57–65.

15. Barnes PJ, Karin M. Nuclear factor-κB: a pivotal transcription factor in chronic inflammatory diseases. N Engl J Med. 1997;336:1066–71.

16. Ridder DA, Schwaninger M. NF-κB signaling in cerebral ischemia. Neuroscience. 2009;158:995–1006.

17. Fang H, Wang PF, Zhou Y, Wang YC, Yang QW. Toll-like receptor 4 signaling in intracerebral hemorrhage-induced inflammation and injury. J Neuroinflammation. 2013;10:27.

18. Kothari RU, Brott T, Broderick JP, Barsan WG, Sauerbeck LR, Zuccarello M, et al. The ABCs of measuring intracerebral hemorrhage volumes. Stroke. 1996;27:1304–5.

19. Barnes JP, Karin M. Nuclear factor-κ B: a pivotal transcription factor in chronic inflammatory diseases. N Engl J Med. 1996;336:1066–71.

20. Bauerle PA, Baltimore D. NF-κB ten years after. Cell. 1996;87:13–20.

21. Kopp EB, Ghosh S. NF-κB and rel proteins in innate immunity. Adv Immunol. 1995;58:1–27.

22. Holmin S, Mathiesen T. Intracerebral administration of interleukin-1β and induction of inflammation, apoptosis and vasogenic edema. J Neurosurg. 2000;92:108–20.

23. Rothwell N. Interleukin-1 and neuronal injury: mechanisms, modification, and therapeutic potential. Brain Behav Immun. 2003;17:152–7.

24. Denes A, Pinteaux E, Rothwell NJ, Allan SM. Interleukin-1 and stroke: biomarker, harbinger of damage, and therapeutic target. Cerebrovasc Dis. 2011;32(6):517–27.

25. Liu T, Clark RK, McDonnell PC, Young PR, White RF, Barone FC, et al. Tumor necrosis factor-α expression in ischemic neurons. Stroke. 1994;25(7):1481–8.

26. Wang HC, Lin WC, Lin YJ, Rau CS, Lee TH, Chang WN, et al. The association between serum adhesion molecules and outcome in acute spontaneous intracerebral hemorrhage. Crit Care. 2011;15(6):R284.

27. Al-Senani FM, Zhao X, Grotta JC, Shirzadi A, Strong R, Aronowski J. Proteasome inhibitor reduces astrocytic iNOS expression and functional deficit after experimental intracerebral hemorrhage in rats. Transl Stroke Res. 2012;3(1):146–53.

28. Zhang Z, Liu Y, Huang Q, Su Y, Zhang Y, Wang G, et al. NF-κB activation and cell death after intracerebral hemorrhage in patients. Neurol Sci. 2014;35(7):1097–102.

29. Lei B, Dawson HN, Roulhac-Wilson B, Wang H, Laskowitz DT, James ML. Tumor necrosis factor α antagonism improves neurological recovery in murine intracerebral hemorrhage. J Neuroinflammation. 2013;10(1):103.

30. Rodrigues CM, Sola S, Nan Z, Castro RE, Ribeiro PS, Low WC, et al. Tauroursodeoxycholic acid reduces apoptosis and protects against neurological injury after acute hemorrhagic stroke in rats. Proc Natl Acad Sci U S A. 2003;100(10):6087–92.

31. Lee S, Chu K, Jung K, Kim S, Kim D, Kang K, et al. Anti-inflammatory mechanism of intravascular neural stem cell transplantation in haemorrhagic stroke. Brain. 2008;131:616–29.

32. Jiang W, Zhang S, Fu F, Zhu H, Hou J. Inhibition of nuclear factor-κB by 6-O-acetyl shanzhiside methyl ester protects brain against injury in a rat model of ischemia and reperfusion. J Neuroinflammation. 2010;7:55.

4

The role of microglia and the TLR4 pathway in neuronal apoptosis and vasospasm after subarachnoid hemorrhage

Khalid A Hanafy

Abstract

Background: Although microglia and the Toll-like receptor (TLR) pathway have long been thought to play a role in the pathogenesis of aneurysmal subarachnoid hemorrhage (aSAH), thus far only correlations have been made. In this study, we attempted to solidify the relationship between microglia and the TLR pathway using depletion and genetic knockouts, respectively.

Methods: Subarachnoid hemorrhage was induced in TLR4−/−, TRIF−/−, MyD88−/− and wild type C57BL/6 mice by injecting 60 µl of autologous blood near the mesencephalon; animals were euthanized 1 to 15 days after SAH for immunohistochemical analysis to detect microglia or apoptotic cells. Lastly, microglial depletion was performed by intracerebroventricular injection of clodronate liposomes.

Results: On post operative day (POD) 7 (early phase SAH), neuronal apoptosis was largely TLR4-MyD88-dependent and microglial-dependent. By POD 15 (late phase SAH), neuronal apoptosis was characterized by TLR4- toll receptor associated activator of interferon (TRIF)-dependence and microglial-independence. Similarly, vasospasm was also characterized by an early and late phase with MyD88 and TRIF dependence, respectively. Lastly, microglia seem to be both necessary and sufficient to cause vasospasm in both the early and late phases of SAH in our model.

Conclusion: Our results suggest that SAH pathology could have different phases. These results could explain why therapies tailored to aSAH patients have failed for the most part. Perhaps a novel strategy utilizing immunotherapies that target Toll like receptor signaling and microglia at different points in the patient's hospital course could improve outcomes.

Keywords: TLR, TRIF, MyD88, SAH, Microglia

Introduction

Aneurysmal subarachnoid hemorrhage (aSAH) is a devastating disease that affects 30,000 Americans each year [1,2]. A total of 30 to 40% of these patients will have delayed cerebral ischemia (DCI) from vasospasm, anywhere from 4 to 14 days after ictus, resulting in increased morbidity and mortality [3]. Few studies have addressed the molecular mechanisms that lead to DCI. The inciting event is the release of oxyhemoglobin from red blood cell lysis in the subarachnoid space [4,5]. The heme that is released from hemoglobin results in a significant cerebral inflammatory response [6]. To dissipate the heme burden, the resident cerebral macrophage or microglia can engulf heme, as demonstrated in mouse intracerebral hemorrhage models, and degrade it via heme oxygenase [7,8]. Furthermore, in primary macrophage culture, heme has been shown to be a specific agonist for the Toll-like receptor 4 (TLR4) [9].

In both SAH patients and mouse models, TLR4 expression is up-regulated in the brain [10-12]. However, little is known about the signal transduction that occurs downstream of TLR4 to cause DCI or what cells mediate DCI. That is, after stimulation of TLR4, the *MyD88* (myeloid differentiation primary response gene) pathway can facilitate further action by phosphorylation and activation of IRAK4 (IL-1 receptor associated kinase 4), which results in NF-kB-dependent inflammation [13].

Correspondence: khanafy@bidmc.harvard.edu
Division of NeuroCritical Care, Department of Neurology, Harvard Medical School, Beth Israel Deaconess Medical Center, The Center for Life Science, 3 Blackfan Circle, Boston, MA 02215, USA

Alternatively, TLR4 signaling can be transduced with the TRIF (toll receptor associated activator of interferon) pathway [13]. TRIF signaling results in a delayed NF-kB activation, similar to MyD88, and facilitates apoptosis [14].

The understanding of the immune cells involved in DCI is in its infancy. Neutrophils may play a role in DCI as systemic depletion resulted in improved cognitive performance and decreased vasospasm; however, their role in cerebral inflammation after SAH is likely indirect [15]. Neutrophils are not endogenous to the brain, nor do they have a published role in aneurysm formation. Resident macrophages of the brain, on the other hand, are first responders to the deluge of heme after SAH, and are necessary for aneurysm formation [9,16]. As of yet, no causal relationship has been elucidated between macrophages and DCI. In this study, we show the critical role that microglia play in facilitating vasospasm and neuronal apoptosis. Furthermore, we establish a temporal role for the TLR4 pathway in the induction of apoptosis and vasospasm using both *in vivo* and *in vitro* models.

Materials and methods
Materials
Hemin was purchased from Sigma Aldrich (St. Louis, MO, USA) and dissolved in dimethyl sulfoxide (DMSO).

Animals
All animal experiments were approved for use by the Beth Israel Deaconess Medical Center Institutional Animal Care and Use Committee and performed in accordance with the National Institutes of Health Guide for the Care and Use of Laboratory Animals. All mice were 10- to 12-week-old males on a C57BL/6 background: TLR4-/-, MyD88-/-, TRIF-/- and wild type (Jackson Laboratory, Bar Harbor, ME, USA).

Primary microglial culture
This method is described in detail elsewhere [17]. Briefly, microglia were harvested from neonatal mice (P0-P5) using the Papain Dissociation System (Worthington Biomedical Corporation, Lakewood Township, NJ, USA). The tissue was minced and triturated, then incubated at 37°C for one hour. The suspension was subjected to a discontinuous gradient separation, followed by re-suspension in DMEM-10% FBS containing 1 ng/ml macrophage colony-stimulating factor (M-CSF). The flask was intermittently shaken over the next two to three weeks to obtain a confluent microglial culture.

TNF-α ELISA
Primary microglial culture was incubated with 40 μm hemin for 24 hours and TNF-α was measured in supernatant per protocol from BD Biosciences (San Jose, CA, USA).

In vitro vasospasm
C57BL/6 mice were anesthetized with isoflurane followed by careful dissection of a 3 cm length of the descending aorta. The aorta was then secured to a vibrotome (Leica Biosystems, Buffalo Grove, IL, USA) plate with glue and 100 μm thick slices were acquired. The aortic slices were incubated in modified Krebs-Henseleit solution containing (mmol/L): NaCl 120, KCl 4.5, MgSO$_4$ 1, NaHCO$_3$ 27, KH$_2$PO$_4$ 1, CaCl$_2$ 2.5 and dextrose 10. The rings were equilibrated for 90 minutes at 37°C 5% CO$_2$ and the medium was replaced every 20 minutes, as described previously [18].

In vitro and in vivo vasospasm measurement
Coronal cross sections were dehydrated using alcohol and stained with hematoxylin and eosin for *in vivo* slices. *In vitro* slices of mouse aorta were imaged directly. Images were acquired with Spot Advanced Software (SPOT Imaging Solutions, Sterling Heights, MI, USA). Using measurement tools provided in the software, the inner and outer perimeters were measured and the lumen radius to wall thickness ratio was calculated from these measurements. Three consecutive slices were measured and averaged to obtain the final lumen to wall ratio.

SAH
The subarachnoid hemorrhage model was previously described with several modifications detailed below [19]. Mice were anesthetized with xylazine (10 mg/kg) and ketamine (12 mg/kg) and placed in a stereotax where a midline scalp incision was performed. A burr hole was drilled 3.5 mm anterior to the bregma until dural penetration was achieved. A 27-gauge spinal needle was advanced ventrally at 40° to a depth of 5 mm dorsoventral. A total of 60 μl of arterial blood from a donor mouse was injected over 10 seconds.

ICV injections
Mice were anesthetized as described above. Two burr holes were drilled 0.22 mm posterior to the bregma, 1 mm lateral, and 2.25 mm in depth to enter the bilateral ventricles. Pulled glass capillaries were used to inject 8 μl of clodronate (a generous gift provided by Prof. Reto Schwendener) or PBS liposomes were divided equally between the ventricles, over 12.5 minutes. The capillaries were held in place for 2.5 minutes thereafter to prevent any regurgitation, followed by skin closure. Intracerebroventricular (ICV) injections were performed on post-operative days (PODs) 1 to 2 after SAH procedure. ICV injections of 5 μg of LPS (lipopolysaccharide) at a concentration of 1 μg/μl were performed at the coordinates noted above in the right lateral ventricle only, as previously described [20]. No SAH surgeries were done in these mice.

Immunohistochemistry and TUNEL staining

Adult male C57BL/6 were sedated with an Avertin overdose (250 mg/kg), followed by perfusion with ice-cold PBS. The brains were fixed and then cut into 12 µm coronal serial sections with a Leica CM3050 S cryostat. TUNEL staining was performed as per instructions (Roche Diagnostics, Indianapolis, IN, USA). Primary antibodies for Isolectin B1 (Sigma-Aldrich, St. Louis, MO, USA), Glial Fibrillary Acidic Protein (Dako, Carpinteria, CA, USA Toll-like receptor 4 (Santa Cruz Biotechnology, Santa Cruz, CA, USA), or β-III Tubulin (Abcam, Cambridge, MA) were applied at a dilution of 1:250, followed by secondary incubation with Alexa Fluor antibodies at a dilution of 1:250. Fluorescent microscopy was done on a Zeiss Axio Scope (Carl Zeiss, Inc., Thornwood, NY, USA). Brightness and contrast of images were adjusted in Image J software (National Institutes of Health, USA).

Statistics

Continuous variables were assessed for normality with skewness and kurtosis. All variables measured in this study were normally distributed and groups were compared with the Student's t-test or ANOVA. If comparisons were made among groups analyzed by ANOVA, the Bonferroni correction was used. All statistical analyses were performed using SPSS 19 software (SPSS Inc., Chicago, IL, USA). $P < 0.05$ was considered statistically significant.

Results

To determine the optimal time to visualize vasospasm, we performed a time course of subarachnoid hemorrhage from PODs 1 through 15 (Figure 1). The dimensions of the middle cerebral artery were analyzed at the level of the hippocampus for consistency, as shown in Figure 1C. We found that the difference between sham and wild type (WT) SAH vasospasm was maximal on days 3 and 10. There was no difference between sham and WT SAH on POD 5, indicating resolution of vasospasm by Day 5, followed by delayed vasospasm beginning on Day 7 and plateauing on Day 10 (Figure 1). To determine if neuronal cell death correlated with vasospasm in our model, we quantified TUNEL positive cells from days 1 through 15 in the dentate gyrus of the hippocampus. Similarly, cell death also had a bimodal distribution, peaking on PODs 7 and 15 (Figure 2).

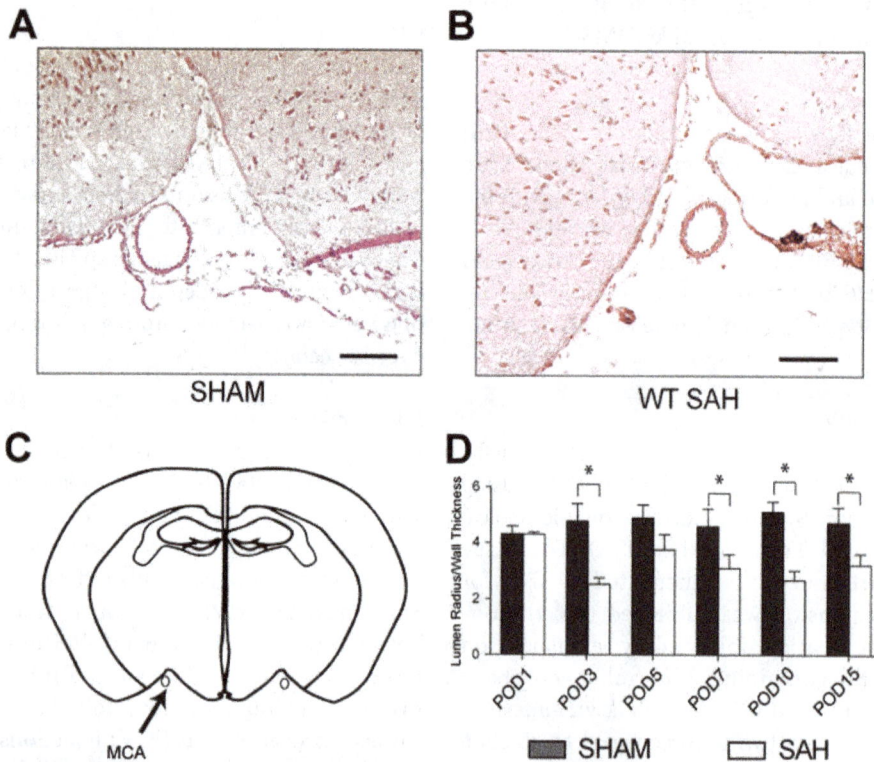

Figure 1 Vasospasm time course in subarachnoid hemorrhage model. A. Hematoxylin and Eosin (H&E) stain of coronal section through middle cerebral artery (MCA) in sham from post-operative day (POD) 7. Scale Bars are all: 10 µm. **B**. H&E of MCA stain after subarachnoid hemorrhage (SAH) induction on POD 7. **C**. Shows a diagram of the coronal section where MCA dimensions were measured for vasospasm analysis. **D**. Lumen radius/wall thickness was measured to determine the degree of vasospasm. Student's t-test was done for each POD and significant differences between sham and SAH were noted for POD 3, 7, 10 and 15 with P-values of <0.001, <0.04, <0.001 and <0.01, respectively. Error bars are standard deviations and N = 4 per group.

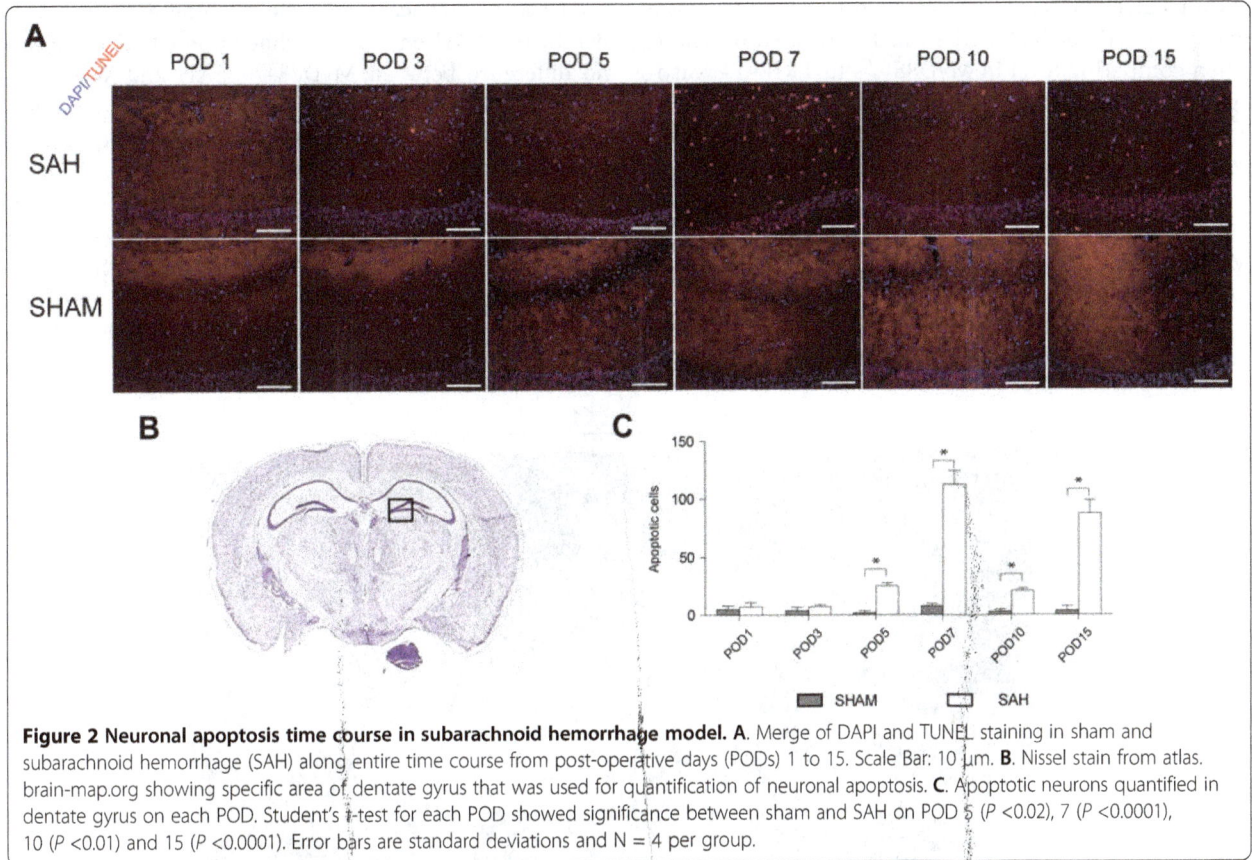

Figure 2 Neuronal apoptosis time course in subarachnoid hemorrhage model. A. Merge of DAPI and TUNEL staining in sham and subarachnoid hemorrhage (SAH) along entire time course from post-operative days (PODs) 1 to 15. Scale Bar: 10 μm. **B.** Nissel stain from atlas. brain-map.org showing specific area of dentate gyrus that was used for quantification of neuronal apoptosis. **C.** Apoptotic neurons quantified in dentate gyrus on each POD. Student's *t*-test for each POD showed significance between sham and SAH on POD 5 (*P* <0.02), 7 (*P* <0.0001), 10 (*P* <0.01) and 15 (*P* <0.0001). Error bars are standard deviations and N = 4 per group.

We focused on PODs 7 and 15 because neuronal cell death was maximal at these two time points, and it correlated well with human vasospasm peaking on post-bleed Day 7, with continued risk of vasospasm through post-bleed Day 14 [21]. We then set out to determine the role of the TLR4 signaling cascade as it relates to vasospasm and neuronal apoptosis on PODs 7 and 15 (Figure 3). On PODs 7 and 15, vasospasm in the WT SAH was significantly increased compared to the TLR4–/– SAH (Figure 3A). Intracerebroventricular injection of LPS, a

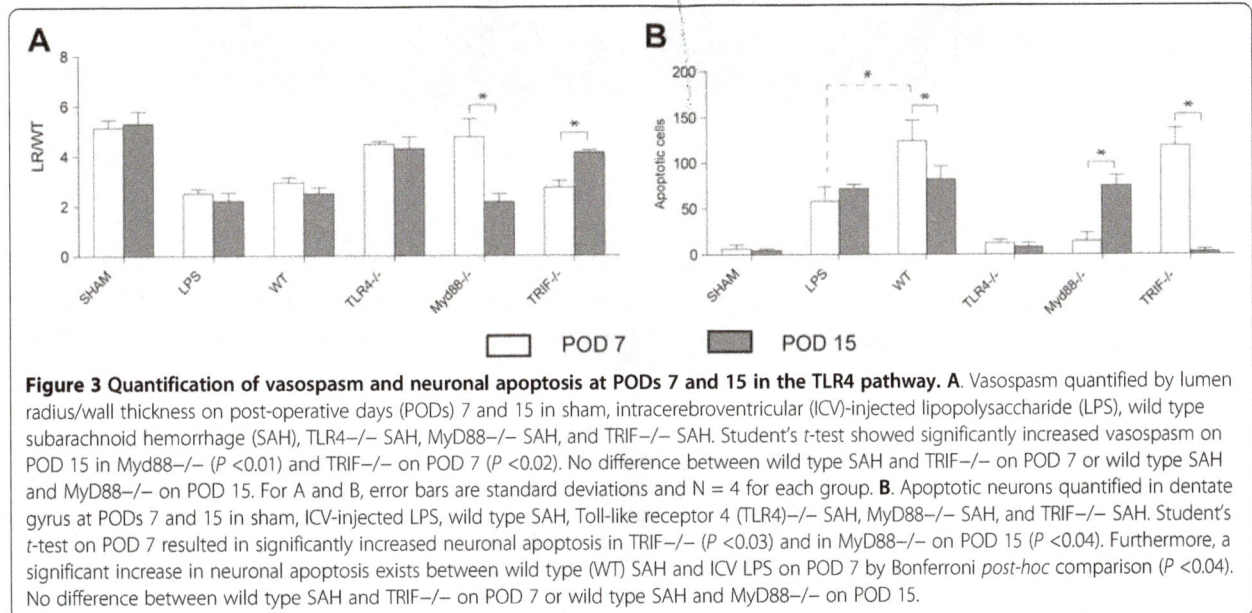

Figure 3 Quantification of vasospasm and neuronal apoptosis at PODs 7 and 15 in the TLR4 pathway. A. Vasospasm quantified by lumen radius/wall thickness on post-operative days (PODs) 7 and 15 in sham, intracerebroventricular (ICV)-injected lipopolysaccharide (LPS), wild type subarachnoid hemorrhage (SAH), TLR4–/– SAH, MyD88–/– SAH, and TRIF–/– SAH. Student's *t*-test showed significantly increased vasospasm on POD 15 in Myd88–/– (*P* <0.01) and TRIF–/– on POD 7 (*P* <0.02). No difference between wild type SAH and TRIF–/– on POD 7 or wild type SAH and MyD88–/– on POD 15. For A and B, error bars are standard deviations and N = 4 for each group. **B.** Apoptotic neurons quantified in dentate gyrus at PODs 7 and 15 in sham, ICV-injected LPS, wild type SAH, Toll-like receptor 4 (TLR4)–/– SAH, MyD88–/– SAH, and TRIF–/– SAH. Student's *t*-test on POD 7 resulted in significantly increased neuronal apoptosis in TRIF–/– (*P* <0.03) and in MyD88–/– on POD 15 (*P* <0.04). Furthermore, a significant increase in neuronal apoptosis exists between wild type (WT) SAH and ICV LPS on POD 7 by Bonferroni *post-hoc* comparison (*P* <0.04). No difference between wild type SAH and TRIF–/– on POD 7 or wild type SAH and MyD88–/– on POD 15.

known TLR4 agonist, showed similar degrees of vasospasm to the WT SAH on both PODs 7 and 15 [22]. Furthermore, when comparing SAH in MyD88–/– to TRIF–/–, vasospasm was significantly greater in the TRIF–/– on POD 7, while the opposite was true at POD 15. Of note, when comparing maximal vasospasm on PODs 7 and 15, there was no difference between WT SAH and TRIF–/– SAH on POD 7, and WT SAH and MyD88–/– SAH on POD 15. Minimal vasospasm was seen in the sham and TLR4–/– SAH on both days.

Additionally, we measured neuronal apoptosis in these groups, as described in Figure 2. Interestingly, TRIF–/–

SAH had a statistically equivalent neural apoptotic burden to WT SAH on POD 7, while on POD 15, there was no difference between MyD88–/– SAH and WT SAH. In terms of minimal apoptotic burden, there was no difference between the number of apoptotic neurons quantified in sham, TLR4–/– SAH, and MyD88 –/– SAH on POD 7. At POD 15, there was no difference between the number of apoptotic neurons quantified in sham, TLR4–/– SAH and TRIF–/– SAH (Figure 3B). Of note, the LPS injected mice, demonstrated significantly less neuronal apoptosis at POD 7, compared to WT SAH; however at POD 15 there was no difference between these groups. With the

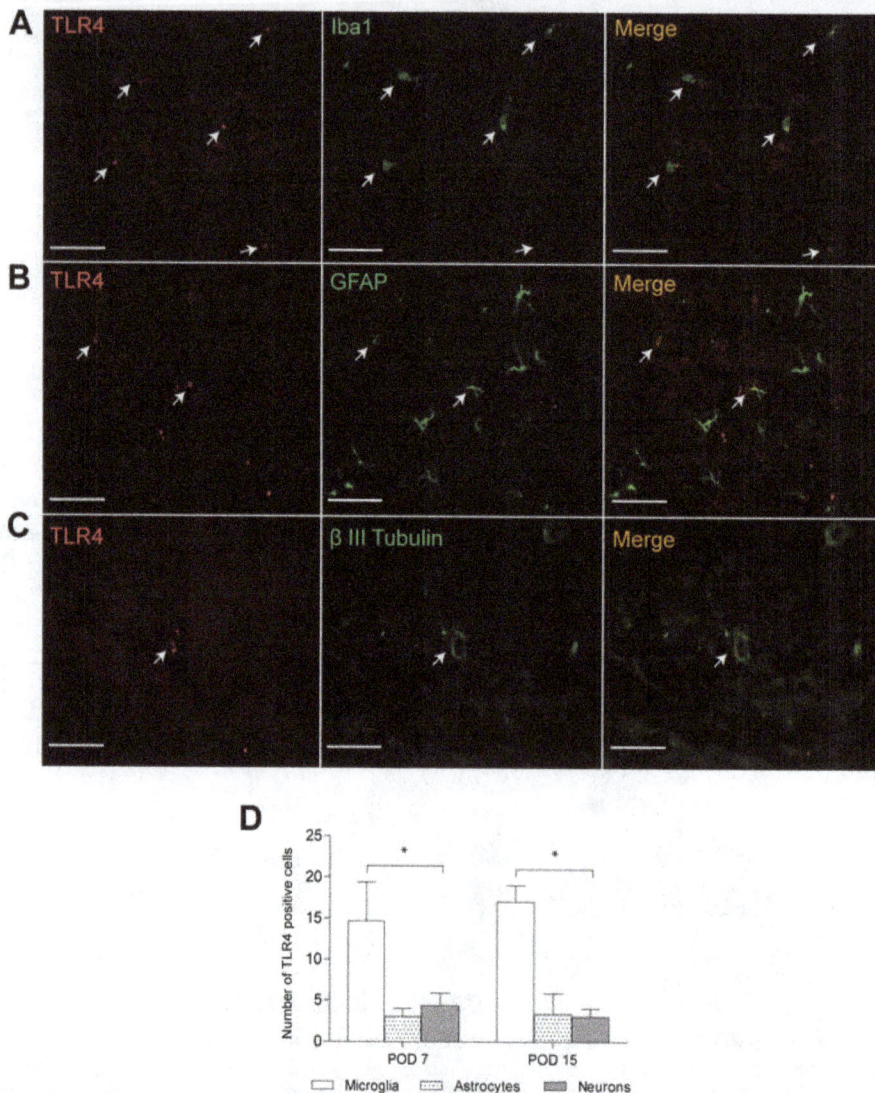

Figure 4 **Immunohistochemistry of TLR4 co-localization among the different cell types of the murine brain.** Representative images from four mice per group and four different fields of view on post-operative day (POD) 7 **A**. Immunohistochemistry across shows staining with Toll-like receptor 4 (TLR4) in the first panel, Iba1 (for microglia) in the second panel, and the merge in the third panel. Arrows delineate co-localization. **B**. Immunohistochemistry showing individual panels and merge for astrocytes with Glial Fibrillary acidic protein. **C**. Immunohistochemistry for β III Tubulin reflecting co-localization of TLR4 and neurons. Scale Bars: 15 μm. **D**. Quantification based on four mice and four different fields of view at POD 7 and POD 15 showing microglia express the most Toll-like receptor 4 (TLR4) by ANOVA at both time points (P <0.001).

understanding that the TLR4 pathway may play a role in vasospasm and neuronal apoptosis, we wanted to identify what type of cell was expressing TLR4. Microglia, astrocytes and neurons were examined for TLR4 expression with representative images shown in Figure 4A-C and quantification of TLR4 co-localization in Figure 4D. Based on these results, we found that the majority of TLR4 is expressed in microglia at both POD 7 and 15 after SAH.

To further elucidate the relationship between microglia and vasospasm, we modified an *in vitro* assay [18] where we incubated neonatal primary microglial (PMG) culture with hemin for 24 hours to simulate the *in vivo* environment after subarachnoid hemorrhage. After 24 hours, the supernatant from the cultures was taken and incubated with axial sections of wild type mouse aortic rings for 5 minutes and vasospasm was measured. PMG from all genotypes, except the TLR4-/- mice, were able to induce vasospasm and secrete TNF-α (Figure 5A, B). Based on these results, the TLR4 receptor is necessary for microglia to secrete some factor into the media that causes vasospasm in mouse aortic slice culture. To exclude endotoxin contamination in our hemin preparation, endotoxin was measured by ELISA and found to be <0.001 ng/μl (data not shown).

The *in vitro* data suggest that the microglial TLR4 receptor is necessary for vasospasm, as well as the *in vivo* data which indicate that the TLR4 receptor is necessary for vasospasm. To resolve whether microglia are necessary for vasospasm *in vivo*, we depleted microglia *in vivo* via intraventricular injection of clodronate liposomes into WT SAH. Immunohistochemistry for microglia shows virtually complete depletion with clodronate compared to PBS liposomes (Figure 6A-C). Additionally, when

vasospasm was measured at PODs 7 and 15, the depletion of microglia with clodronate resulted in significant amelioration of vasospasm at both time points (Figure 6D).

Finally, we determined whether microglial depletion effected neuronal apoptosis in Figure 7, and found a similar bimodal theme. At POD 7, the depletion of microglia resulted in a significant decrease in neuronal apoptosis (Figure 7A, C); while at POD 15, microglial depletion had no effect (Figure 7B, D).

Discussion

In this study, we have elucidated possible roles for microglia and the TLR4 pathway with respect to vasospasm and neuronal apoptosis. Many have suggested a role for TLR4 in SAH and more recently a modulatory role for peroxisome proliferator-activated receptor gamma (PPAR-γ) via the TLR4 pathway [10-12,23]. However, our study is unique in that we attempted to ascertain the roles of different signaling pathways downstream of TLR4 activation and followed the mice out to 15 days to better parallel the human condition where delayed cerebral ischemia can occur up to 21 days from ictus [24].

It is interesting that two phases of vasospasm were observed, one beginning on POD 3, resolving by POD 5, and then another phase beginning on POD 7 and plateauing by Day 10 (Figure 1). This is important to note because it is similar to the human condition in that vasospasm is bimodal, with an early ictal phase followed by a delayed phase; it is the delayed vasospasm that is associated with increased neuronal cell death or delayed cerebral ischemia (DCI) [3,21,25].

Furthermore, our *in vivo* immunohistochemistry data suggest that TLR4 is necessary for neuronal apoptosis.

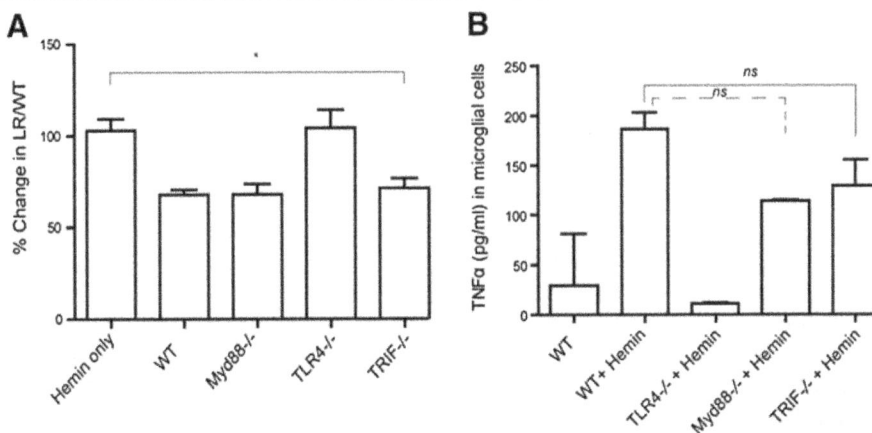

Figure 5 In vitro vasospasm assay and cytokine production in response to hemin. A. *In vitro* vasospasm of mouse aortic ring slice after 5-minute incubation with supernatant from primary microglial cell culture (PMG) exposed to 40 μM hemin for 24 hours. Each PMG culture was exposed to one mouse aortic ring and this was repeated four times. Error bars are standard deviations. **B**. TNF-α was measured in the PMG supernatant after 24 hours of hemin exposure. This was repeated four times to get standard deviations in this graph. No difference was seen between wild type (WT), TRIF-/-, and MyD88-/- PMG per the Bonferroni correction. One way ANOVA for both vasospasm and TNF-α secretion were significant (*P* <0.03, *P* <0.02, respectively).

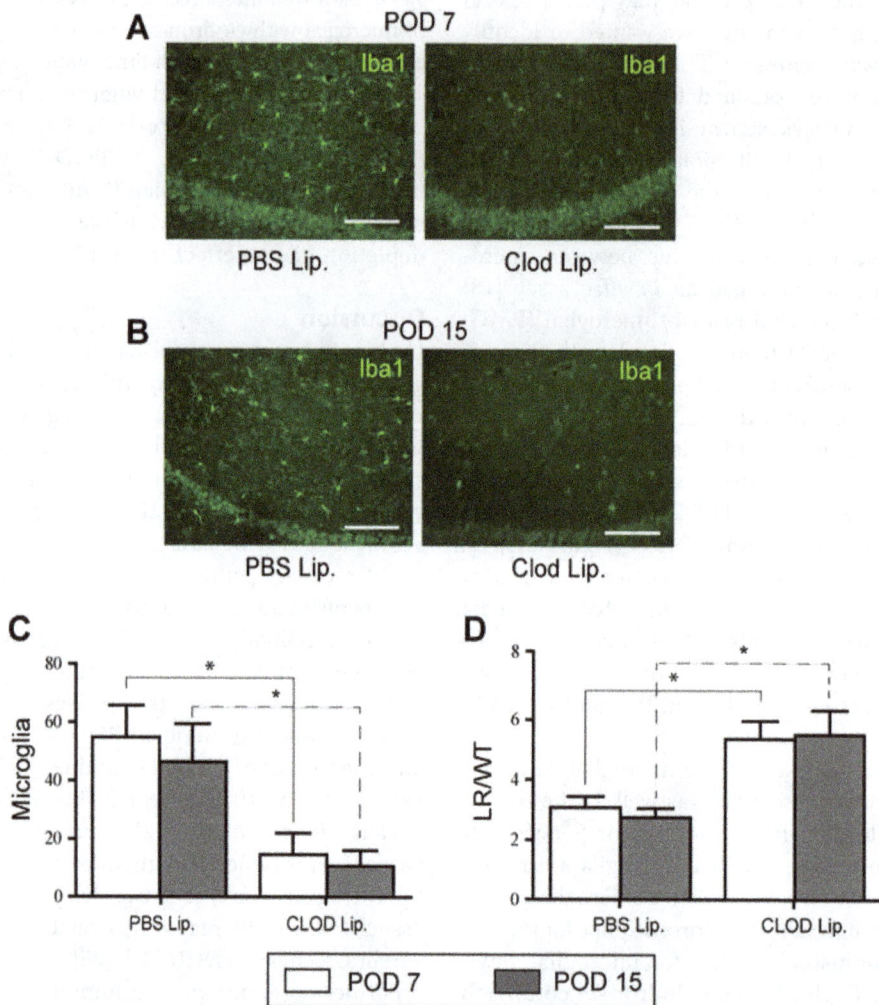

Figure 6 The effects of microglial ablation on vasospasm. A. Top panels: microglial staining with Iba1 at the level of the hippocampus of wild type subarachnoid hemorrhage SAH on post-operative days (PODs) 7 and 15 after intracerebroventricular (ICV) injection of control PBS liposomes. **B**. Bottom panels: microglial depletion in wild type SAH on PODs 7 and 15 after ICV injection with clodronate liposomes. Scale Bars: 10 μm in all panels. **C**. Quantification of microglial cells in the hippocampal area of wild type SAH mice with ICV injections of PBS liposomes and clodronate liposomes. N = 3 for each group and error bars are standard deviations. Comparison by Student's t-test on POD 7 and POD 15 between clodronate and PBS liposomes injections shows significant depletion on both days (P <0.03). **D**. Measurement of vasospasm shows significant ablation of vasospasm at both time points after microglial depletion by Student's t-test: POD 7 (P <0.001) and POD 15 (P <0.001). N = 3 mice for each group.

It is interesting to note that neuronal apoptosis seen in WT SAH and TRIF−/− SAH was significantly greater than that seen in LPS on POD 7, despite equivalent degrees of vasospasm (Figure 3). On POD 7, one can infer that some product from red blood cell breakdown is able to induce increased cell-death in the dentate gyrus through the TLR4-MyD88 pathway and downstream signal transduction systems that LPS cannot; however, an insufficient amount of LPS could also be the case. Because there was no difference between neuronal apoptosis and vasospasm in WT SAH and TRIF−/− SAH at POD 7, we conclude that some portion of the neuronal damage and vasospasm occurring on POD 7 (early SAH)

is TLR4-MyD88-dependent. Likewise, because there was no difference between neuronal apoptosis and vasospasm observed in WT SAH, MyD88−/− SAH and LPS on POD15, neuronal damage and vasospasm on POD 15 (late SAH) are largely TLR4-TRIF-dependent. Based on our results in Figure 3, we see that vasospasm is, for the most part, directly correlated with neuronal apoptosis. Given that vasospasm is either constant or increasing with time, it is expected that the apoptotic burden will not change or decrease only slightly as resolution of the insult occurs. The exception is the TRIF−/− SAH where vasospasm decreases with time and, therefore, we believe that the clearance of the apoptotic burden results

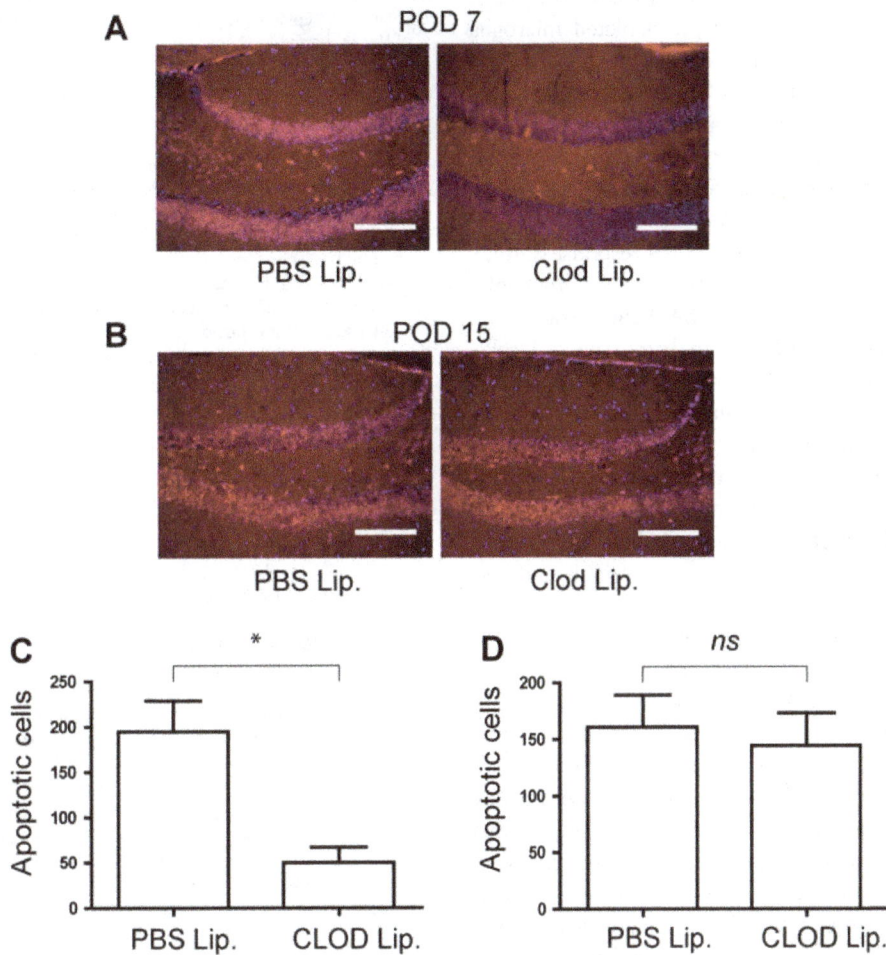

Figure 7 The effects of microglial ablation on neuronal apoptosis. A. Top panel: merge of DAPI and TUNEL staining from dentate gyrus of wild type subarachnoid hemorrhage (SAH) after intracerebroventricular (ICV) PBS liposome injection on POD 7 and 15. **B**. Bottom panel: merge of DAPI and TUNEL staining in wild type SAH after ICV clodronate injection on POD 7 and 15. Scale Bars: 10 μm in all panels. **C**. Quantification of apoptotic neurons on POD 7 displaying significant reduction, by Student's t-test (P <0.03), after ICV clodronate injection and microglial ablation. **D**. Quantification of apoptotic neurons on POD 15 revealing no change between ICV PBS and clodronate injections. N = 3 for each group and error bars are standard deviations.

in virtually no apoptotic cells by Day 15. Furthermore, the temporal relationship between TLR4-MyD88 activation and TLR4-TRIF activation is not unprecedented. Expression of NF-kB is seen in two phases after LPS stimulation of TLR4 [14]. MyD88 is responsible for the early phase and TRIF, the later phase, similar to our results. Because the role for microglia in DCI and SAH is largely unknown with respect to TLR4, we performed immunohistochemistry to verify that microglia do indeed express a majority of TLR4 *in vivo* after SAH at both POD 7 and 15. Although astrocytes and neurons express less TLR4, their role in DCI and cerebral inflammation may still be significant (Figure 4). To verify the relationship between the TLR4 pathway and microglia with respect to vasospasm, we performed *in vitro* vasospasm assays that confirmed a necessary role for the TLR4 receptor (Figure 5). While other groups have implicated microglia and heme in

the pathogenesis of intracerebral hemorrhage and shown that TLR4−/− was protective, the downstream mediators of TLR4 were never examined with respect to cytokine production or vasospasm [26].

We found that the TRIF and MyD88 pathways elicited equal degrees of vasospasm, as well as TNF-α secretion, compared to WT microglia. Because vasospasm and TNF-α secretion were not additive in WT microglia stimulated by heme, the temporal theme of sequential activation of MyD88 and TRIF is supported, although not necessarily in that order based on this *in vitro* experiment. A plateau effect is also possible where despite simultaneous activation of the MyD88 and TRIF pathways in WT microglia, the mouse aortic slice cannot constrict further. The other possible explanation is that the determination of the dominant pathway is influenced by the external chemical and cellular milieu of the brain, which is lacking in culture.

To elucidate the role of microglia *in vivo*, with respect to vasospasm and neuronal apoptosis, we depleted microglia using clodronate liposomes and showed that in both early and late phases of SAH, microglia are necessary for vasospasm. Also of note, neuronal apoptosis was abrogated by microglial depletion in early SAH only (Figure 7). With respect to a role for microglia in SAH, to our knowledge, we are the first to effectively deplete this specific cell type in the brain and demonstrate a functional response. Others have noted proliferation and activation of microglia after hemorrhagic stroke, specifically SAH and intracerebral hemorrhage [26,27]. Interestingly, in hemorrhagic stroke, microglia seem to be detrimental by some accounts, whereas in neonatal stroke and neurodegenerative diseases they have a more beneficial role [26,28,29]. The caveat is that effects of microglial depletion were only examined at one time point after depletion. Perhaps, if other time points after microglial depletion had been studied, the role of microglia in the pathogenesis of these diseases would also change with time.

Taken together, our model suggests that there could be different phases of SAH. The early phase of SAH, where neuronal apoptosis is largely TLR4-MyD88-dependent and microglial-dependent, followed by a late phase that is characterized by a TLR4-TRIF dependent, microglial-independent neuronal apoptosis. Furthermore, vasospasm is characterized by an early and late phase response that depends on MyD88 and TRIF, respectively. Finally, microglia seem to be both necessary and sufficient to cause vasospasm in both the early and late phases of SAH, based on our *in vitro* and *in vivo* models (Figures 5 and 6).

These findings may explain why therapies tailored to aSAH patients have failed for the most part. If these data can be translated to the SAH patient population, novel immunotherapies could be conceived that target different components of Toll like receptor signaling and microglia at different points in the patient's hospital course to alleviate the cerebral inflammatory burden and improve outcomes.

Abbreviations

aSAH: Aneurysmal subarachnoid hemorrhage; DCI: Delayed cerebral ischemia; DMEM: Dulbecco's modified eagle medium; DMSO: Dimethyl sulfoxide; FBS: Fetal bovine serum; ICV: Intracerebroventricular; IRAK4: IL-1 receptor associated kinase 4; LPS: Lipopolysaccharide; MCA: Middle cerebral artery; MCSF: Macrophage colony-stimulating factor; MyD88: Myeloid differentiation primary response gene; NF-κB: Nuclear factor kappa-light-chain-enhancer of activated B cells; PBS: Phosphate-buffered saline; PMG: Primary microglial; POD: Post-operative day; PPAR-γ: Peroxisome proliferator-activated receptor gamma; SAH: Subarachnoid hemorrhage; TLR4: Toll-like receptor 4; TNF-α: Tumor necrosis factor-alpha; TRIF: Toll receptor associated activator of interferon; TUNEL: Terminal deoxynucleotidyl transferase dUTP nick end labeling; WT: Wild type.

Competing interests

The author declares that he has no competing interests.

Acknowledgements

I would like to thank Rambhau Pandit and Justin Oh for technical assistance. KAH.

References

1. King JT Jr: **Epidemiology of aneurysmal subarachnoid hemorrhage.** *Neuroimaging Clin N Am* 1997, **7:**659–668.
2. Graf CJ, Nibbelink DW: **Cooperative study of intracranial aneurysms and subarachnoid hemorrhage. Report on a Randomized Treatment Study III. Intracranial Surgery.** *Stroke* 1974, **5:**557–601.
3. Vergouwen MD, Ilodigwe D, Macdonald RL: **Cerebral infarction after subarachnoid hemorrhage contributes to poor outcome by vasospasm-dependent and -independent effects.** *Stroke* 2011, **42:**924–929.
4. Aoki T, Takenaka K, Suzuki S, Kassell NF, Sagher O, Lee KS: **The role of hemolysate in the facilitation of oxyhemoglobin-induced contraction in rabbit basilar arteries.** *J Neurosurg* 1994, **81:**261–266.
5. Pluta RM, Afshar JK, Boock RJ, Oldfield EH: **Temporal changes in perivascular concentrations of oxyhemoglobin, deoxyhemoglobin, and methemoglobin after subarachnoid hemorrhage.** *J Neurosurg* 1998, **88:**557–561.
6. Crowley RW, Medel R, Kassell NF, Dumont AS: **New insights into the causes and therapy of cerebral vasospasm following subarachnoid hemorrhage.** *Drug Discov Today* 2008, **13:**254–260.
7. Zhao X, Grotta J, Gonzales N, Aronowski J: **Hematoma resolution as a therapeutic target: the role of microglia/macrophages.** *Stroke* 2009, **40**(3 Suppl)**:**S92–S94.
8. Barbagallo I, Marrazzo G, Frigiola A, Zappala A, Li Volti G: **Role of carbon monoxide in vascular diseases.** *Curr Pharm Biotechnol* 2012, **13:**787–796.
9. Figueiredo RT, Fernandez FL, Mourao-Sa DS, Porto BN, Dutra FF, Alves LS, Oliveira MF, Oliveira PL, Graça-Souza AV, Bozza MT: **Characterization of heme as activator of Toll-like receptor 4.** *J Biol Chem* 2007, **282:**20221–20229.
10. Ma C, Yin W, Cai B, Wu J, Wang J, He M, Sun H, Ding JL, You C: **Toll-like receptor 4/nuclear factor-kappa B signaling detected in brain after early subarachnoid hemorrhage.** *Chin Med J* 2009, **122:**1575–1581.
11. Zhou ML, Wu W, Ding YS, Zhang FF, Hang CH, Wang HD, Cheng HL, Yin HX, Shi JX: **Expression of Toll-like receptor 4 in the basilar artery after experimental subarachnoid hemorrhage in rabbits: a preliminary study.** *Brain Res* 2007, **1173:**110–116.
12. Kurki MI, Häkkinen S-K, Frösen J, Tulamo R, von und zu Fraunberg M, Wong G, Tromp G, Niemelä M, Hernesniemi J, Jääskeläinen JE, Ylä-Herttuala S: **Upregulated signaling pathways in ruptured human saccular intracranial aneurysm wall: an emerging regulative role of Toll-like receptor signaling and nuclear factor-κB, hypoxia-inducible factor-1A, and ETS transcription factors.** *Neurosurgery* 2011, **68:**1667–1675. discussion 1675–1676.
13. Zhang G, Ghosh S: **Toll-like receptor-mediated NF-kappaB activation: a phylogenetically conserved paradigm in innate immunity.** *J Clin Invest* 2001, **107:**13–19.
14. O'Neill LA, Bowie AG: **The family of five: TIR-domain-containing adaptors in Toll-like receptor signalling.** *Nat Rev Immunol* 2007, **7:**353–364.
15. Provencio JJ, Altay T, Smithason S, Moore SK, Ransohoff RM: **Depletion of Ly6G/C(+) cells ameliorates delayed cerebral vasospasm in subarachnoid hemorrhage.** *J Neuroimmunol* 2011, **232:**94–100.
16. Aoki T, Kataoka H, Shimamura M, Nakagami H, Wakayama K, Moriwaki T, Ishibashi R, Nozaki K, Morishita R, Hashimoto N: **NF-kappaB is a key mediator of cerebral aneurysm formation.** *Circulation* 2007, **116:**2830–2840.
17. Moussaud S, Draheim HJ: **A new method to isolate microglia from adult mice and culture them for an extended period of time.** *J Neurosci Methods* 2010, **187:**243–253.
18. Zubkov AY, Rollins KS, McGehee B, Parent AD, Zhang JH: **Relaxant effect of U0126 in hemolysate-, oxyhemoglobin-, and bloody cerebrospinal fluid-induced contraction in rabbit basilar artery.** *Stroke* 2001, **32:**154–161.
19. Sabri M, Jeon H, Ai J, Tariq A, Shang X, Chen G, Macdonald RL: **Anterior circulation mouse model of subarachnoid hemorrhage.** *Brain Res* 2009, **1295:**179–185.
20. Aid S, Langenbach R, Bosetti F: **Neuroinflammatory response to lipopolysaccharide is exacerbated in mice genetically deficient in cyclooxygenase-2.** *J Neuroinflammation* 2008, **5:**17.
21. Heros RC, Zervas NT, Varsos V: **Cerebral vasospasm after subarachnoid hemorrhage: an update.** *Ann Neurol* 1983, **14:**599–608.
22. Sasai M, Yamamoto M: **Pathogen recognition receptors: ligands and signaling pathways by Toll-like receptors.** *Int Rev Immunol* 2013, **32:**116–133.
23. Wu Y, Tang K, Huang R-Q, Zhuang Z, Cheng H-L, Yin H-X, Shi JX: **Therapeutic potential of peroxisome proliferator-activated receptor γ agonist rosiglitazone in cerebral vasospasm after a rat experimental subarachnoid hemorrhage model.** *J Neurol Sci* 2011, **305:**85–91.
24. Bederson JB, Connolly ES Jr, Batjer HH, Dacey RG, Dion JE, Diringer MN, Duldner JE Jr, Harbaugh RE, Patel AB, Rosenwasser RH, American Heart

Association: Guidelines for the management of aneurysmal subarachnoid hemorrhage: a statement for healthcare professionals from a special writing group of the Stroke Council, American Heart Association. *Stroke* 2009, **40**:994–1025.

25. Baldwin ME, Macdonald RL, Huo D, Novakovic RL, Novakovia RL, Goldenberg FD, Frank JI, Rosengart AJ: **Early vasospasm on admission angiography in patients with aneurysmal subarachnoid hemorrhage is a predictor for in-hospital complications and poor outcome.** *Stroke* 2004, **35**:2506–2511. Erratum in: *Stroke* 2005, **36**:175. Novakovia, Roberta L [corrected to Novakovic, Roberta L].

26. Lin S, Yin Q, Zhong Q, Lv F-L, Zhou Y, Li J-Q, Wang JZ, Su BY, Yang QW: **Heme activates TLR4-mediated inflammatory injury via MyD88/TRIF signaling pathway in intracerebral hemorrhage.** *J Neuroinflammation* 2012, **9**:46.

27. Simard JM, Tosun C, Ivanova S, Kurland DB, Hong C, Radecki L, Gisriel C, Mehta R, Schreibman D, Gerzanich V: **Heparin reduces neuroinflammation and transsynaptic neuronal apoptosis in a model of subarachnoid hemorrhage.** *Transl Stroke Res* 2012, **3**(Suppl 1):155–165.

28. Faustino JV, Wang X, Johnson CE, Klibanov A, Derugin N, Wendland MF, Vexler ZS: **Microglial cells contribute to endogenous brain defenses after acute neonatal focal stroke.** *J Neurosci* 2011, **31**:12992–13001.

29. Hawkes CA, McLaurin J: **Selective targeting of perivascular macrophages for clearance of beta-amyloid in cerebral amyloid angiopathy.** *Proc Natl Acad Sci U S A* 2009, **106**:1261–1266.

The inhibitory effect of mesenchymal stem cell on blood–brain barrier disruption following intracerebral hemorrhage in rats: contribution of TSG-6

Min Chen[1], Xifeng Li[1], Xin Zhang[1], Xuying He[1], Lingfeng Lai[1], Yanchao Liu[2], Guohui Zhu[1], Wei Li[1], Hui Li[1], Qinrui Fang[1], Zequn Wang[1] and Chuanzhi Duan[1*]

Abstract

Background: Mesenchymal stem cells (MSCs) are well known having beneficial effects on intracerebral hemorrhage (ICH) in previous studies. The therapeutic mechanisms are mainly to investigate proliferation, differentiation, and immunomodulation. However, few studies have used MSCs to treat blood–brain barrier (BBB) leakage after ICH. The influence of MSCs on the BBB and its related mechanisms were investigated when MSCs were transplanted into rat ICH model in this study.

Methods: Adult male Sprague–Dawley (SD) rats were randomly divided into sham-operated group, PBS-treated (ICH + PBS) group, and MSC-treated (ICH + MSC) group. ICH was induced by injection of IV collagenase into the rats' brains. MSCs were transplanted intravenously into the rats 2 h after ICH induction in MSC-treated group. The following factors were compared: inflammation, apoptosis, behavioral changes, inducible nitric oxide synthase (iNOS), matrix metalloproteinase 9 (MMP-9), peroxynitrite ($ONOO^-$), endothelial integrity, brain edema content, BBB leakage, TNF-α stimulated gene/protein 6 (TSG-6), and nuclear factor-κB (NF-κB) signaling pathway.

Results: In the ICH + MSC group, MSCs decreased the levels of proinflammatory cytokines and apoptosis, downregulated the density of microglia/macrophages and neutrophil infiltration at the ICH site, reduced the levels of iNOS and MMP-9, attenuated $ONOO^-$ formation, and increased the levels of zonula occludens-1 (ZO-1) and claudin-5. MSCs also improved the degree of brain edema and BBB leakage. The protective effect of MSCs on the BBB in ICH rats was possibly invoked by increased expression of TSG-6, which may have suppressed activation of the NF-κB signaling pathway. The levels of iNOS and $ONOO^-$, which played an important role in BBB disruption, decreased due to the inhibitory effects of TSG-6 on the NF-κB signaling pathway.

Conclusions: Our results demonstrated that intravenous transplantation of MSCs decreased the levels of $ONOO^-$ and degree of BBB leakage and improved neurological recovery in a rat ICH model. This strategy may provide a new insight for future therapies that aim to prevent breakdown of the BBB in patients with ICH and eventually offer therapeutic options for ICH.

Keywords: Mesenchymal stem cell, Intracerebral hemorrhage, Blood–brain barrier, Peroxynitrite, TNF-α stimulated gene/protein 6, Nuclear factor-κB, Inducible nitric oxide synthase

* Correspondence: duanchuanzhi_zj@126.com
[1]The National Key Clinic Specialty, The Neurosurgery Institute of Guangdong Province, Guangdong Provincial Key Laboratory on Brain Function Repair and Regeneration, Department of Neurosurgery, Zhujiang Hospital, Southern Medical University, Guangzhou 510282, China
Full list of author information is available at the end of the article

Background

Intracerebral hemorrhage (ICH) has high mortality and accounts for 10% to 20% of all strokes [1]. ICH, which occurs when a blood vessel within the brain ruptures, causes the accumulation of blood within the extracellular space. ICH always has the following features: compression of adjacent brain tissue due to hematoma, reduction of cerebral blood flow, disruption of blood–brain barrier (BBB) function, and increased brain edema, which all contribute to neurological deterioration [2,3]. In particular, BBB leakage, which is closely associated with brain edema formation, may cause secondary brain damage in ICH patients and lead to disability or death.

The BBB is mainly formed by endothelial cells with complex tight junctions which are governed by intracellular proteins, zonula occludens (ZO) as well as essential transmembrane proteins including occludin, claudins, and junctional adhesion molecules [4]. The BBB maintains the neural microenvironment by regulating the passage of molecules into and out of the brain and protects the brain against microorganisms and toxins in the blood [5]. Disruption of the BBB is an important pathophysiological change after ICH and contributes to formation of vasogenic brain edema, which plays an important role in secondary neuronal death and neurological dysfunction [6,7].

Peroxynitrite (ONOO$^-$), which is formed by the diffusion-controlled reaction between nitric oxide (NO) and superoxide [8], can exert a devastating effect on the BBB in several diseases including ICH. Upregulation of three isoforms of NOS, which are essential for ONOO$^-$ formation, may be correlated with BBB disruption [9]. Under some circumstances, microglia and astrocyte in the central nervous system can generate NO radicals from inducible NOS (iNOS) activation [10,11]. NO is produced in large quantities by iNOS and leads to ONOO$^-$ formation and is thought to be a damaging radical that is responsible for brain injury [12]. ONOO$^-$ can disrupt BBB integrity by several mechanisms such as impairing cellular energy metabolism, inhibiting Na$^+$/K$^+$-ATPase activity, which lead to cytotoxic brain edema, and activating the matrix metalloproteinases (MMPs), which can compromise BBB integrity [13-16]. In addition, sites of enhanced 3-nitrotyrosine (3-NT), which is a hallmark of ONOO$^-$, are co-localized with tight junction proteins such as zonula occludens-1 (ZO-1) and claudin-5, indicate the direct disruptive effect of ONOO$^-$ on BBB integrity [9].

Although mesenchymal stem cells (MSCs) have been successfully used for treatment of experimental ICH, to the best of our knowledge, no previous studies have investigated the possible protective effect of MSCs on the BBB after ICH. Previous studies have indicated that transplanted MSCs are recruited to the site of injury and contribute to repair by transdifferentiation [17,18]. However, recent investigations have shown that paracrine signaling is the primary mechanism accounting for the beneficial effects of MSCs in response to injury [19,20]. After intravenous infusion of MSCs, the cells trapped as emboli in the lung are activated to express the anti-inflammatory factor TNF-α stimulated gene/protein 6 (TSG-6) and eventually reduce inflammatory responses and infarct size in mice with myocardial infarction [21]. The potential mechanism by which MSCs exert their therapeutic effect involves TSG-6 and has been reported in traumatic brain injury [20], renal tubular inflammation and fibrosis [22], corneal injury [23], and dendritic cell maturation [24]. However, whether intravenous transplantation of MSCs improves BBB function after disruption and whether the mechanism is, at least in part, related to secretion of TSG-6, which inhibits the nuclear factor-κB (NF-κB) signaling pathway and decreases of ONOO$^-$ in ICH, remain unclear.

Therefore, the effects of MSCs on BBB leakage in a rat ICH model and their potential mechanisms of action were investigated in this study.

Materials and methods

BMMSC isolation, culture, and identification

The steps of bone marrow mesenchymal stem cell (BMMSC) isolation were prepared as described previously [25]. MSCs were isolated from the bone marrow of the femur and tibia of the 5-week-old male Sprague–Dawley (SD) rats. The femur and tibia from both knees were isolated with sterile forceps and surgical scissors, and both ends of the long bones were cut away. Mononuclear cells were isolated by Ficoll-Hypaque density gradient centrifugation for 20 minutes at 1,500 rpm. The collected mononuclear cells were plated at 1×10^6 cells/25 cm^2 in culture flasks in 5 ml DMEM/F12 (1:1) with 10% fetal bovine serum. Non-adherent cells were removed from the cultures after incubation. When the cells reached 90% confluence, adherent cells were harvested and expanded. MSCs that had undergone three passages were used in this study. Flow cytometry analysis was used for MSCs identification. The antibodies were as follows: FITC-CD29, PE-CD34, FITC-CD44, FITC-CD45, and PE-CD90 (Becton-Dickinson Biosciences, San Jose, CA, USA).

Animals and experimental groups

Our animal study and protocol was approved by the Southern Medical University Ethics Committee. All animal procedures were performed to minimize pain or discomfort in accordance with current protocols. Adult male SD rats weighting 250 to 300 g were purchased from the Animal Experiment Center of Southern Medical University (Guangzhou, China). Animals were housed under a 12-h light/dark cycle with free access to food and water. The SD rats were randomly assigned to three experimental groups: sham-operated group, PBS-treated group (ICH + PBS), and MSC-treated group (ICH + MSC).

Intracerebral hemorrhage animal model

ICH was induced via the stereotaxic intrastriatal injection of collagenase type IV (Sigma-Aldrich, St. Louis, MO, USA) as described previously with modifications [26]. In brief, the rats were anesthetized with 10% chloral hydrate (0.3 ml/100 g, i.p.; Sigma-Aldrich, St. Louis, MO, USA). Rectal temperature was maintained at 37°C throughout the surgical procedure using a heating lamp. Animals were placed in a stereotaxic frame and under aseptic conditions, and an incision was made exposing the bregma. A 10-uL microsyringe was inserted stereotactically through the burr hole and into the right striatum which coordinates are 0.2 mm anterior, 5.8 mm ventral, and 3.0 mm lateral to the bregma. Collagenase type IV (0.5 IU) in 2 µl saline was injected over a period of 5 min. After placement for another 5 min, the microsyringe was slowly removed. The burr hole was sealed with bone wax, and the wound was sutured. The sham-operated rats were treated the same way except that they were administered 2 µl sterile saline into the right striatum.

MSC transplantation

Two hours after ICH induction, MSCs were administered intravenously into the rats as previously described with slight modification [27]. The jugular vein was exposed and then isolated with blunt dissection. A 250-µl Hamilton syringe attached with a 31-gauge needle (Hamilton, Princeton, NJ, USA) was laid into the lumen and fixed in place. The cells (5×10^6) in 200 µl PBS (Invitrogen, Carlsbad, CA, USA) were delivered over 10 min. Then, the needle was withdrawn carefully and incision was closed. As a comparison, an equal amount of PBS without MSCs was administered via jugular vein to animals in the PBS-treated group.

TUNEL assay

Terminal deoxynucleotidyl transferase-mediated biotinylated-dUTP nick-end labeling (TUNEL) staining was performed 72 h after ICH as previously described with minor modifications [28], by use of the in situ cell death detection kit (Roche, Nutley, NJ, USA) according to the manufacturer's instruction. The slides were analyzed with fluorescence microscopy (Bx51, Olympus Corporation, Shinjuku-ku, Japan).

Behavioral testing

Behavioral testing was conducted 24 and 72 h after ICH according to the previous study [29]. Briefly, the modified neurological severity score (mNSS) test includes motor, sensory, reflex, and balance tests. The mNSS test is graded on a scale of 0 to 18, where a total score of 18 points indicates severe neurological deficit and a score of 0 indicates normal performance, 13 to 18 points indicate severe injury, 7 to 12 indicate moderate injury, and 1 to 6 indicate mild injury. The mNSS test was monitored by two investigators and both of whom had been blinded to groups.

Analysis of brain water content

Brain water content was measured 24 and 72 h after ICH as described earlier [3,30]. The brains of the rats were removed immediately after anesthetization followed by decapitation, and the brain was divided into two hemispheres along the midline, and the cerebellum and brain stem were removed. Two hemispheres were weighed on an electronic analytical balance to obtain wet weights and then dried in an electric oven at 100°C for 24 h to obtain dry weight. The brain water percentage was calculated as the following formula: ([wet weight – dry weight] / wet weight) × 100 (%).

Immunohistochemistry

For immunohistochemistry, the rats were anesthetized and transcardially perfused with cold PBS and 4% paraformaldehyde at 72 h after ICH. Slides were incubated with primary antibodies: anti-MPO antibody (1:100, Abcam, Cambridge, MA, USA), anti-Iba-1 antibody (1:100, Abcam, Cambridge, MA, USA) at 4°C overnight. Following primary antibody incubation, the slides were incubated in secondary antibody. Finally, the nucleus was counterstained with hematoxylin. Images were observed with the use of a microscope (Bx51, Olympus Corporation, Shinjuku-ku, Japan).

ELISA

The rats were killed at 1, 3, and 7 days after ICH or sham operation, the brain tissues were obtained, and the following cytokine levels were quantified by enzyme-linked immunosorbent assay (ELISA): IL-1β, IL-6, IL-10, tumor necrosis factor (TNF)-α, interferon (IFN)-γ, and transforming growth factor (TGF)-β1. Photometric measurements were conducted at 450 nm using microplate reader (Bio-Rad, Hercules, MA, USA). In the process of ELISA, commercial ELISA kits (Bio-Rad, Hercules, MA, USA) were used following the manufacturer's instructions.

Quantitative analysis of blood–brain barrier permeability

BBB leakage was assessed as previously described with slight modification [31]. The rats received 100 µl of a 5% solution of Evan's blue (EB) in saline administered intravenously 24 and 72 h following ICH. Two hours after EB injection, cardiac perfusion was performed under deep anesthesia with 200 ml of saline to clear the cerebral circulation of EB. The brain was removed and sliced. The two hemispheres were isolated and mechanically homogenized in 750 µl of N,N-dimethylformamide (DMF). The suspension obtained was kept at room temperature in the dark for 72 h. It was centrifuged at $10,000 \times g$ for 25 min and the supernatant was spectrofluorimetrically analyzed (λ_{ex} 620 nm, λ_{em} 680 nm) to determine EB content.

Imnunofluorescence analysis

Immunofluorescence was performed at 72 h after ICH as previously described [9,32]. After antigen retrieval by heat treatment, the sections were incubated at 4°C overnight with primary antibodies: anti-iNOS antibody (Abcam, Cambridge, MA, USA), anti-3-Nitrotyrosine antibody (Abcam, Cambridge, MA, USA), anti-ZO-1 antibody (Invitrogen, Carlsbad, CA, USA). It was then incubated with the appropriate fluorescence conjugated secondary antibodies for 1.5 h at room temperature. Nuclei were stained by Hoechst 33258 (Sigma-Aldrich, St. Louis, MO, USA) for 10 min at room temperature. The slices were observed underneath a fluorescence microscope (Bx51, Olympus Corporation, Shinjuku-ku, Japan).

NF-κB assay in brain

Cytosolic and nuclear extracts were prepared as previously described [33,34] with slight modifications. Briefly, the brain tissues from rats were suspended in extraction buffer A containing 0.2 mM phenylmethanesulfonyl fluoride (PMSF), 0.15 µM pepstatin A, 20 µM leupeptin, and 1 mM sodium orthovanadate, homogenized at the highest setting for 2 min, and centrifuged at $1,000 \times g$ for 10 min at 4°C. Supernatants represented the cytosolic fraction. The pellets, containing enriched nuclei, were resuspended in buffer B containing 1% Triton X-100, 150 mM NaCl, 10 mM Tris–HCl, pH 7.4, 1 mM EGTA, 1 mM EDTA, 0.2 mM PMSF, 20 µM leupeptin, and 0.2 mM sodium orthovanadate. After centrifugation for 30 min at $15,000 \times g$ at 4°C, the supernatants containing the nuclear protein were stored at –80°C for further analysis. The levels of IκB-α and phospho-NF-κB p65 (serine 536) were quantified in the cytosolic fraction from the brain tissue collected 24 and 72 h after ICH, while NF-κB p65 levels were quantified in the nuclear fraction. The filters were blocked with 1× PBS, 5% (w/v) nonfat dried milk for 40 min at room temperature and subsequently probed with specific Abs IκB-α (1:1000, Santa Cruz Biotechnology, Santa Cruz, CA, USA), or phospho-NF-κB p65 (serine 536) (1:1000, Cell Signaling Technology, Beverly, MA, USA), or anti-NF-κB p65 (1:1000, Santa Cruz Biotechnology, Santa Cruz, MA, USA) in 1× PBS, 5% w/v nonfat dried milk, 0.1% Tween-20 (PMT) at 4°C overnight. Membranes were incubated with goat anti-mouse IgG (1:1000, Invitrogen, Carlsbad, CA, USA) or goat anti-rabbit IgG (1:1000, Invitrogen, Carlsbad, CA, USA) secondary antibody for 1 h at room temperature. Immunoblots were

detected using an enhanced chemiluminescence (ECL) kit (Thermo Fisher Scientific, Waltham, MA, USA) and GAPDH (1:1000, Cell Signaling Technology, Beverly, MA, USA) was employed as the loading control.

Total RNA extraction and real-time PCR

Total RNA extraction and real-time PCR of TSG-6 was performed as previously described [20]. Total RNA was extracted from tissues around the lesional sites 24 and 72 h after ICH using Trizol reagent (Invitrogen, Carlsbad, CA, USA). One microgram of total RNA was reverse transcribed to cDNA with High Capacity cDNA Reverse Transcription Kits (Applied Biosystems, Foster City, CA, USA). Gene transcription was detected by real-time PCR in an ABI Prism 7500 sequence detection system (Applied Biosystems, Foster City, CA, USA) using specific primers designed from known sequences. GAPDH (1:1000, Cell Signaling Technology) was used as an endogenous control. Sequence-specific primers for TSG-6 and GADPH were showed as follows:

TSG-6, 5′-GCAGCTAGAAGCAGCCAGAAAG-3′ (forward primer),
TSG-6, 5′-TTGTAGCAATAGGCGTCCCACC-3′ (reverse primer);
GAPDH, 5′-AAGGTGAAGGTCGGAGTCAA-3′ (forward primer),
GAPDH, 5′-AATGAAGGGGTCATTGATGG-3′ (reverse primer).

Western blotting analysis

Rats were sacrificed 24 and 72 h after ICH by injecting overdose of chloral hydrate. Total tissue protein was isolated from ipsilateral lesional brain tissues using ice-cold RIPA buffer. Protein concentrations were measured with the BCA Protein Assay Kit (Thermo Fisher Scientific, Waltham, MA, USA). The samples were subjected to SDS-polyacrylamide gel electrophoresis and transferred to a polyvinylidene diflouride (PVDF) filter membrane. The membranes were blocked with 5% nonfat milk and incubated with primary antibody (rabbit polyclonal anti-iNOS 1:800, Abcam, USA; mouse monoclonal anti-3-nitrotyrosine, 1:1000, Abcam, USA; mouse monoclonal anti-ZO-1, 1:200, Invitrogen, USA; rabbit polyclonal anti-Claudin-5, 1:800, Novus, USA; rabbit polyclonal anti-matrix metalloproteinase-9 (MMP-9), 1:250, Abcam, USA; mouse monoclonal anti-TSG-6, 1:800, Santa Cruz Biotechnology, USA) overnight. The blots were incubated with secondary antibodies after washing with Tris-buffered saline. Immunoblots were detected using an enhanced chemiluminescence (ECL) kit (Thermo Fisher Scientific), and GAPDH (1:1000, Cell Signaling Technology) was employed as the loading control.

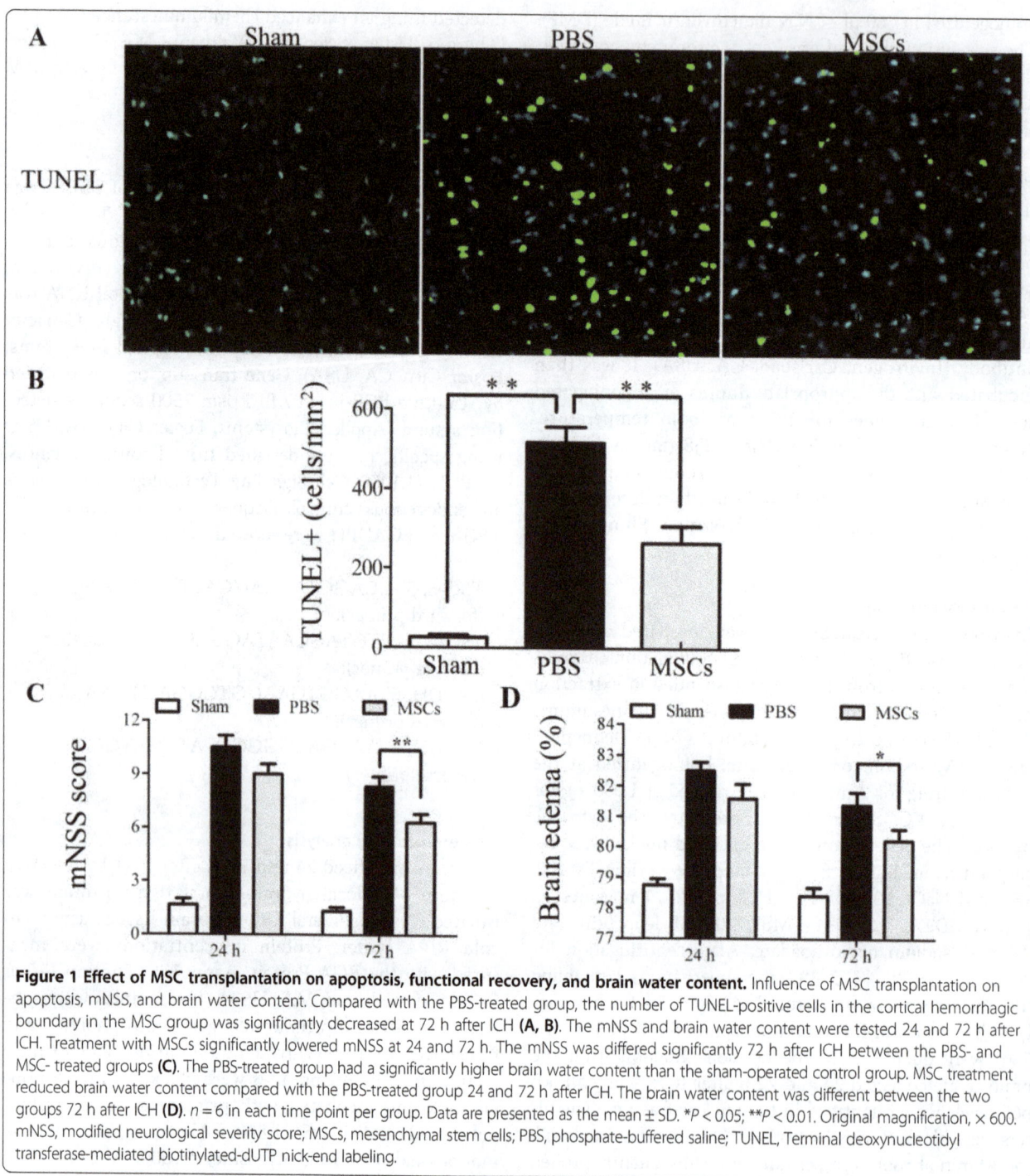

Figure 1 Effect of MSC transplantation on apoptosis, functional recovery, and brain water content. Influence of MSC transplantation on apoptosis, mNSS, and brain water content. Compared with the PBS-treated group, the number of TUNEL-positive cells in the cortical hemorrhagic boundary in the MSC group was significantly decreased at 72 h after ICH **(A, B)**. The mNSS and brain water content were tested 24 and 72 h after ICH. Treatment with MSCs significantly lowered mNSS at 24 and 72 h. The mNSS was differed significantly 72 h after ICH between the PBS- and MSC- treated groups **(C)**. The PBS-treated group had a significantly higher brain water content than the sham-operated control group. MSC treatment reduced brain water content compared with the PBS-treated group 24 and 72 h after ICH. The brain water content was different between the two groups 72 h after ICH **(D)**. $n = 6$ in each time point per group. Data are presented as the mean ± SD. *$P < 0.05$; **$P < 0.01$. Original magnification, × 600. mNSS, modified neurological severity score; MSCs, mesenchymal stem cells; PBS, phosphate-buffered saline; TUNEL, Terminal deoxynucleotidyl transferase-mediated biotinylated-dUTP nick-end labeling.

Statistical analysis

Data are presented as means ± SD and analyzed by SPSS 13.0 software (SPSS, Chicago, IL, USA). Comparison between groups was assessed by Student's t test or one-way analysis of variance (ANOVA). A P-value of <0.05 was considered to indicate a statistically significant result.

Results

Isolation and characterization of MSCs

The MSCs used in our study were isolated from SD rats' bone marrow and were analyzed for cell surface antigens at passage three. The results gained by using flow cytometry showed that MSCs were positive for CD29 (99.52%), CD44 (94.63%), and CD90 (99.65%)

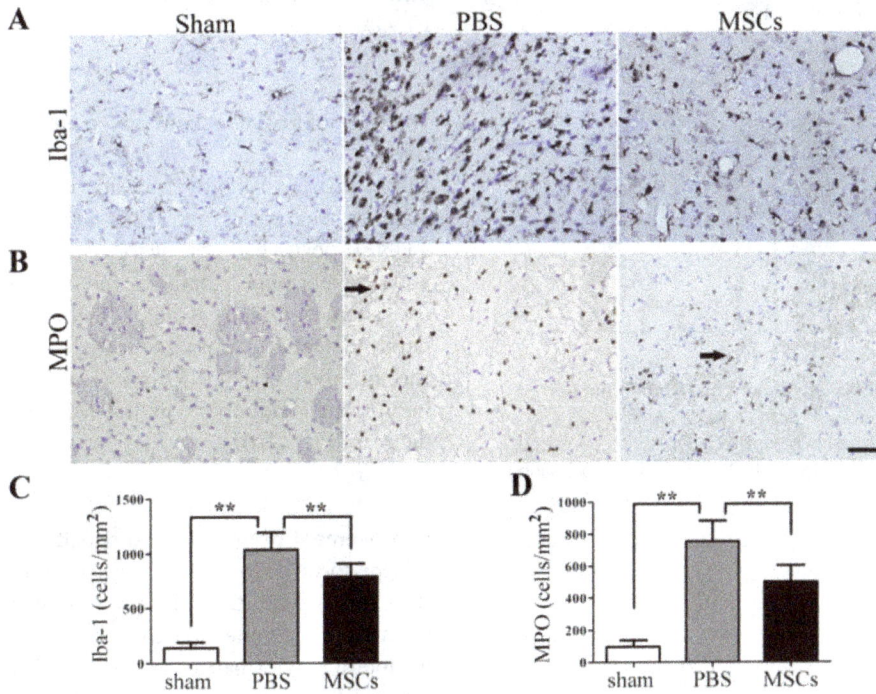

Figure 2 The influence of MSC on brain inflammatory cell infiltration and microglia numbers. Iba-1[+] microglia cells/macrophages and MPO[+] neutrophils were identified by immunohistochemistry 72 h after ICH to test the effects of MSC treatment on the number of peripheral infiltrating and brain-resident immune cells. Both the numbers of Iba-1[+] microglia cells/macrophages **(A, C)** and infiltrated MPO[+] neutrophils **(B, D)** were reduced in the MSC-treated group when compared with the PBS-treated group. The sign of arrow indicates the edge of the hematoma. $n = 6$ per group. Data are presented as the mean ± SD. Bar = 50 μm. **$P < 0.01$. MPO, myeloperoxidase; MSCs, mesenchymal stem cells; PBS, phosphate-buffered saline.

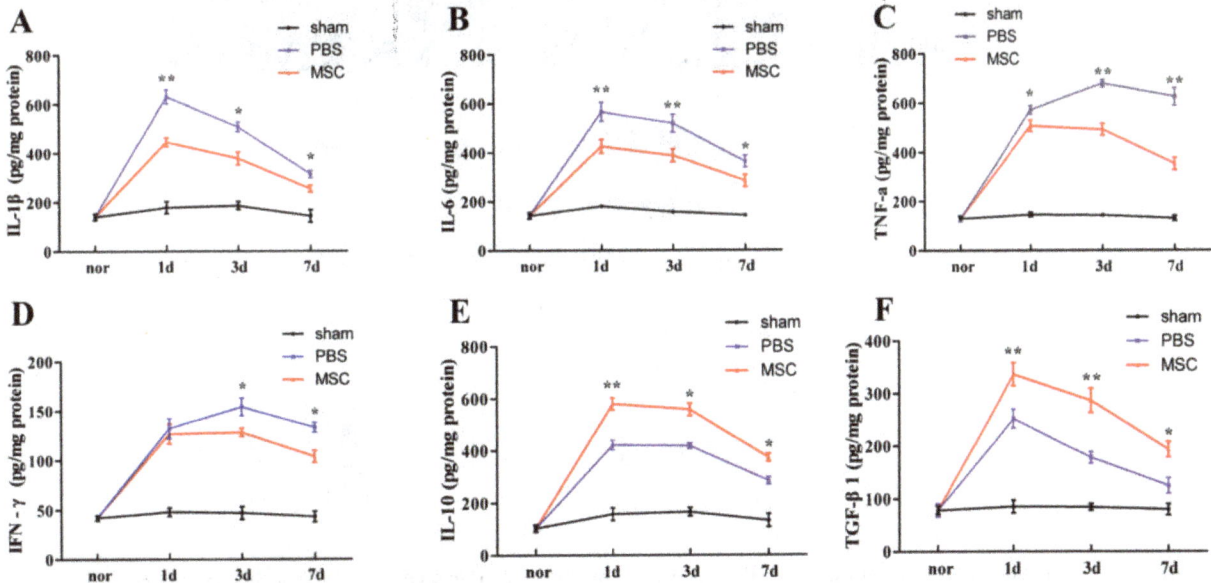

Figure 3 Influence of MSC treatment on cytokine concentrations. Levels of the proinflammatory cytokines IL-1β (at 1, 3, and 7 days), IL-6 (at 1, 3, and 7 days), TNF-α (at 1, 3, and 7 days), and IFN-γ (at 3 and 7 days) were decreased in the MSC-treated group compared with the PBS-treated group **(A-D)**. Levels of the anti-inflammatory cytokines IL-10 (at 1, 3, and 7 days) and TGF-β1 (at 1, 3, and 7 days) were increased in the MSC-treated group compared with the PBS-treated group **(E-F)**. $n = 6$ in each time point per group. Data are presented as the mean ± SD. *$P < 0.05$; **$P < 0.01$. MSCs, mesenchymal stem cells; PBS, phosphate-buffered saline.

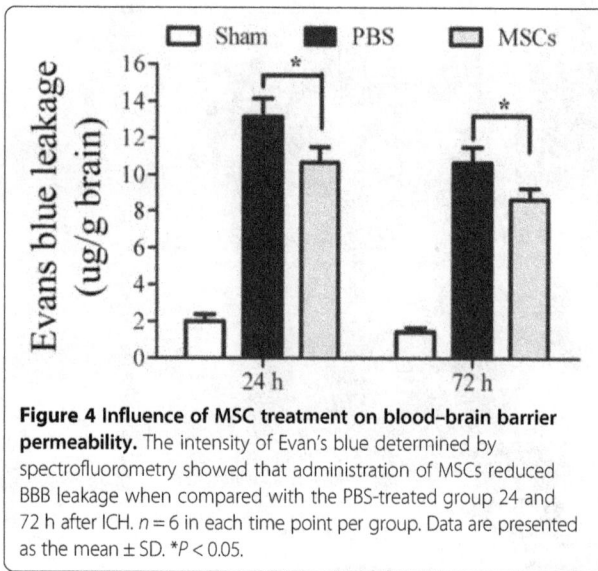

Figure 4 Influence of MSC treatment on blood–brain barrier permeability. The intensity of Evan's blue determined by spectrofluorometry showed that administration of MSCs reduced BBB leakage when compared with the PBS-treated group 24 and 72 h after ICH. $n = 6$ in each time point per group. Data are presented as the mean ± SD. *$P < 0.05$.

and were negative for CD34 (1.61%) and CD45 (0.95%).

The effect of MSC treatment on the number of TUNEL-positive cells

In order to investigate apoptotic cells after ICH, TUNEL staining was performed 72 h after ICH (Figure 1A,B). TUNEL-positive cells were detected in the center and the peripheral area of the hemorrhagic lesion. In the sham-operated group, TUNEL-positive cells were barely detected. Compared with the PBS-treated group, the number of TUNEL-positive cells in the cortical hemorrhagic boundary in the MSC-treated group were decreased ($P < 0.01$).

Improvement of neurological deficits with MSC treatment

We performed the mNSS tests in purpose of examining the effect of MSC transplantation on neurological function. Compared with the PBS-treated group, the improvement in motor performance in the MSC-treated group was statistically significantly different 72 h after ICH ($P < 0.01$) (Figure 1C).

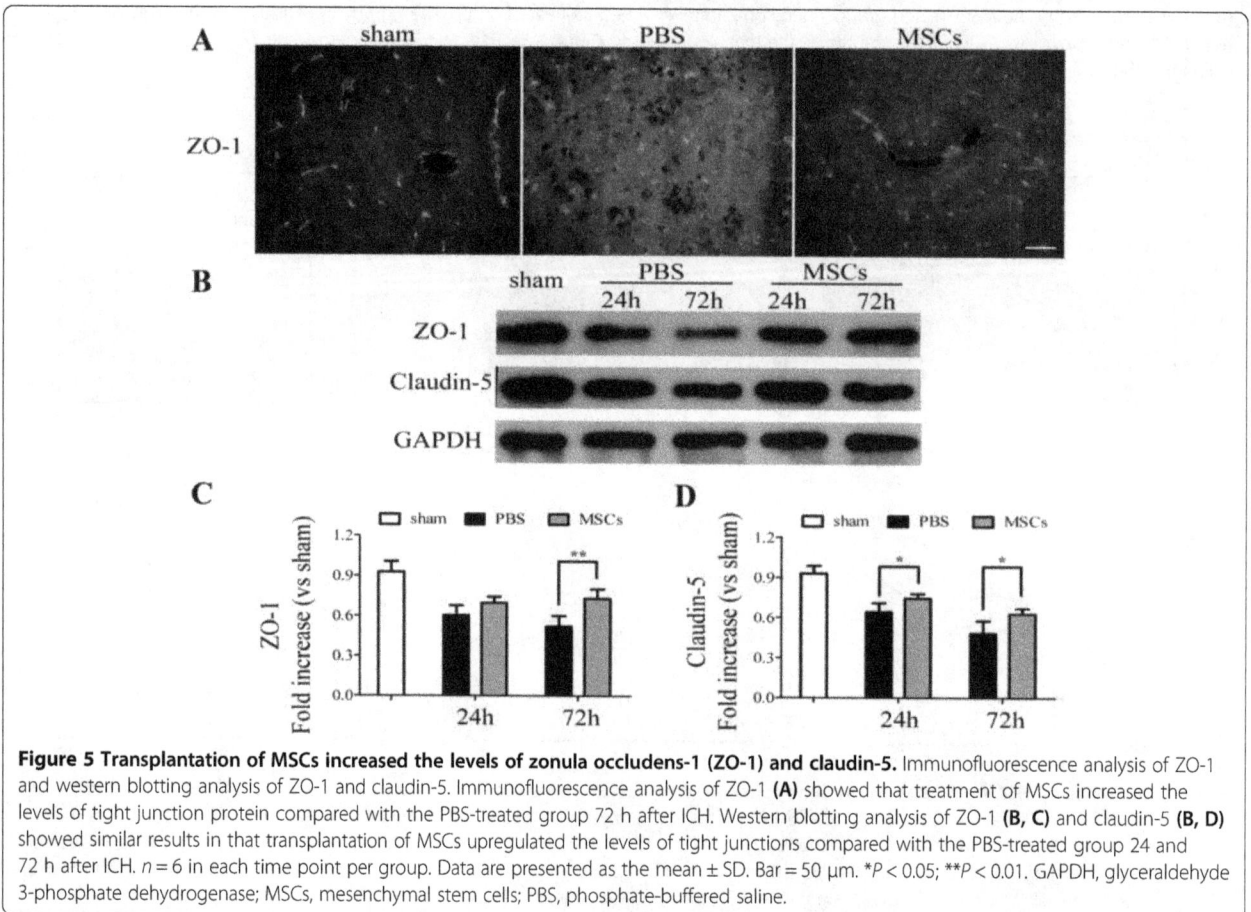

Figure 5 Transplantation of MSCs increased the levels of zonula occludens-1 (ZO-1) and claudin-5. Immunofluorescence analysis of ZO-1 and western blotting analysis of ZO-1 and claudin-5. Immunofluorescence analysis of ZO-1 **(A)** showed that treatment of MSCs increased the levels of tight junction protein compared with the PBS-treated group 72 h after ICH. Western blotting analysis of ZO-1 **(B, C)** and claudin-5 **(B, D)** showed similar results in that transplantation of MSCs upregulated the levels of tight junctions compared with the PBS-treated group 24 and 72 h after ICH. $n = 6$ in each time point per group. Data are presented as the mean ± SD. Bar = 50 μm. *$P < 0.05$; **$P < 0.01$. GAPDH, glyceraldehyde 3-phosphate dehydrogenase; MSCs, mesenchymal stem cells; PBS, phosphate-buffered saline.

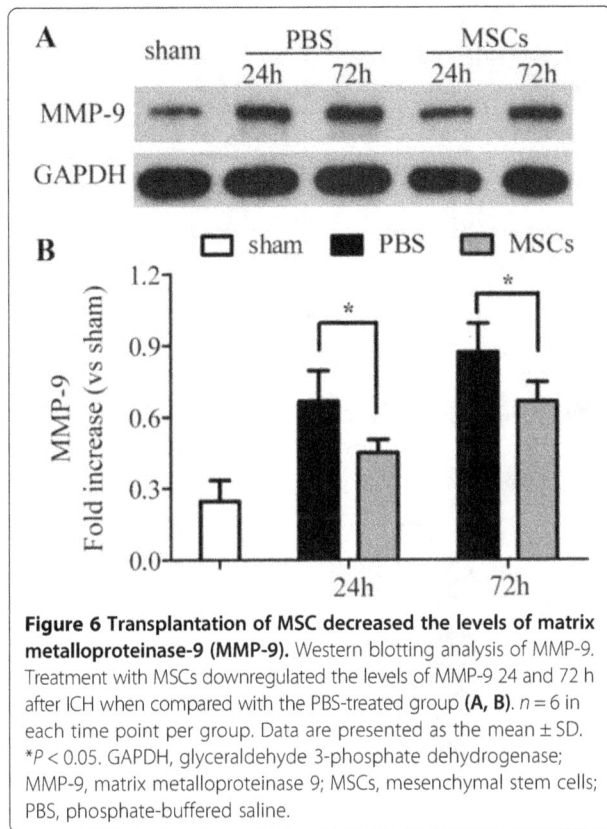

Figure 6 Transplantation of MSC decreased the levels of matrix metalloproteinase-9 (MMP-9). Western blotting analysis of MMP-9. Treatment with MSCs downregulated the levels of MMP-9 24 and 72 h after ICH when compared with the PBS-treated group **(A, B)**. $n = 6$ in each time point per group. Data are presented as the mean ± SD. *$P < 0.05$. GAPDH, glyceraldehyde 3-phosphate dehydrogenase; MMP-9, matrix metalloproteinase 9; MSCs, mesenchymal stem cells; PBS, phosphate-buffered saline.

MSC treatment reduced brain water content

The brain water content was tested to represent the brain edema in hemorrhagic hemispheres and to investigate the effect of MSC treatment on BBB leakage. At 24 and 72 h after ICH, the PBS-treated group had a higher brain water content than the sham-operated group, and brain water content was reduced in the MSC-treated group when compared with the PBS-treated group. The brain water content was statistically significantly different at 72 h between the PBS- and MSC-treated group ($P < 0.05$) (Figure 1D).

The influence of MSC on brain inflammatory cell infiltration and microglia numbers

Iba-1$^+$ microglia cells/macrophages and MPO$^+$ neutrophils were identified by immunohistochemistry to test the effect of MSC treatment on the number of peripheral infiltrating and brain-resident immune cells. Both the numbers of Iba-1$^+$ microglia cells/macrophages (Figure 2A,C) and infiltrated MPO$^+$ neutrophils (Figure 2B,D) were reduced in the MSC-treated group when compared with the PBS-treated group ($P < 0.01$).

Cytokine levels detected by ELISA

To further assess the microenvironment in the brain which may closely relate to the BBB disruption, we examined the expression of inflammatory-associated cytokines in hemorrhagic lesion at 1, 3, and 7 days after ICH. The levels of IL-1β (at 1, 3, and 7 days), IL-6 (at 1, 3, and 7 days), TNF-a (at 1, 3, and 7 days), and IFN-γ (at 3 and 7 days) were all substantially downregulated in the MSC-treated group when compared with the PBS-treated group, whereas the levels of anti-inflammatory cytokines IL-10 (at 1, 3, and 7 days) and TGF-β1 (at 1, 3, and 7 days) were upregulated ($P < 0.05$) (Figure 3).

Effect of treatment with MSCs on recovery of BBB integrity

Disruption of the BBB and edema formation is associated with endothelial dysfunction [35]. To investigate the neurovascular protective action of MSCs on ICH, we compared the MSC group to the PBS group in relation to the intensity of Evan's blue 24 and 72 h after ICH. The intensity of Evan's blue determined by spectrofluorometric estimation showed that administration of MSCs reduced BBB leakage when compared with the PBS-treated group 24 and 72 h after ICH ($P < 0.05$) (Figure 4).

In addition, tight junction molecules were studied to assess microvascular integrity. As shown in Figure 5, compared with the PBS-treated group, blood vessels in the MSC-treated group were surrounded by more intense and continuous reactivity for ZO-1, which was analyzed by fluorescence microscopy (Figure 5A) and western blotting (Figure 5B,C). Western blotting analysis of claudin-5 (Figure 5B,D) showed similar results in that tight junctions were decreased in the PBS-treated group but increased in the MSC-treated group. The activity of MMP-9, which is also closely related to BBB integrity, was analyzed by western blotting. As shown in Figure 6, transplantation of MSCs reduced the expression of MMP-9, compared with that of the PBS-treated group 24 and 72 h after ICH (Figure 6A, B) ($P < 0.05$).

The influence of MSCs treatment on the expression of 3-NT and iNOS

Since ONOO$^-$ is unstable, the nitration of tyrosine residues in proteins by ONOO$^-$ to 3-NT is a reliable hallmark of the presence of ONOO$^-$ [36], so its detection through 3-NT expression is an index of the levels of ONOO$^-$ [37]. As shown in Figures 7 and 8, the MSC-treated group decreased the expression of iNOS (Figure 7) and 3-NT (Figure 8A,C,D) obviously when compared with the PBS-treated group. The western blotting analysis of iNOS and 3-NT showed the similar results in that administration of MSCs downregulated the levels of iNOS (Figure 7B,C) and 3-NT (Figure 8C,D) 24 and 72 h after ICH ($P < 0.05$).

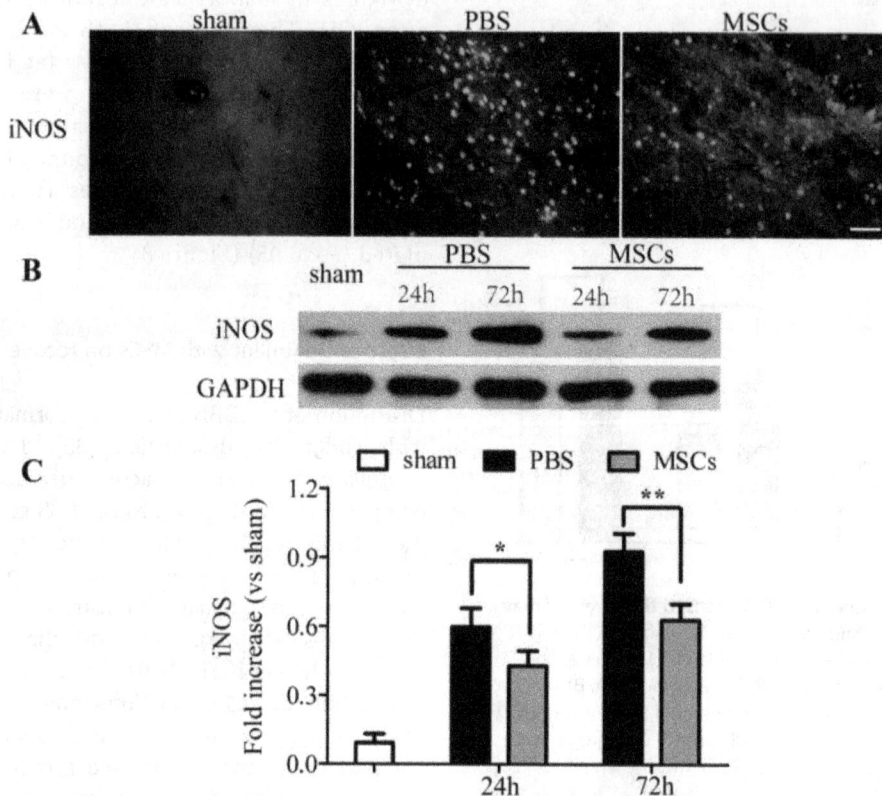

Figure 7 Transplantation of MSC decreased the levels of inducible nitric oxide synthase (iNOS). Immunofluorescence and western blotting analysis of iNOS. Immunofluorescence analysis of iNOS **(A)** showed that treatment with MSCs decreased the levels of iNOS compared with the PBS-treated group 72 h after ICH. Western blotting **(B, C)** analysis of iNOS showed similar results in that transplantation of MSCs downregulated the levels of iNOS compared with the PBS-treated group 24 and 72 h after ICH. $n = 6$ in each time point per group. Data are presented as the mean ± SD. Bar = 50 μm. *$P < 0.05$; **$P < 0.01$. GAPDH, glyceraldehyde 3-phosphate dehydrogenase; iNOS, inducible nitric oxide synthase; MSCs, mesenchymal stem cells; PBS, phosphate-buffered saline.

The influence of MSC treatment on the expression of TSG-6

The expression of TSG-6 was detected by western blotting and real-time polymerase chain reaction in order to assess the potential mechanisms which may relate to the protective effect of MSCs on the BBB disruption. As the result of western blotting shown (Figure 9A,B), the treatment of MSC in ICH have upregulated the expression of the inhibitory factors TSG-6 24 and 72 h after ICH ($P < 0.05$); similar results were obtained at the mRNA levels (Figure 9C) ($P < 0.01$).

Effects of MSC on IκB-α degradation, phosphorylation of Ser536 on p65, expression of NF-κB p65, and NF-κB translocation

To further investigate the mechanisms by which may attenuate BBB leakage, we evaluated IκB-α degradation, phosphorylation of Ser536 on the NF-κB subunit p65, and total NF-κB p65 by western blotting. Compared with a basal level of IκB-α in the sham-operated group, the levels of IκB-α in the PBS-treated group were reduced; on the contrary, treatment with MSCs inhibited the degradation of IκB-α 24 and 72 h after ICH ($P < 0.05$) (Figure 10A,B). Unlike the levels of IκB-α, phosphorylation of Ser536 on p65 was increased in the PBS-treated group 24 and 72 h post-ICH when compared with the sham-operated group, whereas the treatment of MSC inhibited its increase ($P < 0.05$) (Figure 10C,D). The same as phosphorylation of Ser536 on p65, MSC treatment reduced NF-κB p65 levels in the nuclear fractions of the ICH tissue when compared with the PBS-treated group 24 and 72 h after ICH ($P < 0.01$) (Figure 10E,F).

Discussion

The main pathophysiological factors of ICH include hematoma size and edema [38]. The formation of edema, which is mainly caused by disruption of the BBB following ICH, is associated with patient outcome. The BBB is composed of endothelial cells, tight junction proteins, astrocyte end-feet, and pericytes, which have the function of maintaining homeostasis of the neuro-parenchymal microenvironment [6]. Loss of BBB integrity is an important pathophysiological change that contributes to initiation of the inflammatory cascade, edema formation, and ultimately

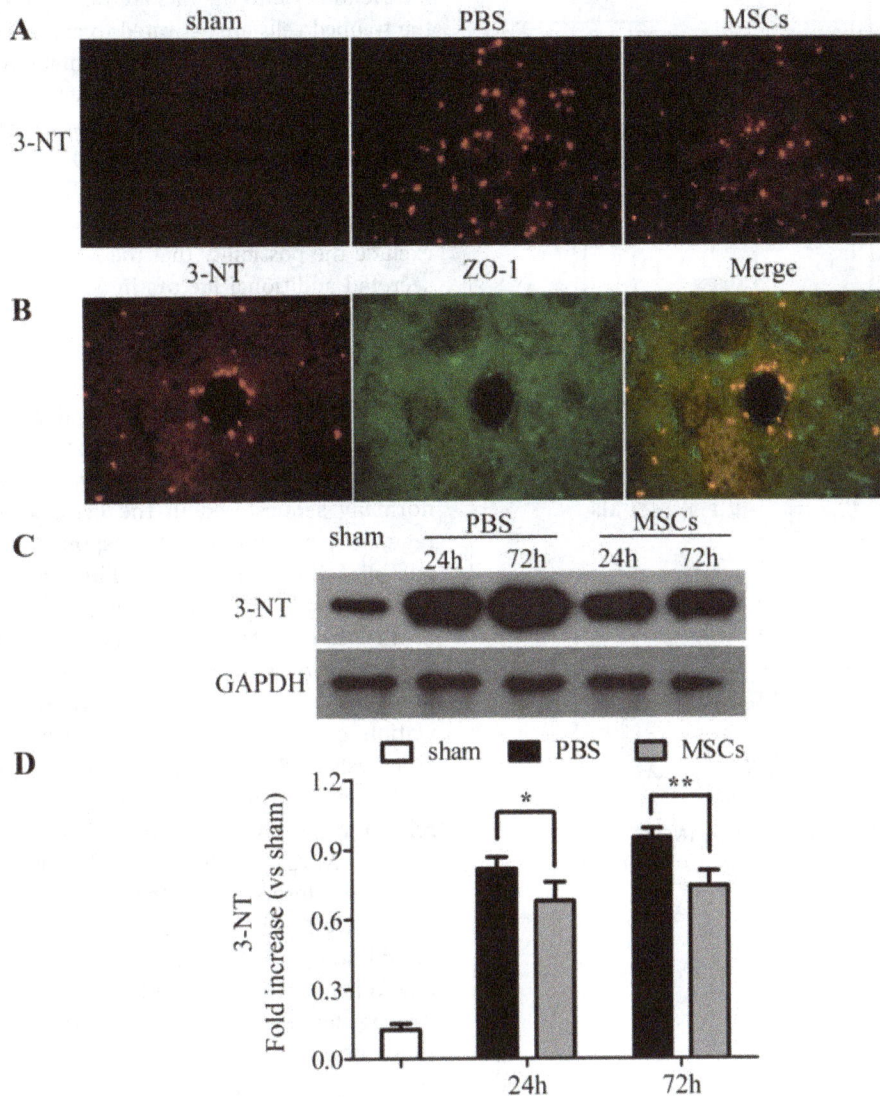

Figure 8 Transplantation of MSCs decreased the levels of 3-nitrotyrosine (3-NT). Immunofluorescence and western blotting analysis of 3-NT. Immunofluorescence analysis of 3-NT **(A)** showed that the treatment with MSCs decreased the levels of 3-NT compared with the PBS-treated group 72 h after ICH. Western blotting **(C, D)** analysis of 3-NT showed the similar results in that transplantation of MSCs downregulated the levels of 3-NT compared with the PBS-treated group 24 and 72 h after ICH. The double labeling of 3-NT and ZO-1 indicated that 3-NT and vascular damage are closely related **(B)**. $n = 6$ in each time point per group. Data are presented as the mean ± SD. Bar = 50 μm. *$P < 0.05$; **$P < 0.01$. GAPDH, glyceraldehyde 3-phosphate dehydrogenase; MSCs, mesenchymal stem cells; PBS, phosphate-buffered saline.

poor outcome [39]. In this study, the effect of MSCs on BBB leakage in ICH rats and relevant mechanisms were investigated after intravenous transplantation of MSCs.

Besides endothelial cell activation, vascular ONOO⁻, which is formed by NO and superoxide anion, is closely related to BBB leakage [37]. Studies have already shown that ONOO⁻ alone is sufficient to induce BBB leakage, endothelial dysfunction, and neurodegeneration [40,41]. Several tight junction proteins, such as claudin-5 [42], occludin [43], and ZO-1 [44], are critical determinants of BBB permeability in rats. In the process of BBB damage, the formation of ONOO⁻ may play an important role by reducing the tight junction proteins. In addition to the impact on the tight junction proteins, ONOO⁻-mediated increased expression of MMP-9 is reported to exacerbate BBB leakage [45]. MMPs are important for normal physiological brain function, but in the early stage of ICH, they can be detrimental [7]. Previous studies have established the link between MMP-9 and degradation of tight junction proteins, BBB disruption, inflammation, and tissue injury [46,47]. Our study showed that the increase in ONOO⁻ in ICH rats may have caused harmful effects, such as BBB disruption and brain edema formation. In addition, the levels of tight junction proteins, including

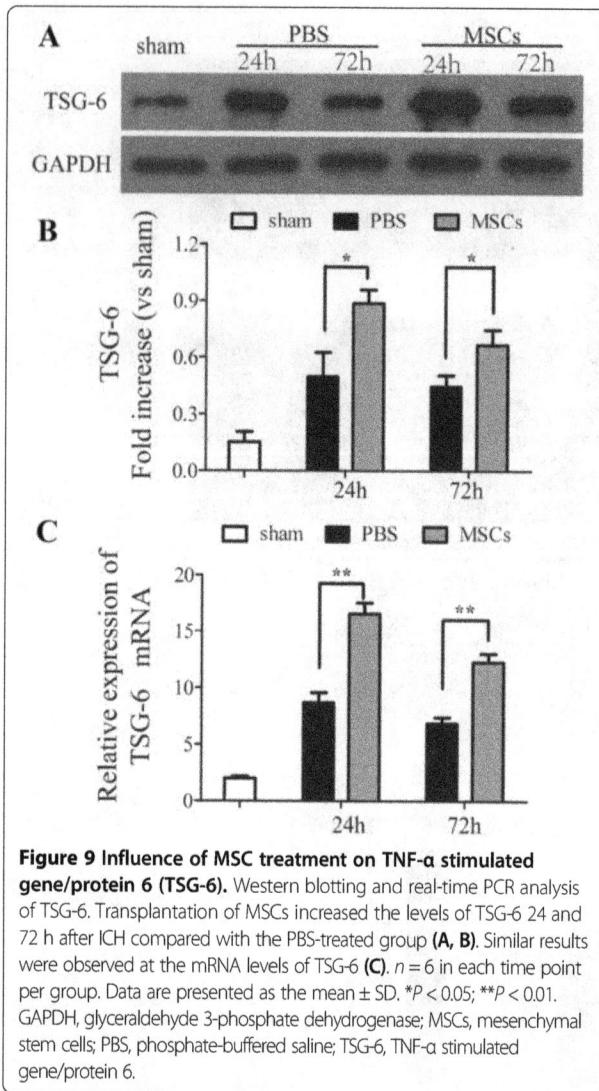

Figure 9 Influence of MSC treatment on TNF-α stimulated gene/protein 6 (TSG-6). Western blotting and real-time PCR analysis of TSG-6. Transplantation of MSCs increased the levels of TSG-6 24 and 72 h after ICH compared with the PBS-treated group **(A, B)**. Similar results were observed at the mRNA levels of TSG-6 **(C)**. $n = 6$ in each time point per group. Data are presented as the mean ± SD. *$P < 0.05$; **$P < 0.01$. GAPDH, glyceraldehyde 3-phosphate dehydrogenase; MSCs, mesenchymal stem cells; PBS, phosphate-buffered saline; TSG-6, TNF-α stimulated gene/protein 6.

ZO-1 and claudin-5, were decreased whereas MMP-9 was increased. MSC treatment restored the reduced expression of BBB integrity proteins such as claudin-5 and ZO-1 and attenuated BBB leakage. Considering that ONOO⁻ formation is closely related to BBB disruption, our results indicated that MSC blocked BBB leakage by suppressing ONOO⁻.

Several studies have elaborated the effect of MSCs on ICH. The potential mechanisms include increase of immature neurons and synaptogenesis [48], enhancement of survival and differentiation of neural cells [49], reduction of inflammatory infiltration, and promotion of angiogenesis [50,51]. However, recent studies indicate that the capacity of MSCs is related to some soluble factors such as interleukin (IL)-10 [52], indoleamine 2,3-dioxygenase [53,54], prostaglandin E2 [52,55], which is a so-called bystander mechanism of MSCs. More recently, TSG-6, one of the anti-inflammatory factors, has attracted increased attention. Although most MSCs which were infused

intravenously into the rats are rapidly trapped in the lung, the trapped cells are activated to express amount of TSG-6 [21]. TSG-6 can play a role by inhibiting components in the inflammatory network of proteases [56], suppressing neutrophil migration into the site of inflammation [57], and interacting through the CD44 receptor on resident macrophages to decrease nuclear translocation of the NF-κB complex [58]. Although published literatures do not exclude the possibility that the MSCs trapped in the lung secreted additional factors in addition to TSG-6, an increasing number of results have suggested that the beneficial effect of MSCs are related to the inhibitory effect of TSG-6 on NF-κB [20,24]. Previous studies have indicated that NF-κB is activated as early as 15 min after ICH, reaching a maximum between 1 and 3 days, and remaining elevated for several weeks [59]. NF-κB is normally sequestered in the cytoplasm and bound to regulatory protein IκBs. In response to a wide range of stimuli, IκB is phosphorylated by the enzyme IκB kinase and the result is the release of the NF-κB dimer, which is then free to translocate into the nucleus [60]. Our study showed that in this ICH model, MSC treatment prevented IκB-α degradation and attenuated phosphorylation of Ser536 in the cytoplasm. Likewise, NF-κB p65 levels in the nuclear fraction were also decreased.

The downstream gene products of NF-κB are closely related to NF-κB signal activity. Therefore, the inhibitory effect of MSCs on NF-κB signaling pathway, via TSG-6, may affect formation of the relevant downstream products. Since MSCs can produce some bioactive molecules in addition to TSG-6, we cannot exclude the possibility that other factors augmented the effect of the TSG-6. Among the downstream gene products of NF-κB, iNOS, which plays a significant role in ONOO⁻ formation, may be closely correlated with BBB disruption. In the brain, there is a close relation between iNOS and ONOO⁻ in brain ischemia [61-63], septic animals [64], and Alzheimer's disease [65]. Our results confirmed the original hypothesis that along with increased levels of TSG-6 and subsequent inhibition of NF-κB activity, the levels of iNOS and ONOO⁻ were clearly decreased.

Besides exacerbation of edema formation, disruption of BBB integrity by ONOO⁻ is a critical event in the initiation of the inflammatory cascade [39]. Our results indicate that MSCs reduce infiltration of microglia cells and neutrophils, increase the levels of anti-inflammatory cytokines, whereas decrease the levels of proinflammatory cytokines, suggesting that they could act also through attenuating the inflammatory response, thus decreasing BBB disruption.

Taken as a whole, we investigated the properties of MSCs in ONOO⁻ formation and BBB protection in a rat ICH model. By transplantation of bone marrow MSCs from the jugular vein, the MSCs were trapped in the

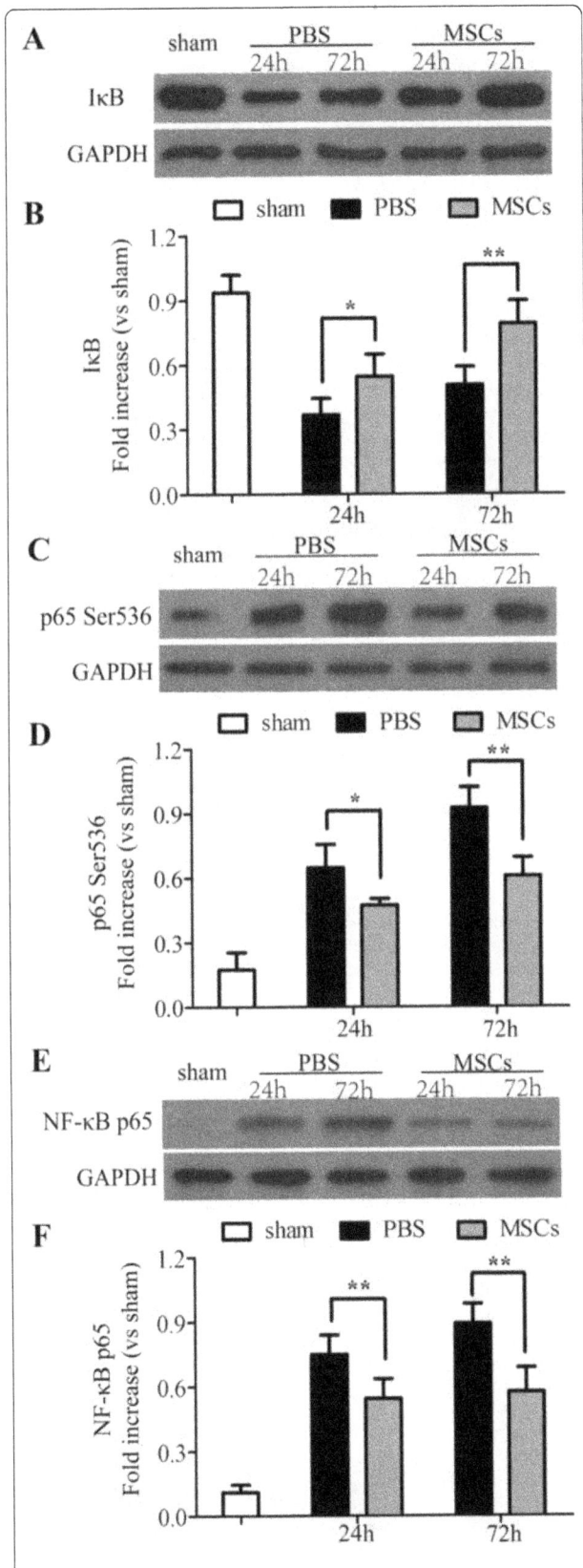

Figure 10 Effects of MSC on NF-κB signaling pathway.
Treatment with MSCs suppressed activation of the NF-κB signaling pathway 24 and 72 h after ICH. By Western blotting analysis, a basal level of IκB-α (**A, B**) was detected in the brain tissue from sham-operated rats, whereas in the PBS-treated rats, IκB-α levels were substantially reduced. MSC treatment prevented the degradation of IκB-α in the PBS-treated group. Phosphorylation of Ser536 (**C, D**) in the cytoplasm and phosphorylation of NF-κB p65 (**E, F**) levels in nuclear fractions were increased in the PBS-treated group when compared with the sham-operated group. MSC treatment significantly reduced the phosphorylation of p65 on Ser536 and NF-κB p65 levels. $n = 6$ in each time point per group. Data are presented as the mean ± SD. *$P < 0.05$; **$P < 0.01$. GAPDH, glyceraldehyde 3-phosphate dehydrogenase; MSCs, mesenchymal stem cells; NF-κB, nuclear factor-κB; PBS, phosphate-buffered saline.

lungs and produced a large amount of TSG-6, which acted by suppressing activation of the NF-κB signaling pathway. In ICH, ONOO⁻ is formed around the vessels that attenuate BBB integrity, destroy tight junction proteins, and suppress tissue inhibitor of metalloproteinases-1 (TIMP-1) to initiate a damage cascade. TIMP-1 is one of the naturally occurring inhibitors of MMPs and inhibits multiple MMP activation [66]. INOS, which is regulated by the NF-κB signaling pathway, is of major importance during ONOO⁻ formation. This study focused on the protective effect of MSCs on BBB disruption in a rat ICH model and indicated that the mechanism of MSCs in ICH rats was related to TSG-6, which improved BBB disruption by inhibiting the NF-κB signaling pathway. The levels of iNOS and ONOO⁻ decrease after the inhibitory effect of TSG-6 on the NF-κB signaling pathway. Although there may be also other factors involved in the decrease in iNOS and ONOO⁻, the inhibitory effect of TSG-6 on the NF-κB signaling pathway, at least in part, was a critical contributor to it in ICH rats.

Conclusions

In summary, our results indicated that MSCs block ONOO⁻-induced BBB disruption in ICH. This strategy may be useful for future therapies targeting prevention of BBB disruption in clinical ICH patients. However, further studies are required to investigate the mechanisms in more detail.

Abbreviations
3-NT: 3-nitrotyrosine; BBB: Blood–brain barrier; BMMSC: Bone marrow mesenchymal stem cell; ICH: Intracerebral hemorrhage; iNOS: Inducible nitric oxide synthase; MMP-9: Matrix metalloproteinase-9; mNSS: modified neurological severity score; MSC: mesenchymal stem cell; NF-κB: nuclear factor-κB; NO: nitric oxide; ONOO⁻: peroxynitrite; SD: Sprague–Dawley; TIMP-1: tissue inhibitor of metalloproteinases-1; TSG-6: TNF-α stimulated gene/protein 6; ZO-1: zonula occludens-1..

Competing interests
The authors declare that they have no competing interests.

Authors' contributions

MC and CZD conceived and designed the experiments. MC performed the experiments, analyzed the data, and wrote the paper. CZD revised the paper. XFL, XZ, XYH, LFL, YCL, GHZ, WL, HL, QRF, and ZQW provided the experimental technical support and assisted in completing the study at different stages. All authors read and approved the final manuscript.

Acknowledgements

This study was supported by the National Natural Science Foundation of China (Nos. 81271315)

Author details

[1]The National Key Clinic Specialty, The Neurosurgery Institute of Guangdong Province, Guangdong Provincial Key Laboratory on Brain Function Repair and Regeneration, Department of Neurosurgery, Zhujiang Hospital, Southern Medical University, Guangzhou 510282, China. [2]Department of Neurosurgery, The First People's Hospital of Foshan and Foshan Hospital of Sun Yat Sen University, Foshan, Guangdong 528000, China.

References

1. Butcher K, Laidlaw J. Current intracerebral haemorrhage management. J Clin Neurosci. 2003;10:158–67.
2. Xi G, Keep RF, Hoff JT. Erythrocytes and delayed brain edema formation following intracerebral hemorrhage in rats. J Neurosurg. 1998;89:991–6.
3. Yang GY, Betz AL, Chenevert TL, Brunberg JA, Hoff JT. Experimental intracerebral hemorrhage: relationship between brain edema, blood flow, and blood–brain barrier permeability in rats. J Neurosurg. 1994;81:93–102.
4. Abbott NJ, Patabendige AA, Dolman DE, Yusof SR, Begley DJ. Structure and function of the blood–brain barrier. Neurobiol Dis. 2010;37:13–25.
5. Kim KS. Mechanisms of microbial traversal of the blood–brain barrier. Nat Rev Microbiol. 2008;6:625–34.
6. Chu H, Ding H, Tang Y, Dong Q. Erythropoietin protects against hemorrhagic blood–brain barrier disruption through the effects of aquaporin-4. Lab Invest. 2014;94:1042–53.
7. Wang T, Chen X, Wang Z, Zhang M, Meng H, Gao Y, et al. Poloxamer-188 can attenuate blood–brain barrier damage to exert neuroprotective effect in mice intracerebral hemorrhage model. J Mol Neurosci. 2014;55:240–50.
8. Beckman JS, Beckman TW, Chen J, Marshall PA, Freeman BA. Apparent hydroxyl radical production by peroxynitrite: implications for endothelial injury from nitric oxide and superoxide. Proc Natl Acad Sci U S A. 1990;87:1620–4.
9. Ding R, Chen Y, Yang S, Deng X, Fu Z, Feng L, et al. Blood–brain barrier disruption induced by hemoglobin in vivo: involvement of up-regulation of nitric oxide synthase and peroxynitrite formation. Brain Res. 2014;1571:25–38.
10. Marcus JS, Karackattu SL, Fleegal MA, Sumners C. Cytokine-stimulated inducible nitric oxide synthase expression in astroglia: role of Erk mitogen-activated protein kinase and NF-kappaB. Glia. 2003;41:152–60.
11. Candolfi M, Jaita G, Zaldivar V, Zarate S, Pisera D, Seilicovich A. Tumor necrosis factor-alpha-induced nitric oxide restrains the apoptotic response of anterior pituitary cells. Neuroendocrinology. 2004;80:83–91.
12. Chang CC, Wang YH, Chern CM, Liou KT, Hou YC, Peng YT, et al. Prodigiosin inhibits gp91(phox) and iNOS expression to protect mice against the oxidative/nitrosative brain injury induced by hypoxia-ischemia. Toxicol Appl Pharmacol. 2011;257:137–47.
13. Qayyum I, Zubrow AB, Ashraf QM, Kubin J, Delivoria-Papadopoulos M, Mishra OP. Nitration as a mechanism of Na+, K+ –ATPase modification during hypoxia in the cerebral cortex of the guinea pig fetus. Neurochem Res. 2001;26:1163–9.
14. Cassina A, Radi R. Differential inhibitory action of nitric oxide and peroxynitrite on mitochondrial electron transport. Arch Biochem Biophys. 1996;328:309–16.
15. Wang W, Sawicki G, Schulz R. Peroxynitrite-induced myocardial injury is mediated through matrix metalloproteinase-2. Cardiovasc Res. 2002;53:165–74.
16. Suofu Y, Clark J, Broderick J, Wagner KR, Tomsick T, Sa Y, et al. Peroxynitrite decomposition catalyst prevents matrix metalloproteinase activation and neurovascular injury after prolonged cerebral ischemia in rats. J Neurochem. 2010;115:1266–76.
17. Li J, Zhang L, Xin J, Jiang L, Li J, Zhang T, et al. Immediate intraportal transplantation of human bone marrow mesenchymal stem cells prevents death from fulminant hepatic failure in pigs. Hepatology. 2012;56:1044–52.
18. Shi LL, Liu FP, Wang DW. Transplantation of human umbilical cord blood mesenchymal stem cells improves survival rates in a rat model of acute hepatic necrosis. Am J Med Sci. 2011;342:212–7.
19. Liu L, Yu Y, Hou Y, Chai J, Duan H, Chu W, et al. Human umbilical cord mesenchymal stem cells transplantation promotes cutaneous wound healing of severe burned rats. PLoS One. 2014;9:e88348.
20. Zhang R, Liu Y, Yan K, Chen L, Chen XR, Li P, et al. Anti-inflammatory and immunomodulatory mechanisms of mesenchymal stem cell transplantation in experimental traumatic brain injury. J Neuroinflammation. 2013;10:106.
21. Lee RH, Pulin AA, Seo MJ, Kota DJ, Ylostalo J, Larson BL, et al. Intravenous hMSCs improve myocardial infarction in mice because cells embolized in lung are activated to secrete the anti-inflammatory protein TSG-6. Cell Stem Cell. 2009;5:54–63.
22. Wu HJ, Yiu WH, Li RX, Wong DW, Leung JC, Chan LY, et al. Mesenchymal stem cells modulatealbumin-induced renal tubular inflammation and fibrosis. PLoS One. 2014;9:e90883.
23. Oh JY, Roddy GW, Choi H, Lee RH, Ylostalo JH, Rosa RJ, et al. Anti-inflammatory protein TSG-6 reduces inflammatory damage to the cornea following chemical and mechanical injury. Proc Natl Acad Sci U S A. 2010;107:16875–80.
24. Liu Y, Zhang R, Yan K, Chen F, Huang W, Lv B, et al. Mesenchymal stem cells inhibit lipopolysaccharide-induced inflammatory responses of BV2 microglial cells through TSG-6. J Neuroinflammation. 2014;11:135.
25. Jung Y, Kim SH, Kim YH, Kim SH. The effects of dynamic and three-dimensional environments on chondrogenic differentiation of bone marrow stromal cells. Biomed Mater. 2009;4:55009.
26. Rosenberg GA, Mun-Bryce S, Wesley M, Kornfeld M. Collagenase-induced intracerebral hemorrhage in rats. Stroke. 1990;21:801–7.
27. Garbuzova-Davis S, Willing AE, Zigova T, Saporta S, Justen EB, Lane JC, et al. Intravenous administration of human umbilical cord blood cells in a mouse model of amyotrophic lateral sclerosis: distribution, migration, and differentiation. J Hematother Stem Cell Res. 2003;12:255–70.
28. Ke K, Rui Y, Li L, Zheng H, Xu W, Tan X, et al. Upregulation of EHD2 after intracerebral hemorrhage in adult rats. J Mol Neurosci. 2014;54:171–80.
29. Chen J, Li Y, Wang L, Zhang Z, Lu D, Lu M, et al. Therapeutic benefit of intravenous administration of bone marrow stromal cells after cerebral ischemia in rats. Stroke. 2001;32:1005–11.
30. Song EC, Chu K, Jeong SW, Jung KH, Kim SH, Kim M, et al. Hyperglycemia exacerbates brain edema and perihematomal cell death after intracerebral hemorrhage. Stroke. 2003;34:2215–20.
31. Khan M, Sakakima H, Dhammu TS, Shunmugavel A, Im YB, Gilg AG, et al. S-nitrosoglutathione reduces oxidative injury and promotes mechanisms of neurorepair following traumatic brain injury in rats. J Neuroinflammation. 2011;8:78.
32. Yang S, Chen Y, Deng X, Jiang W, Li B, Fu Z, et al. Hemoglobin-induced nitric oxide synthase overexpression and nitric oxide production contribute to blood–brain barrier disruption in the rat. J Mol Neurosci. 2013;51:352–63.
33. Bethea JR, Castro M, Keane RW, Lee TT, Dietrich WD, Yezierski RP. Traumatic spinal cord injury induces nuclear factor-kappaB activation. J Neurosci. 1998;18:3251–60.
34. Genovese T, Mazzon E, Esposito E, Muia C, Di Paola R, Bramanti P, et al. Beneficial effects of FeTSPP, a peroxynitrite decomposition catalyst, in a mouse model of spinal cord injury. Free Radic Biol Med. 2007;43:763–80.
35. Shlosberg D, Benifla M, Kaufer D, Friedman A. Blood–brain barrier breakdown as a therapeutic target in traumatic brain injury. Nat Rev Neurol. 2010;6:393–403.
36. Muijsers RB, Folkerts G, Henricks PA, Sadeghi-Hashjin G, Nijkamp FP. Peroxynitrite: a two-faced metabolite of nitric oxide. Life Sci. 1997;60:1833–45.
37. Pacher P, Beckman JS, Liaudet L. Nitric oxide and peroxynitrite in health and disease. Physiol Rev. 2007;87:315–424.
38. Arima H, Wang JG, Huang Y, Heeley E, Skulina C, Parsons MW, et al. Significance of perihematomal edema in acute intracerebral hemorrhage: the INTERACT trial. Neurology. 2009;73:1963–8.
39. Chen HY, Chen TY, Lee MY, Chen ST, Hsu YS, Kuo YL, et al. Melatonin decreases neurovascular oxidative/nitrosative damage and protects against early increases in the blood–brain barrier permeability after transient focal cerebral ischemia in mice. J Pineal Res. 2006;41:175–82.

40. Parathath SR, Parathath S, Tsirka SE. Nitric oxide mediates neurodegeneration and breakdown of the blood–brain barrier in tPA-dependent excitotoxic injury in mice. J Cell Sci. 2006;119:339–49.

41. Phares TW, Fabis MJ, Brimer CM, Kean RB, Hooper DC. A peroxynitrite-dependent pathway is responsible for blood–brain barrier permeability changes during a central nervous system inflammatory response: TNF-alpha is neither necessary nor sufficient. J Immunol. 2007;178:7334–43.

42. Nitta T, Hata M, Gotoh S, Seo Y, Sasaki H, Hashimoto N, et al. Size-selective loosening of the blood–brain barrier in claudin-5-deficient mice. J Cell Biol. 2003;161:653–60.

43. Zhang GS, Tian Y, Huang JY, Tao RR, Liao MH, Lu YM, et al. The gamma-secretase blocker DAPT reduces the permeability of the blood–brain barrier by decreasing the ubiquitination and degradation of occludin during permanent brain ischemia. CNS Neurosci Ther. 2013;19:53–60.

44. Anderson JM, Fanning AS, Lapierre L, Van Itallie CM. Zonula occludens (ZO)-1 and ZO-2: membrane-associated guanylate kinase homologues (MAGuKs) of the tight junction. Biochem Soc Trans. 1995;23:470–5.

45. Gursoy-Ozdemir Y, Can A, Dalkara T. Reperfusion-induced oxidative/nitrative injury to neurovascular unit after focal cerebral ischemia. Stroke. 2004;35:1449–53.

46. Wang J, Tsirka SE. Neuroprotection by inhibition of matrix metalloproteinases in a mouse model of intracerebral haemorrhage. Brain. 2005;128:1622–33.

47. Wang J, Dore S. Inflammation after intracerebral hemorrhage. J Cereb Blood Flow Metab. 2007;27:894–908.

48. Seyfried D, Ding J, Han Y, Li Y, Chen J, Chopp M. Effects of intravenous administration of human bone marrow stromal cells after intracerebral hemorrhage in rats. J Neurosurg. 2006;104:313–8.

49. Wang SP, Wang ZH, Peng DY, Li SM, Wang H, Wang XH. Therapeutic effect of mesenchymal stem cells in rats with intracerebral hemorrhage: reduced apoptosis and enhanced neuroprotection. Mol Med Rep. 2012;6:848–54.

50. Bao XJ, Liu FY, Lu S, Han Q, Feng M, Wei JJ, et al. Transplantation of Flk-1+ human bone marrow-derived mesenchymal stem cells promotes behavioral recovery and anti-inflammatory and angiogenesis effects in an intracerebral hemorrhage rat model. Int J Mol Med. 2013;31:1087–96.

51. Liao W, Zhong J, Yu J, Xie J, Liu Y, Du L, et al. Therapeutic benefit of human umbilical cord derived mesenchymal stromal cells in intracerebral hemorrhage rat: implications of anti-inflammation and angiogenesis. Cell Physiol Biochem. 2009;24:307–16.

52. Nemeth K, Leelahavanichkul A, Yuen PS, Mayer B, Parmelee A, Doi K, et al. Bone marrow stromal cells attenuate sepsis via prostaglandin E(2)-dependent reprogramming of host macrophages to increase their interleukin-10 production. Nat Med. 2009;15:42–9.

53. Meisel R, Zibert A, Laryea M, Gobel U, Daubener W, Dilloo D. Human bone marrow stromal cells inhibit allogeneic T-cell responses by indoleamine 2,3-dioxygenase-mediated tryptophan degradation. Blood. 2004;103:4619–21.

54. Spaggiari GM, Capobianco A, Abdelrazik H, Becchetti F, Mingari MC, Moretta L. Mesenchymal stem cells inhibit natural killer-cell proliferation, cytotoxicity, and cytokine production: role of indoleamine 2,3-dioxygenase and prostaglandin E2. Blood. 2008;111:1327–33.

55. Aggarwal S, Pittenger MF. Human mesenchymal stem cells modulate allogeneic immune cell responses. Blood. 2005;105:1815–22.

56. Milner CM, Higman VA, Day AJ. TSG-6: a pluripotent inflammatory mediator? Biochem Soc Trans. 2006;34:446–50.

57. Getting SJ, Mahoney DJ, Cao T, Rugg MS, Fries E, Milner CM, et al. The link module from human TSG-6 inhibits neutrophil migration in a hyaluronan- and inter-alpha -inhibitor-independent manner. J Biol Chem. 2002;277:51068–76.

58. Choi H, Lee RH, Bazhanov N, Oh JY, Prockop DJ. Anti-inflammatory protein TSG-6 secreted by activated MSCs attenuates zymosan-induced mouse peritonitis by decreasing TLR2/NF-kappaB signaling in resident macrophages. Blood. 2011;118:330–8.

59. Zhao X, Zhang Y, Strong R, Zhang J, Grotta JC, Aronowski J. Distinct patterns of intracerebral hemorrhage-induced alterations in NF-kappaB subunit, iNOS, and COX-2 expression. J Neurochem. 2007;101:652–63.

60. Bowie A, O'Neill LA. Oxidative stress and nuclear factor-kappaB activation: a reassessment of the evidence in the light of recent discoveries. Biochem Pharmacol. 2000;59:13–23.

61. Bredt DS. Endogenous nitric oxide synthesis: biological functions and pathophysiology. Free Radic Res. 1999;31:577–96.

62. Ohtaki H, Funahashi H, Dohi K, Oguro T, Horai R, Asano M, et al. Suppression of oxidative neuronal damage after transient middle cerebral artery occlusion in mice lacking interleukin-1. Neurosci Res. 2003;45:313–24.

63. Walford GA, Moussignac RL, Scribner AW, Loscalzo J, Leopold JA. Hypoxia potentiates nitric oxide-mediated apoptosis in endothelial cells via peroxynitrite-induced activation of mitochondria-dependent and -independent pathways. J Biol Chem. 2004;279:4425–32.

64. Yokoo H, Chiba S, Tomita K, Takashina M, Sagara H, Yagisita S, et al. Neurodegenerative evidence in mice brains with cecal ligation and puncture-induced sepsis: preventive effect of the free radical scavenger edaravone. PLoS One. 2012;7:e51539.

65. Luth HJ, Munch G, Arendt T. Aberrant expression of NOS isoforms in Alzheimer's disease is structurally related to nitrotyrosine formation. Brain Res. 2002;953:135–43.

66. Murphy G, Willenbrock F, Crabbe T, O'Shea M, Ward R, Atkinson S, et al. Regulation of matrix metalloproteinase activity. Ann N Y Acad Sci. 1994;732:31–41.

Roles of programmed death protein 1/ programmed death-ligand 1 in secondary brain injury after intracerebral hemorrhage in rats: selective modulation of microglia polarization to anti-inflammatory phenotype

Jie Wu[†], Liang Sun[†], Haiying Li, Haitao Shen, Weiwei Zhai, Zhengquan Yu[*] and Gang Chen[*]

Abstract

Background: Microglia and its polarization play critical roles in intracerebral hemorrhage-induced secondary brain injury. Programmed death protein 1/programmed death-ligand 1 has been reported to regulate neuroimmune cell functions. Signal transducers and activators of transcription 1 participate in microglia polarization, and programmed death protein 1/programmed death-ligand 1 could regulate the activation of signal transducers and activators of transcription 1. We herein show the critical role of programmed death protein 1/programmed death-ligand 1 in the polarization of microglia during intracerebral hemorrhage-induced secondary brain injury in rat models.

Methods: An autologous blood intracerebral hemorrhage model was established in Sprague Dawley rats (weighing 250–300 g), and primary cultured microglia was exposed to oxyhemoglobin to mimic intracerebral hemorrhage in vitro. Specific siRNAs and pDNA for programmed death protein 1 and programmed death-ligand 1 were exploited both in vivo and in vitro.

Results: In the brain tissue around hematoma, the protein levels of programmed death protein 1 and programmed death-ligand 1 and the interaction between them, as well as the phosphorylation of signal transducers and activators of transcription 1, were higher than that of the sham group and collectively peaked at 24 h after intracerebral hemorrhage. Overexpression of programmed death protein 1 and programmed death-ligand 1 ameliorated intracerebral hemorrhage-induced secondary brain injury, including brain cell death, neuronal degeneration, and inflammation, while their knockdown induced an opposite effect. In addition, overexpression of programmed death protein 1 and programmed death-ligand 1 selectively promoted microglia polarization to anti-inflammation phenotype after intracerebral hemorrhage and inhibited the phosphorylation of signal transducers and activators of transcription 1, suggesting that intracerebral hemorrhage-induced increases in programmed death protein 1 and programmed death-ligand 1 maybe a self-help.

Conclusions: Enhancing the expressions of programmed death protein 1 and programmed death-ligand 1 may induce a selective modulation of microglia polarization to anti-inflammation phenotype for intracerebral hemorrhage treatment.

Keywords: Intracerebral hemorrhage, Secondary brain injury, Programmed death protein 1, Programmed death-ligand 1, Microglia polarization

* Correspondence: 13280008348@163.com; nju_neurosurgery@163.com
Jie Wu and Liang Sun are co-first authors.
Gang Chen and Zhengquan Yu are co-corresponding authors.
[†]Equal contributors
Department of Neurosurgery & Brain and Nerve Research Laboratory, The First Affiliated Hospital of Soochow University, 188 Shizi Street, Suzhou, Jiangsu Province 215006, China

Background

Intracerebral hemorrhage (ICH) accounts for ~15% of stroke cases in developed countries and ~50% or more in developing countries, especially in regions of Asia with high incidence of hypertension [1–3]. And ICH severely reduces the quality of life of patients, with a 5-year survival rate of ~30% [4, 5]. Beside blood clot-induced primary injury in the early phase [6], a series of chemical and immune responses known as secondary brain injury (SBI) seriously affect the prognosis of patients and is likely to be subjected to intervention [7–9].

Recent reports have shown that microglia/macrophages are the main regulatory cells in the immune defense response of the central nervous system (CNS) that affect subsequent inflammatory processes [10, 11]. After brain injury, a large number of microglia and macrophages around the hematoma rapidly respond and release effector molecules [12, 13]. Numerous recent studies have shown that in response to brain injury, different phenotypes of microglia/macrophages are observed and play various roles based on signals released in the microenvironment [11, 13]. Two main phenotypes of microglia/macrophages are pro-inflammatory phenotype and anti-inflammatory phenotype. Pro-inflammatory phenotype promotes inflammation and kills microorganisms, while anti-inflammatory inhibits inflammation and is involved in tissue repair and reconstruction [13]. Microglia activation and polarization during experimental intracerebral hemorrhage has been reported [14, 15].

Programmed death-1 (PD-1; also known as CD279 or PDCD1), which is a transmembrane glycoprotein of the CD28/cytotoxic T lymphocytes associated antigen-4 (CTLA-4) immunoglobulin superfamily, was first discovered in 1992 [16]. Its ligands, programmed death-ligand 1 (PD-L1) (B7-H1) and PD-L2 (B7-CD), are type I transmembrane proteins of the B7 family. PD-1 inhibits phosphatidylinositol-3-kinase (PI3K) and protein kinase B (Akt) activities [17]. The PI3K-Akt signaling pathway is involved in mediating phosphorylation of signal transducers and activators of transcription 1 (STAT1) [18], which has been reported to promote pro-inflammatory phenotype polarization of microglia [19]. PD-L2, another ligand of PD-1, was reported to have a threefold higher affinity for PD-1 compared with PD-L1 [20]. However, studies of the PD-1/PD-L2 signaling pathway have been rarely reported. Numerous studies have shown that PD-1/PD-Ls play important roles in mediating CNS disorders such as ischemic stroke [21], multiple sclerosis [22], and Alzheimer's disease [23].

In conclusion, accumulating researches suggested a therapeutic potential of PD-1/PD-Ls in ICH-induced SBI via regulating microglia polarization. However, until now, no study has investigated the contribution of PD-1/PD-Ls to microglia polarization. Therefore, the aim of this study was to investigate the role of PD-1/PD-Ls and to assess the therapeutic potential of PD-1/PD-Ls in ICH-induced SBI.

Methods

Experimental animals

Adult male Sprague Dawley rats weighing 250–300 g were purchased from the Laboratory Animal Center, Medical College of Soochow University, Suzhou, Jiangsu, China. The animal experimental protocols were approved by the Animal Care and Use Committee of Soochow University and complied with the ARRIVE guidelines. All animals were housed in a quiet environment maintained at 18–22 °C with stable humidity, and animals had free access to food and water.

ICH modeling in rats

As described by Deinsberger et al., ICH modeling in rats was performed by injecting autologous arterial blood into the basal ganglia [24]. Rats were anesthetized by intraperitoneal injection of 10% chloral hydrate (36 mg/100 g bodyweight). After successful anesthesia, rats were placed in the prone position, and their heads were fixed with a stereotaxic frame (ZH-Lanxing B-type stereotaxic frame, Anhui Zhenghua Biological Equipment Co., Ltd. Anhui, China). The drill site of each animal was determined according to the stereotaxic atlas of the rat brain (arterial blood injection in this experiment was unified in the right basal ganglia) and was located 0.2 mm rostral to and 3.5 mm lateral to the anterior fontanelle (bregma). After stereotaxic positing, a cranial drill was used to drill a ~1-mm-diameter hole through the skull to the dura mater. A 100 μL microsyringe (Hamilton Company, Reno, NV) was fixed to a vertical position on the stereotaxic frame, and the needle head and dental drill were then aligned. The position of the stereotactic frame was fixed, and the microsyringe was removed. The hind limbs of the rat were then repositioned to face upward. The abdominal skin was disinfected, and a ventral midline laparotomy incision of ~2–3 mm in length was made. The caudal artery was carefully separated and exposed under a dissecting microscope. The region was rinsed with normal saline, and the caudal artery was punctured with a microsyringe needle to collect 100 μL of arterial blood without anticoagulant. After repositioning the animal in the stereotaxic frame, the microsyringe needle was slowly and vertically inserted through the dental drill until it reached a depth of ~5.5 mm. Next, 100 μL of autologous arterial blood was injected into the basal ganglia at a rate of 20 μL/min. After the injection, the needle was retained for 10 min to prevent bleeding. The microsyringe needle was slowly withdrawn, and sterilized bone wax was used to seal the hole in the skull. After confirming that there was no hemorrhage, the incision and head skin were sutured, and the tail incision was bandaged with pressure. Each animal received a subcutaneous injection of 5 ml normal saline for postoperative fluid replacement to prevent excessive loss of body fluid. Heart rate, blood pressure, and real-time body and rectal temperature were monitored for approximately 2 h, and temperature was maintained at 37.5 °C, until recovery from anesthesia. According to the four-level evaluation of neurological symptoms described by Bederson et al. [25], rats with neurological symptoms up to one to three level(s) were considered successfully established ICH models. Brain tissues were sampled 1 mm away from the hematoma to avoid potential red blood cell contamination for further study (Fig. 1a).

Intracerebroventricular injection of pDNA or siRNA

The drilling site of the intracerebroventricular region for each rat was determined as described in previous studies [26, 27]. The relevant dosage of pDNA or small interfering RNA (siRNA) for intracerebroventricular injection was in accordance with manufacturer instructions. The drilling site was located 0.2 mm caudal to and 1.6 mm lateral to the anterior fontanelle (bregma). The depth of the drilling site was 4.5 mm.

Microglia culture

Primary microglia-enriched cultures were prepared from the whole brains of 1-day-old pups as described previously [28]. Rats were fixed on a dissection platform and disinfected using 75% alcohol. The skin and skull were opened, and brain tissues were collected. Brain tissues were washed once in PBS and isolated from the brain stem. The meninges and blood vessels were removed, and the brain tissues were placed in serum-free DMEM/F12 culture medium. The tissues were cut into small pieces and transferred to centrifuge tubes. Next, 0.125% trypsin was added, and the brain tissue was digested in a water bath at 37 °C for 15 min. Trypsinization was terminated by adding a serum solution. After the tissue was precipitated, the supernatant was collected, and the remaining tissue was homogenized and trypsinized before filtering the tissue lysate. The filtered solution was centrifuged at 1500 rpm for 5 min. The supernatant was removed, and the cells were resuspended in complete culture medium before cell counting. The culture medium was changed every 2 days, and stratified cell layers were observed ~10 days later. Cells in the upper layer, which were mainly microglia, and a small number of oligodendrocytes, were semi-adherent and round with

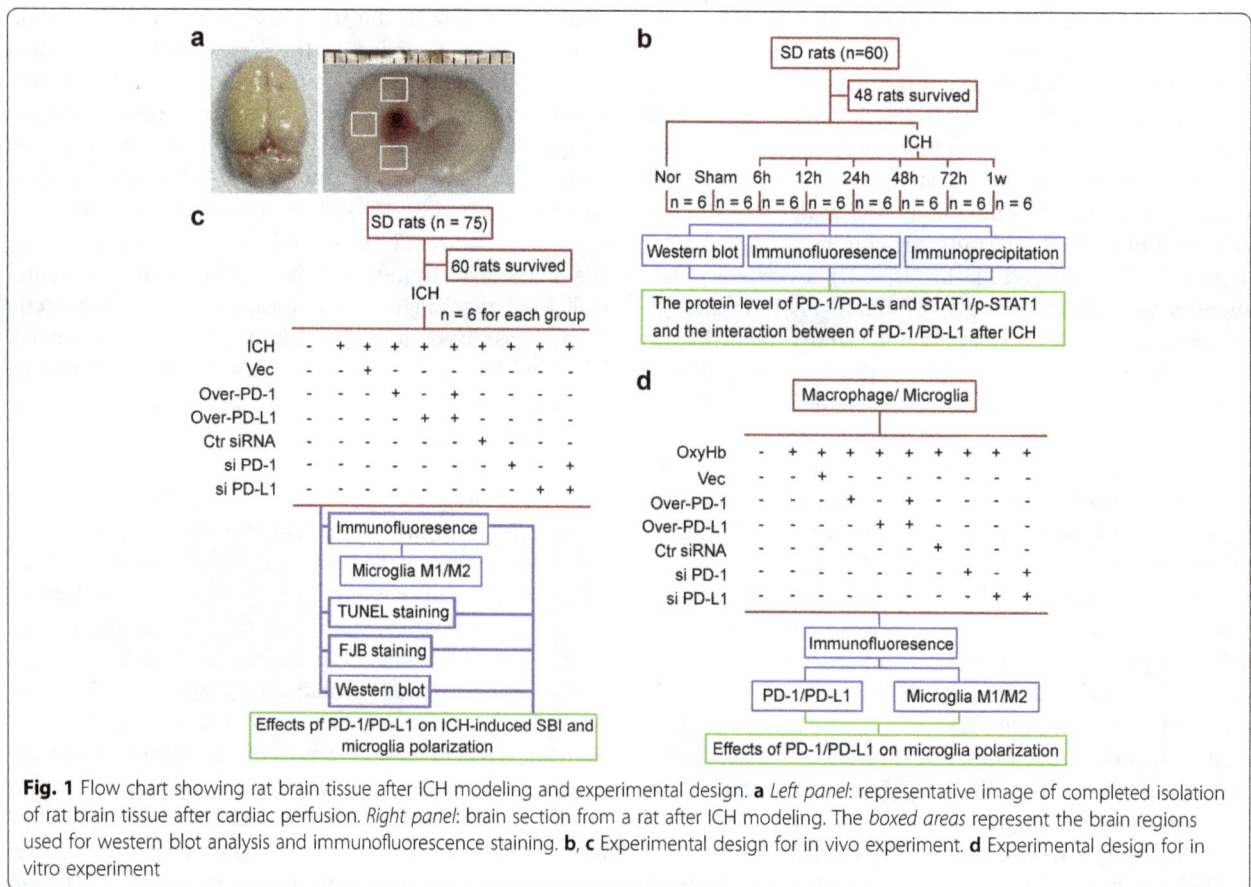

Fig. 1 Flow chart showing rat brain tissue after ICH modeling and experimental design. **a** *Left panel*: representative image of completed isolation of rat brain tissue after cardiac perfusion. *Right panel*: brain section from a rat after ICH modeling. The *boxed areas* represent the brain regions used for western blot analysis and immunofluorescence staining. **b**, **c** Experimental design for in vivo experiment. **d** Experimental design for in vitro experiment

good light transmission. Cells in the lower layer were mainly astrocytes and neurons. Subsequently, culture flasks covered with glial cells/neurons were placed on a shaker and mixed at 180 rpm for 15 min. The culture medium was then collected, non-adherent cells were washed once with PBS, and the cells were centrifuged at 1500 rpm for 5 min. After removing the supernatant, cell pellets were resuspended with complete culture medium and incubated with 5% CO_2 at 37 °C for 15–30 min. After changing the culture medium, the adhered cells in the culture flasks were purified microglia.

Experimental groups

To examine PD-1 and PD-Ls expression at different time points after ICH, rats were divided into three groups: normal control group ($n = 6$), sham group ($n = 6$), and ICH group ($n = 36$) (Fig. 1b). Normal control group animals were not subjected to a procedure. Sham group animals underwent withdrawal of tail artery blood and sphenotresia via microsyringe needle puncture reaching basal ganglia but not blood vessels. ICH group animals were subjected to successful ICH modeling. The ICH group was randomly subdivided into six groups ($n = 6$ each) to collect brain samples at the indicated time points: post-ICH 6 h, post-ICH 12 h, post-ICH 24 h, post-ICH 48 h, post-ICH 72 h, and post-ICH 7 d. Rat brain tissues in the sham group were collected 48 h after sphenotresia.

To assess the effect of PD-1/PD-L1 on brain injury, rats were grouped as follows 24 h after ICH modeling (Fig. 1c). Seventy-five rats were randomly divided into ten groups: sham group ($n = 6$); ICH group ($n = 6$); vector group ($n = 6/7$, number of successful ICH models/total number of ICH models, same below); ICH + PD-1 overexpression group ($n = 6/7$); ICH + PD-L1 overexpression group ($n = 6/9$), ICH + PD-1 overexpression + PD-L1 overexpression group ($n = 6/7$); ICH + control siRNA group ($n = 6/7$); ICH + PD-1 siRNA group ($n = 6/8$); ICH + PD-L1 siRNA group ($n = 6/8$); and ICH + PD-1 siRNA + PD-L1 siRNA ($n = 6/10$). pDNA or siRNA was intracerebroventricularly injected into the rats 12 h before modeling. Animals were killed to collect brain tissue 24 h after ICH onsets. The serum was collected for enzyme-linked immunosorbent assay (ELISA). DNA and siRNA transfection efficiencies of each sample were verified using western blot analysis. Subsequently, effects of PD-1/PD-L1 on SBI and microglia polarization after ICH were determined using terminal dexynucleotidyl transferase(TdT)-mediated dUTP nick end labeling (TUNEL) staining, Fluoro-Jade B (FJB) staining, western blot analysis, and immunofluorescence staining.

To examine the effect of PD-1/PD-L1 on microglia polarization in vitro (Fig. 1d), cultured microglia were randomly divided into ten groups: control group, OxyHb group, OxyHb + vector group, OxyHb + PD-1 overexpression group, OxyHb + PD-L1 overexpression group, OxyHb + PD-1 overexpression + PD-L1 overexpression group, OxyHb + control siRNA group, OxyHb + PD-1 siRNA group, OxyHb + PD-L1 siRNA group, and OxyHb + PD-1 siRNA + PD-L1 siRNA group. pDNA or siRNA was transfected to the cultured microglia populations, and after 24 h, the cells were fixed with 4% formaldehyde. pDNA and siRNA transfection efficiencies of each sample were verified using western blot analysis, followed by microglia polarization analysis.

pDNA and siRNA for PD-1/PD-L1 and transfection

Specific pDNA and siRNA for PD-1 and PD-L1 were obtained from Guangzhou Ribo Biotechnology Co., Ltd. (Guangzhou, China). To improve the knockdown efficiency, the interference efficiency of three different siRNAs (shown below) was test, and the most efficient one (I for PD-1, III for PD-L1) was used in the following study.

PD-1 siRNA sequences:

(I) Sense: 5′ CCACCUUCACCUGCAGUUU dTdT 3′
Antisense: 3′ dTdT GGUGGAAGUGGACGUC AAA 5′
(II) Sense: 5′ CCGCUUCCAGAUCGUACAA dTdT 3′
Antisense: 3′ dTdT GGCGAAGGUCUAGCAU GUU 5′
(III)Sense: 5′ CCUUCUGCUCAACAGGUAU dTdT 3′
Antisense: 3′ dTdT GGAAGACGAGUUGUCC AUA 5′

PD-L1 siRNA sequences:

(I) Sense: 5′ GCAGAUUCCCAGUAGAACA dTdT 3′
Antisense: 3′ dTdT CGUCUAAGGGUCAUCU UGU 5′
(II) Sense: 5′ GCCGAAGUGAUCUGGACAA dTdT 3′
Antisense: 3′ dTdT CGGCUUCACUAGACCU GUU 5′
(III)Sense: 5′ GGUCAACGCAACAGCUAAU dTdT 3′
Antisense: 3′ dTdT CCAGUUGCGUUGUCGA UUA 5′

pDNA and siRNA sequences were dissolved in RNase-free water to a concentration of 500 pmol/10 μL and then diluted with the same volume of transfection reagent. For each rat, 4 g of nucleic acid was injected intracerebroventricularly.

TUNEL staining

Paraffin-embedded brain sections (4–6 μm thick) were incubated at 70 °C for 1 h, followed by dewaxing and rehydrating in xylene and graded ethanol (100, 95, 90, 80, and 70%) solutions. TUNEL fluorescence staining reagents (Roche) were used in accordance with the manufacturer's instructions. Anti-quenching mounting medium was used to seal tissue sections between glass slides and cover slips. Brain sections were observed under a fluorescence microscope, and ImageJ software was used to analyze TUNEL staining. Six microscopic fields in each tissue section and three sections per rat were examined and photographed in parallel for TUNEL-positive cell counting. Microscopy was performed by an experienced pathologist blind to the experimental condition. The number of TUNEL-positive cells was assessed in ≥ 300 cells.

FJB staining
After dewaxing the paraffin-embedded brain sections (described above), the samples were placed in the dark at room temperature and incubated with 0.06% $KMnO_4$ solution for 15 min. Sections were then washed three times with PBS (5 min/wash), incubated with FJB working solution (containing 0.1% acetic acid solvent) for 60 min., and washed three times with PBS (5 min/wash). Brain sections on glass slides were air-dried at room temperature in a dark room and sealed with anti-quenching mounting medium and cover slips. Fluorescence microscopy was used for observation and photography. Six microscopic fields in each tissue section and three sections per rat were examined and photographed in parallel for FJB-positive cell counting. Microscopy was performed by an experienced pathologist blind to the experimental condition. The number of FJB-positive cells was assessed in ≥ 300 cells.

Antibodies
Mouse anti-PD-1 antibody (MA5-15780), rabbit anti-PD-L1 antibody (PA5-20343), and rabbit anti-PD-L2 antibody (PA5-20344) were form Thermo Fisher (USA). p-STAT1 antibody (ab29045), STAT1 antibody (ab31369), rabbit anti-CD16 antibody (ab109223), anti-iNOS antibody (ab15323), anti-TNF alpha antibody (ab6671), anti-IL1 beta antibody (ab9722), anti-IL4 antibody (ab9811), and anti-IL10 antibody (ab9969) were from Abcam (Cambridge, MA, USA). Arginase 1 antibody (GTX109242) was form GeneTex (USA). Mouse anti-CD11b antibody (sc-516102), goat anti-CD206 antibody (sc-34577), mouse anti-β-actin (C4) antibody (sc-47778), normal mouse IgG (sc-2025), normal rabbit IgG (sc-2027), and normal goat IgG (sc-3887) were from Santa Cruz Biotechnology. Secondary antibodies for western blot analysis, including goat anti-rabbit IgG-HRP (sc-2004), goat anti-mouse IgG-HRP (sc-2005), and rabbit anti-goat IgG-HRP (sc-2922) were from Santa Cruz Biotechnology. Secondary antibodies for immunofluorescence microscopy, including Alexa Fluor-555 donkey anti-rabbit IgG antibody (A31572), Alexa Fluor-488 donkey anti-rabbit IgG antibody (A21206), Alexa Fluor-555 donkey anti-mouse IgG antibody (A31570), Alexa Fluor-488 donkey anti-goat IgG antibody (A11055), Alexa Fluor-488 goat anti-mouse IgG antibody (A-11001), Alexa Fluor-555 donkey anti-goat IgG antibody (A-21432), and Alexa Fluor-647 goat anti-rabbit IgG antibody (A32733) were from Invitrogen.

Immunohistochemical study
The brain samples were fixed in 4% paraformaldehyde, embedded in paraffin, cut into 4-μm sections, and examined by immunofluorescence staining. Then, the sections were stained with primary antibodies (all diluted 1:200; from Santa Cruz Biotechnology, Inc.) and appropriate secondary antibodies (1:500 dilution; Santa Cruz Biotechnology, Inc.) as described. Normal rabbit IgG was used as a negative control for immunofluorescence assay (data not shown). Finally, sections were observed by a fluorescence microscope (OLYMPUS BX50/BX-FLA/DP70; Olympus Co., Japan). For fluorescence intensity assay, the relative fluorescence intensity was analyzed by use of ImageJ program by subtracting background. For positive cell counting, six microscopic fields in each tissue section and three sections per rat were examined and photographed in parallel for positive cell counting. Microscopy was performed by an experienced pathologist blind to the experimental condition. The number of positive cells was assessed in ≥ 100 cells.

Western blot analysis
The brain tissue around hematoma was thoroughly ground on ice. RIPA lysis buffer (Beyotime Biotechnology) was used to lyse the brain tissue for 30 min. The lysate was then transferred to a centrifuge tube and centrifuged at 12,000 rpm for 5 min at 4 °C. The supernatant from each sample was collected and stored at −20 °C. Total protein extracted from each sample was quantified using a BSA protein concentration assay kit (Beyotime Biotechnology). Fifty micrograms of total protein from each sample was separated using SDS-PAGE. After transferring the protein gel to a PVDF membrane, corresponding proteins were probed with different antibodies and signals were detected using an ECL kit. ImageJ software was used to analyze optical density of bands.

ELISA
The concentrations of IL-1β and TNF-α in serum were determined by corresponding ELISA kits (R&D Systems Inc., USA). These assays were performed according to manufacturer's instructions, and these data were expressed relative to standard curves prepared for them.

Co-immunoprecipitation (Co-IP)

Protein A + G agarose for IP was washed twice with lysis buffer. Total protein (100 μg) from each sample was diluted in 500 μL lysis buffer. Approximately 1 μg of conventional IgG, which was identical to the IgG used for IP, was added with 25 μL fully resuspended protein A + G agarose and gently mixed on a rocker at 4 °C for 30 min. Samples were then centrifuged at $1000 \times g$ for 5 min at 4 °C, and the supernatant was collected for subsequent IP and removal of nonspecific antigens. Next, protein solution was added with 2 μg of the corresponding primary antibody, and the mixture was incubated on a rocker at 4 °C for 1 h. After thorough binding between antigen and primary antibody, 50 μL of fully resuspended protein A + G agarose was added, and the reaction was gently mixed on a rocker at 4 °C overnight. The mixture was then centrifuged at $1000 \times g$ for 5 min at 4 °C, and the supernatant was discarded. The beads were washed three times with lysis buffer, and 75 μL 4× SDS sample buffer was added. The sample was boiled at 100 °C for 5 min and then centrifuged at $1000 \times g$ for 5 min at 4 °C. The supernatant was collected and placed in a new Eppendorf tube. Each prepared sample was used directly in western blot analysis.

Data analysis

All data are expressed as mean ± SEM. One-way ANOVA for multiple comparisons and Student-Newman-Keuls post hoc test were performed for TUNEL and FJB staining, immunofluorescence staining, immunoprecipitation

analysis, and western blot. $p < 0.05$ was considered statistically significant.

Results

ICH-induced increase in the expressions of PD-1 and PD-L1 and the interaction between them in the brain tissue around hematoma in rats

Expression of PD-1 protein in brain tissues from ICH model rats significantly increased at 24 h after ICH onsets. Results of western blot analysis showed that PD-1 protein expression in post-ICH 24 h, post-ICH 48 h, and post-ICH 72 h subgroups of ICH rats were significantly higher than that in the sham group (Fig. 2a). In addition, PD-L1 protein expression in post-ICH 24 h and post-ICH 48 h subgroups of ICH rats also increased. This enhanced expression of PD-L1 protein decreased in the post-ICH 72 h subgroup, which had similar PD-L1 protein expression levels as the control group (Fig. 2a). No significant changes in PD-L2 protein expression were found in the different groups (Fig. 2a). In addition, ICH also increased the interaction between PD-1 and PD-L1 at post-ICH 12 h, post-ICH 24 h, and post-ICH 48 h (Fig. 1b, c). And the protein levels of PD-1 and PD-L1 and the interaction between them, as well as the phosphorylation of STAT1, collectively peaked at 24 h after ICH. Therefore, we selected the post-ICH 24 h subgroup to study the effect of PD-1/PD-L1 on ICH-induced SBI.

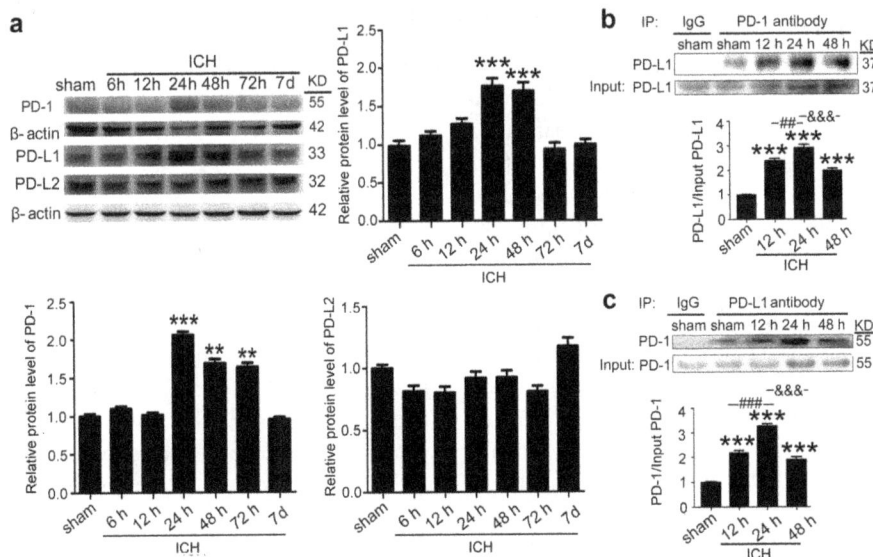

Fig. 2 ICH increased the protein levels of PD-1/PD-Ls and the interaction between PD-1 and PD-L1. **a** Time course of the protein levels of PD-1, PD-L1, and PD-L2 in the brain tissue around hematoma after ICH. Representative western blot bands of PD-1, PD-L1, and PD-L2 and quantitative analysis of the relative protein level were shown. The mean value of sham group was normalized to 1.0. Data are expressed as mean ± SEM, $n = 6$. *Double asterisks* indicate $p < 0.01$, *triple asterisks* indicate $p < 0.001$ vs. sham group. **b, c** Immunoprecipitation analysis of the interaction between PD-1 and PD-L1 at indicated times after ICH. All values are means ± SEM, $n = 6$. *triple asterisks* indicate $p < 0.001$ vs. sham group, *triple pound signs* indicate $p < 0.001$

Effects of overexpression and knockdown of PD-1 and PD-L1 on brain cell death and neuronal degeneration in ICH rats

The experimental group of Fig. 3 is shown in Fig. 3a. Western blot assay showed that the protein levels of PD-1 and PD-L1 were significantly increased by pDNA transfection and decreased by siRNA transfection (Fig. 3b, c). TUNEL assay and FJB staining were used to assess the effects of PD-1/PD-L1 on brain cell death and neuronal degeneration in the brain after ICH modeling (Fig. 3d–g). The numbers of TUNEL- and FJB-positive cells in rat brains 24 h after ICH modeling were significantly higher than those in the sham group. However, overexpression of both PD-1 and PD-L1 significantly inhibited ICH-induced brain cell death and neuronal degeneration, while knockdown of them exerted an opposite effect. In addition, inflammation-associated molecules, including IL-1β and TNF-α, were tested. As shown in Fig. 3h, i, IL-1β and TNF-α were found to be significantly higher in the serum of the ICH group than that in the sham group. Compared with ICH group, the mean inflammatory cytokine contents were lower in overexpression group and higher in knockdown group. The results also showed that there were no significant differences between the vector group and PD-1 plasmid group or PD-L1 plasmid group, while there were significant differences between the control siRNA group and PD-1 siRNA group or PD-L1 siRNA group, suggesting that PD-1 and PD-L1complement each other in modulation of brain cell death and neuronal degeneration in ICH rats.

Effects of PD-1 and PD-L1 on ICH-induced microglia polarization and STAT1 phosphorylation in rats

We next observed the effects of PD-1 and PD-L1 overexpression or knockdown on the microglia polarization in ICH rat brain (Fig. 4). The experimental group of Fig. 4 is shown in Fig. 4a. The results showed that ICH induced microglia polarization to a pro-inflammatory phenotype, as defined by CD16/CD11b-positive, and also to an anti-inflammatory phenotype, as defined by CD206/CD11b-positive (Fig. 4b–e). The results also showed that ICH mainly selectively modulated microglia polarizing to pro-inflammatory phenotype, which was ameliorated by overexpression of PD-1 and PD-L1 and aggravated by knockdown of PD-1 and PD-L1. To further elucidate the role of PD-1 and PD-L1 in microglia polarization, we co-stained brain sections of ICH + PD-1 overexpression + PD-L1 overexpression group for PD1, CD16 and CD11b or PD1, CD206, and CD11b (Fig. 4f). The results demonstrated that almost all of the CD206/CD11b-positive cells were co-labeled with high fluorescence intensity of PD1, while almost all of the CD16/CD11b-positive cells showed almost undetectable fluorescence intensity of PD1.

In addition, we used western blot analysis to measure the phosphorylation level of STAT1. Our results indicated that the phosphorylation level of p-STAT1 after ICH modeling was significantly higher than that in the sham group and peaked at 24 h after ICH onsets (Fig. 4g). And the phosphorylation level of STAT1 was decreased by overexpression of PD-1 and PD-L1 and further increased by knockdown of PD-1 and PD-L1 (Fig. 4h).

Critical role of PD-1 and PD-L1 in microglia polarization in cultured microglia under OxyHb treatment

We next observed the effects of PD-1 and PD-L1 overexpression or knockdown on microglia polarization in cultured microglia under OxyHb treatment (Fig. 5). The experimental group of Fig. 5 is shown in Fig. 5a. Firstly, the expression plasmid-mediated overexpression of PD1 and PD-L1 as well as the efficiency of siRNA-mediated knockdown in cultured microglia is verified by immunofluorescence staining (Fig. 5b). In addition, double-immunofluorescence analysis showed that OxyHb treatment induced microglia polarization both to a pro-inflammatory phenotype and an anti-inflammatory phenotype (Fig. 5c–f). The results also showed that OxyHb treatment mainly selectively modulated microglia polarizing to pro-inflammatory phenotype, which was ameliorated by overexpression of PD-1 and PD-L1 and aggravated by knockdown of PD-1 and PD-L1. To further elucidate the role of PD-1 and PD-L1 in microglia polarization, we co-stained brain sections of OxyHb + PD-1 overexpression + PD-L1 overexpression group for PD1, CD16 and CD11b or PD1, CD206, and CD11b (Fig. 5g). The results demonstrated that almost all of the CD206/CD11b-positive cells were co-labeled with high fluorescence intensity of PD1, while almost all of the CD16/CD11b-positive cells showed almost undetectable fluorescence intensity of PD1.

In addition, as previously reported [29], the use of single phenotypic markers (CD206 and CD16) is not sufficient to identify microglia polarization. Inflammation-associated molecules, including TNF-α, IL-1β, iNOS, arginase1, IL-4, and IL-10, were tested to provide more information on the biological state of microglia after ICH and the roles of PD-1 and PD-L2 in the process (Fig. 6). The results showed that the mean protein levels of pro-inflammation molecules, including TNF-α, IL-1β, and iNOS, in cultured microglia were significantly increased by OxyHb treatment. However, among the anti-inflammation molecules, including arginase1, IL-4 and IL-10, only the protein level of arginase1 was increased after OxyHb treatment. These results suggested that OxyHb induced microglia polarization to a pro-inflammation phenotype. In addition, a significant decrease in the mean protein levels of TNF-α, IL-1β, and iNOS and a significant increase in the mean protein levels

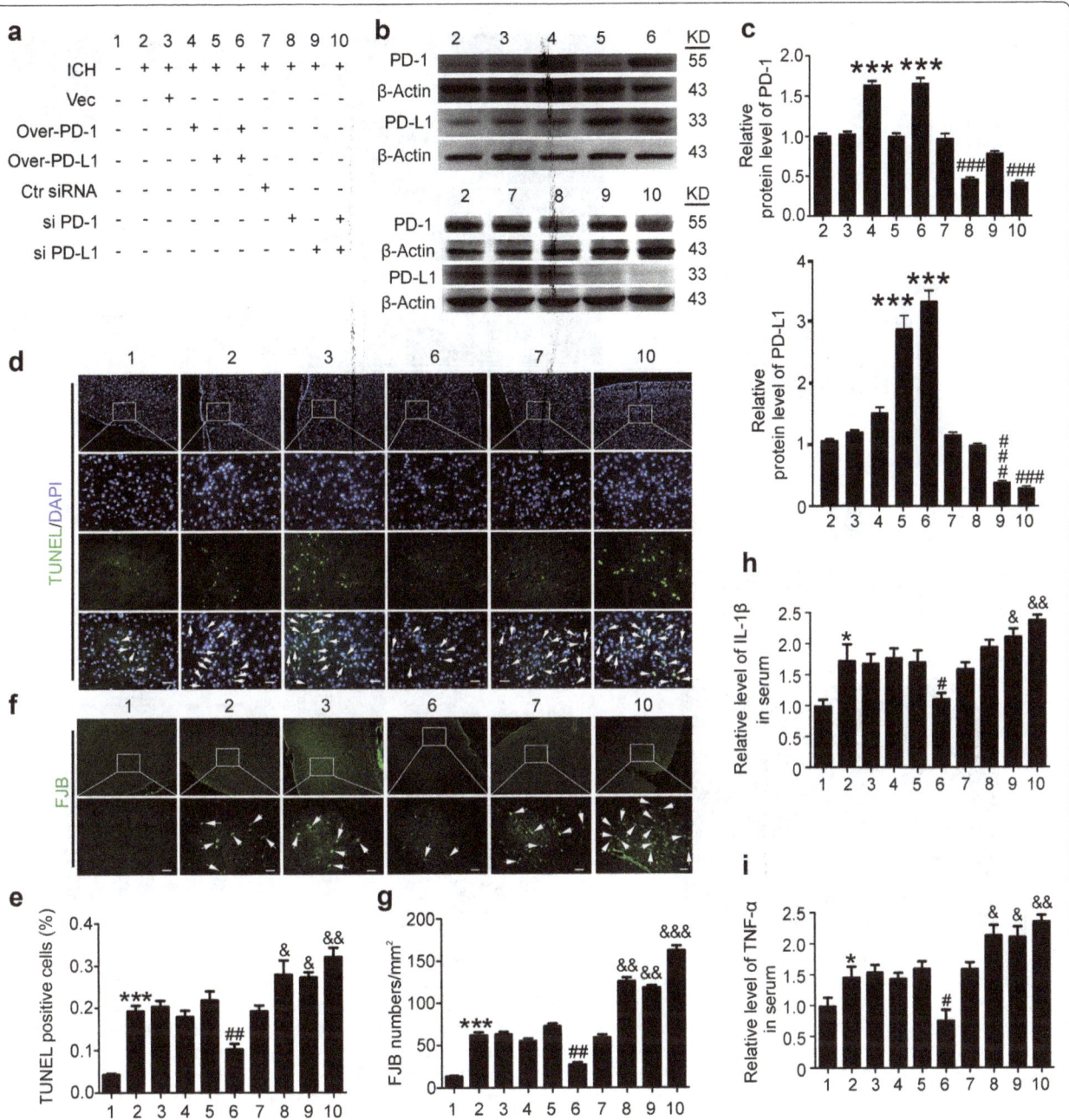

Fig. 3 Effects of PD-1/PD-L1 overexpression and knockdown on brain cell death and neuronal degeneration after ICH. **a** ICH rats accepted intra-cerebroventricular injection of pDNA or siRNAs as indicated. **b** Western blot analysis of the efficiency of PD-1 and PD-L1 overexpression or knockdown in brain of ICH rats. Quantification of relative protein levels of PD-1 and PD-L1 was shown in **c**. **c** Data are expressed as mean ± SEM, $n = 6$. *Triple asterisks* indicate $p < 0.001$ vs. ICH + vector group; *triple pound signs* indicate $p < 0.001$ vs. ICH + control siRNA group. **d** Terminal deoxynu-cleotidyl transferase dUTP nick end labeling (TUNEL) staining. Sections were labeled by TUNEL (*green*) to detect apoptotic brain cells and coun-terstained with DAPI (*blue*) to detect nuclei. *Arrows* point to TUNEL-positive cells. *Scale bar* = 64 μm. **e** Percentage of TUNEL-positive cells. Data are expressed as mean ± SEM, $n = 6$. *Triple asterisks* indicate $p < 0.001$ vs. sham group; *double pound signs* indicate $p < 0.01$ vs. ICH + vector group; *amper-sand* indicates $p < 0.05$, *double ampersands* indicate $p < 0.01$ vs. ICH + control siRNA group. **f** Fluoro-jade B (FJB) staining. *Arrows* point to FJB-positive cells. *Scale bar* = 64 μm. The number of FJB-positive brain cells was calculated. **g** Data are expressed as mean ± SEM, $n = 6$. *Triple asterisks* indicate $p < 0.001$ vs. sham group; *double pound signs* indicate $p < 0.01$ vs. ICH + vector group; *double ampersands* indicate $p < 0.01$, *triple ampersands* indicate $p < 0.001$ vs. ICH + control siRNA group. **h, i** ELISA assay of the contents of IL-1β and TNF-α in the serum. The mean values of the sham group were normalized to 1.0. Data are expressed as mean ± SEM, $n = 6$. *Single asterisk* indicates $p < 0.05$ vs. sham group; *Single pound sign* indicates $p < 0.05$ vs. ICH + vector group; *Single ampersand* indicates $p < 0.05$, *double ampersands* indicate $p < 0.01$ vs. ICH + control siRNA group

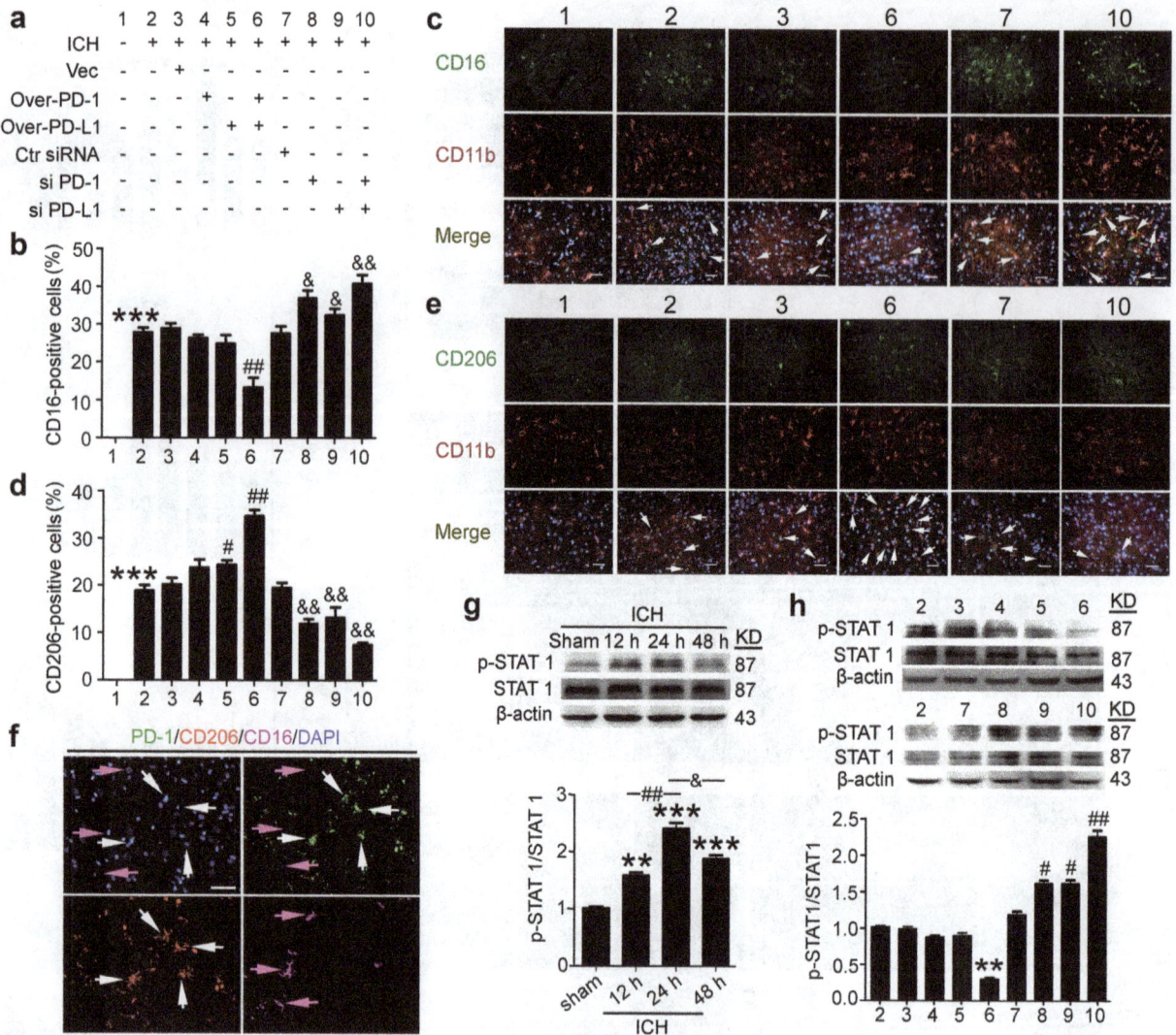

Fig. 4 Effects of PD-1/PD-L1 overexpression and knockdown on ICH-induced microglia polarization and STAT1 phosphorylation. **a** ICH rats accepted intracerebroventricular injection of pDNA or siRNAs as indicated. Sections were stained for CD16/CD11b (pro-inflammatory microglia marker) or CD206/CD11b (anti-inflammatory microglia marker). Percentage of CD16-positive cells or CD206-positive cells was shown in **b** and **d** and representative images were shown in **c** and **e**. *Scale bar* = 64 μm. In **b** and **d**, data are expressed as mean ± SEM, n = 6. *Triple asterisks* indicate $p < 0.001$ vs. sham group; *single pound sign* indicates $p < 0.05$, *double pound signs* indicate $p < 0.01$ vs. ICH + vector group; *single ampersand* indicates $p < 0.05$, *double ampersands* indicate $p < 0.01$ vs. ICH + control siRNA group. **f** Sections of ICH + PD-1 overexpression + PD-L1 overexpression group were stained for PD1/CD16/CD206. *White arrows* point to CD206-positive cells with high fluorescence intensity of PD-1, and *purple arrows* point to CD16-positive cells with low fluorescence intensity of PD-1. *Scale bar* = 64 μm. **g** Western blot analysis and quantification of the phosphorylation level of STAT1. The mean values of the protein levels in the sham group were normalized to 1.0. Data are expressed as mean ± SEM, n = 6. *Double asterisks* indicate $p < 0.01$, *triple asterisks* indicate $p < 0.001$ vs. sham group; *double pound signs* indicate $p < 0.01$, *single ampersand* indicates $p < 0.05$. **h** Western blot analysis and quantification of the phosphorylation level of STAT1. The mean values of the protein levels in the ICH group were normalized to 1.0. Data are expressed as mean ± SEM, n = 6. *Double asterisks* indicate $p < 0.01$ vs. ICH + vector group; *single pound sign* indicates $p < 0.05$, *double pound signs* indicate $p < 0.01$ vs. ICH + control siRNA group

of arginase 1, IL-4, and IL-10 were observed in microglia with PD-1 and PD-L1 overexpression, while opposite trends were shown in microglia with PD-1 and PD-L1 knockdown, suggesting that PD-1 and PD-L1 selectively inhibited OxyHb-induced pro-inflammation polarization of microglia.

In addition, the mean protein levels of pro-inflammatory markers, including TNF-α, IL-1β, and iNOS, in cultured microglia were significantly increased by OxyHb treatment (Fig. 6). However, among the anti-inflammatory markers, including arginase 1, IL-4, and IL-10, only the protein level of arginase1 was increased

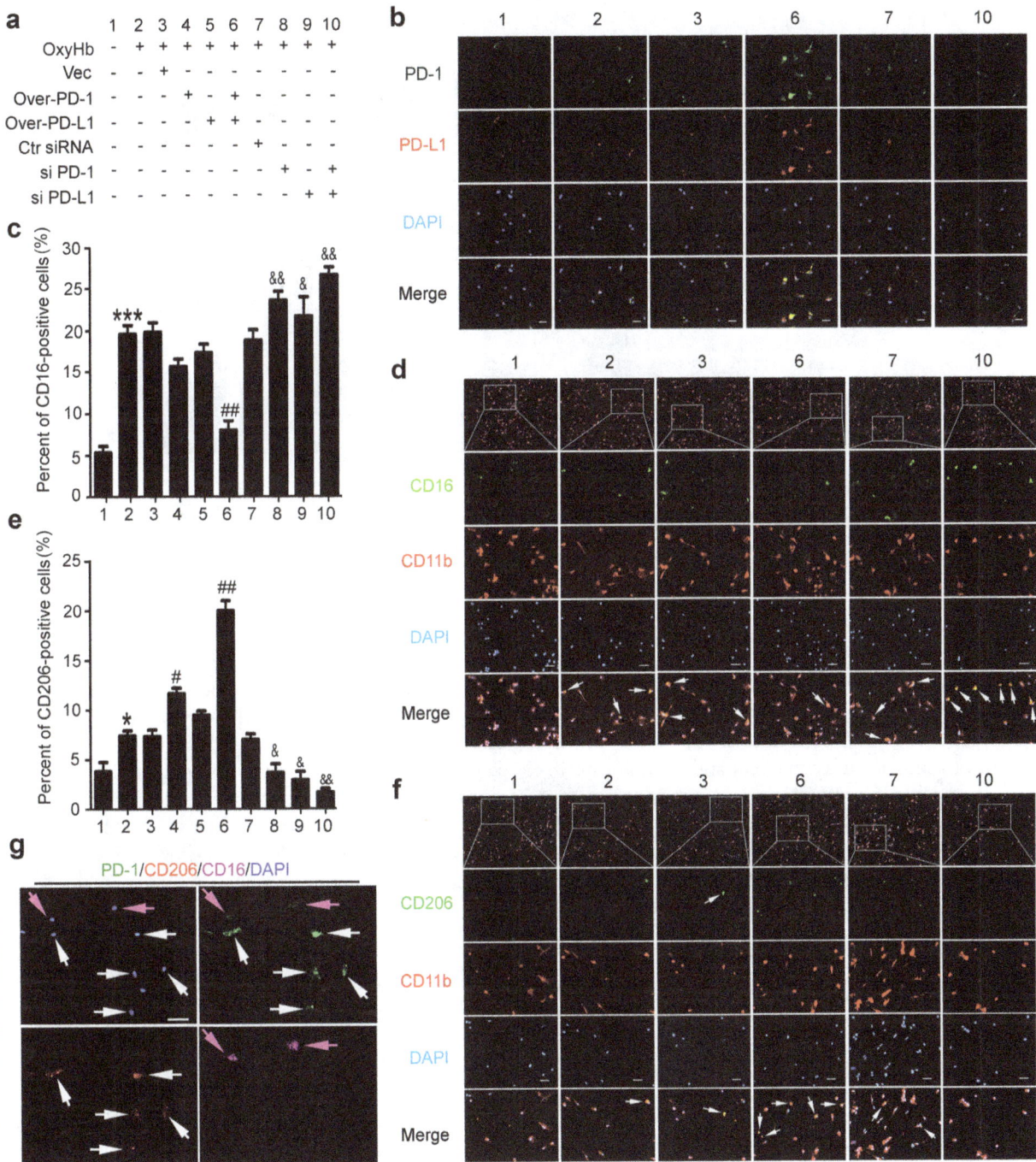

Fig. 5 Effects of PD-1/PD-L1 overexpression and knockdown on the polarization of OxyHb-treated microglia. **a** Cultured microglia accepted transfection of pDNA or siRNAs as indicated. **b** The efficiency of pDNA and siRNA in cultured microglia was verified by immunofluorescence staining. *Scale bar* = 64 μm. Cultured microglia was stained for CD16/CD11b (pro-inflammatory microglia marker) or CD206/CD11b (anti-inflammatory microglia marker). Percentage of CD16-positive cells or CD206-positive cells was shown in **c** and **e** and representative images were shown in **d** and **f**. *Scale bar* = 64 μm. In **c** and **e**, data are expressed as mean ± SEM, n = 6. *Single asterisk* indicates $p < 0.05$, *triple asterisks* indicate $p < 0.001$ vs. sham group; *single pound sign* indicates $p < 0.05$, *double pound signs* indicate $p < 0.01$ vs. ICH + vector group; *single ampersand* indicates $p < 0.05$, *double ampersands* indicate $p < 0.01$ vs. ICH + control siRNA group. **g** Microglia of ICH + PD-1 overexpression + PD-L1 overexpression group was stained for PD1/CD16/CD206. *White arrows* point to CD206-positive cells with high fluorescence intensity of PD-1, and *purple arrows* point to CD16-positive cells with low fluorescence intensity of PD-1. *Scale bar* = 64 μm

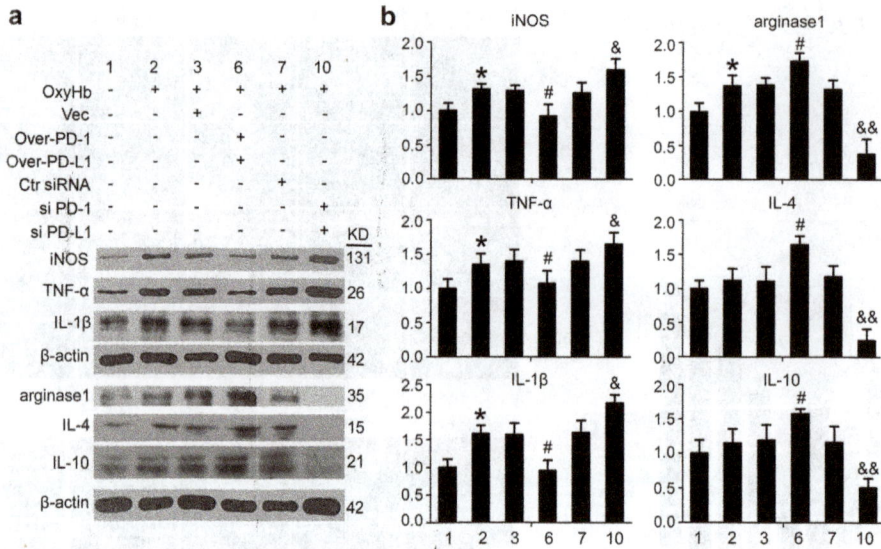

Fig. 6 Changes in the expression of pro-inflammatory- and anti-inflammatory-like polarization markers in microglia under indicated treatment. **a** The immunoblots show TNF-α, IL-1β, iNOS, arginase1, IL-4, and IL-10 produced by microglia under indicated treatment. **b** The quantitative analyses of TNF-α, IL-1β, iNOS, arginase1, IL-4, and IL-10 in the immunoblots in **a**. Date = mean ± SEM, $n = 6$. *Single asterisk* indicates $p < 0.05$ vs. control group; *single pound sign* indicates $p < 0.05$ vs. ICH + vector group; *single ampersand* indicates $p < 0.05$, *double ampersands* indicate $p < 0.01$ vs. ICH + control siRNA group

after OxyHb treatment. These results suggested that OxyHb induced microglia activation and mainly promoted microglia polarization to pro-inflammatory phenotype. A significant decrease in the mean protein levels of pro-inflammatory markers and a significant increase in the mean protein levels of anti-inflammatory markers were observed in microglia with PD-1 and PD-L1 overexpression, while opposite trends were shown in microglia with PD-1 and PD-L1 knockdown, suggesting that PD-1 and PD-L1 selectively inhibited OxyHb-induced pro-inflammatory polarization of microglia.

Discussion

In this study, we established a rat model of ICH to determine whether PD-1/PD-Ls play a role in SBI and to elucidate the potential mechanisms. Our findings showed that PD-1/PD-L1 protein expression in brain tissue significantly increased after ICH. In addition, the proportion of STAT1 phosphorylation increased after ICH. These changes were more significant ~24 h after ICH. Overexpression of PD1 and PD-L1 inhibited STAT1 phosphorylation, which was an important factor for transforming microglia to the pro-inflammatory subtype. Thus, these results suggested that enhancing the expressions of PD-1 and PD-L1 may induce a selective modulation of microglia polarization to anti-inflammatory phenotype via STAT1 for ICH treatment (Fig. 7). This finding has not been reported in previous studies.

In a study of autoimmune encephalomyelitis, Carter et al. [30] showed that PD-1/PD-L1 but not PD-L2 are

involved in T cell activation. In this study, we demonstrated that PD-1 and PD-L1 but not PD-L2 protein expression significantly reduced early brain injury (Fig. 2). Thus, we suggest that the PD-1/PD-L1 signaling pathway plays an important role in regulating the inflammatory response in nervous tissue. In the ICH rat model, PD-1 and PD-L1 protein expression and their binding to each other were elevated 24 h after ICH modeling, further indicating

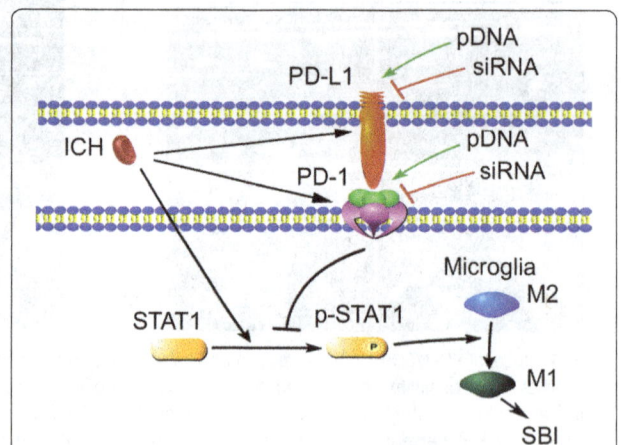

Fig. 7 Possible mechanism of PD-1/PD-L1 in secondary brain injury after ICH modeling. After ICH, PD-1/PD-L1 protein expression in the brain tissue significantly increased. In addition, the proportion of STAT1 phosphorylation increased. Moreover, upregulation of PD-1/PD-L1 expression by overexpression suppressed the phosphorylation of p-STAT1, pro-inflammatory polarization of microglia, and subsequent SBI under ICH condition, while PD-1/PD-L1 knockdown induced an opposite effect

that PD-1/PD-L1 are involved in ICH-induced SBI. The severity of brain injury was alleviated increased protein expression of both PD-1 and PD-L1. In contrast, reduced PD-1 and PD-L1 protein expression increased the severity of brain injury, indicating a causal relationship between PD-1/PD-L1 and brain injury (Fig. 3).

Microglia/macrophages effectively regulate restoration and regeneration of the CNS. However, these molecules can act as double-edged swords, resulting in both destruction and restoration [31]. Further studies have demonstrated that activation of microglia/macrophages can convert the cells into two opposite phenotypes: proinflammatory microglia that release destructive inflammatory cytokines and anti-inflammatory microglia that release cytokines for protection and restoration [25, 32]. In addition, multiple members of the STAT family (i.e., STAT1, STAT3, and STAT6) are involved in morphological typing of microglia/macrophages. For example, STAT1 promotes transformation of microglia into proinflammatory microglia [19, 33], and STAT6 stimulates transformation of microglia into anti-inflammatory microglia [34]. Moreover, STAT1 and STAT6 have a mutually inhibitory relationship [35]. In this study, the ratio of p-STAT1/STAT1 was significantly increased following ICH (Fig. 4g), while ICH did not affect the level of p-STAT6/STAT6 significantly (data not shown). Among the different ICH rat model groups, the proportion of phosphorylated STAT1 was maximal 24 h after ICH. PD-1 reduced phosphorylation of STAT1, which was consistent with the result of a previous study [36]. The possible mechanism may be due to PD-1 blocking the PI3K-Akt pathway, which inhibits promotion of phosphorylation of STAT1 [18]. In a mouse model of spinal cord injury, inhibition of PD-1 promotes transformation of microglia/macrophages into pro-inflammatory microglia [36]. These findings support our hypothesis that PD-1/PD-L1 is involved in inhibiting pro-inflammatory polarization of microglia under conditions of ICH [36].

There are several limitations of this study. In vitro experiment showed OxyHb maybe an incentive for the increase in the expressions of PD-1 and PD-L1. However, due to lacking studies of other contents of hematoma, this study cannot draw the mechanism underlying ICH-induced increase in the expressions of PD-1 and PD-L1. In addition, whether ICH-induced increase in the expressions lead to ICH-induced increase in the interaction between PD-1 and PD-L1 is also not answered in this study. It also reported that the PD-L1-mediated inflammatory response expanded the infarct size in experimental stroke model [37]. The possible mechanism may involve binding between PD-L1 and CTLA-4. CTLA-4 inhibits Akt phosphorylation through activation of protein phosphatase 2 (PP2A) [17, 38]. And a study has shown that PD-1 can inhibit PD-L1 protein expression

by promoting transcription of MicroRNA 513 [39] to negatively regulate PD-L1 and play a neuroprotective effect in nervous tissue. The effect of CTLA-4 and Micro-RNA 513 on microglia polarization in ICH condition deserves further study.

Conclusions

Microglia polarization is part of the basic machinery of brain injury. PD-1/PD-L1, a typical member of immunoglobulin superfamily, plays a critical role in neuroimmune cell functions. On the other hand, much attention has been also paid to the role of STATs in microglia polarization. In this study, using in vivo and in vitro models of relevance to ICH, we found a critical role of PD-1/PD-L1 through STAT1 in the polarization of microglia. These findings suggest PD-1/PD-L1 as promising pharmacological targets for the treatment of hemorrhagic brain injury.

Abbreviations
Akt: Protein kinase B; CNS: Central nervous system; Co-IP: Co-immunoprecipitation; CTLA-4: Cytotoxic T lymphocytes associated antigen-4; FJB: Fluoro-Jade B; ICH: Intracerebral hemorrhage; PD-1: Programmed death protein 1; PD-L1: Programmed death-ligand 1; PI3K: Phosphatidylinositol-3-kinase; SBI: Secondary brain injury; STAT1: Signal transducers and activators of transcription 1; TUNEL: Terminal dexynucleotidyl transferase(TdT)-mediated dUTP nick end labeling

Acknowledgements
None.

Funding
This work was supported by Suzhou Key Medical Center (Szzx201501), grants from the National Natural Science Foundation of China (No. 81571115, 81422013, and 81471196), Scientific Department of Jiangsu Province (No. BL2014045), Suzhou Government (No. LCZX201301, SZS201413, and SYS201332), and a project funded by the Priority Academic Program Development of Jiangsu Higher Education Institutions.

Authors' contributions
GC and ZY conceived and designed the study, including quality assurance and control. JW and LS performed the experiments and wrote the paper. HL designed the study's analytic strategy. HS helped conduct the literature review and prepare the "Methods" section of the text. WZ reviewed and edited the manuscript. All authors read and approved the manuscript.

Competing interests
The authors declare that they have no competing interests.

References
1. Krishnamurthi RV, et al. Global and regional burden of first-ever ischaemic and haemorrhagic stroke during 1990-2010: findings from the Global Burden of Disease Study 2010. Lancet Glob Health. 2013;1(5):e259–81.
2. Behrouz R. Re-exploring tumor necrosis factor alpha as a target for therapy in intracerebral hemorrhage. Transl Stroke Res. 2016;7(2):93–6.

3. Jiang, B., et al., Role of glibenclamide in brain injury after intracerebral hemorrhage. Transl Stroke Res, 2016

4. van Asch CJ, et al. Incidence, case fatality, and functional outcome of intracerebral haemorrhage over time, according to age, sex, and ethnic origin: a systematic review and meta-analysis. Lancet Neurol. 2010;9(2):167–76.

5. Poon MT, Fonville AF, Al-Shahi Salman R. Long-term prognosis after intracerebral haemorrhage: systematic review and meta-analysis. J Neurol Neurosurg Psychiatry. 2014;85(6):660–7.

6. Dang G, et al. Early erythrolysis in the hematoma after experimental intracerebral hemorrhage. Transl Stroke Res. 2016. Pubmed number 27783383. In press.

7. Xi G, Keep RF, Hoff JT. Mechanisms of brain injury after intracerebral haemorrhage. Lancet Neurol. 2006;5(1):53–63.

8. Xiong XY, Yang QW. Rethinking the roles of inflammation in the intracerebral hemorrhage. Transl Stroke Res. 2015;6(5):339–41.

9. Chen S, et al. An update on inflammation in the acute phase of intracerebral hemorrhage. Transl Stroke Res. 2015;6(1):4–8.

10. Venkatesan C, et al. Chronic upregulation of activated microglia immunoreactive for galectin-3/Mac-2 and nerve growth factor following diffuse axonal injury. J Neuroinflammation. 2010;7:32.

11. Loane DJ, Byrnes KR. Role of microglia in neurotrauma. Neurotherapeutics. 2010;7(4):366–77.

12. Amor S, et al. Inflammation in neurodegenerative diseases. Immunology. 2010;129(2):154–69.

13. Jin X, et al. Temporal changes in cell marker expression and cellular infiltration in a controlled cortical impact model in adult male C57BL/6 mice. PLoS One. 2012;7(7):e41892.

14. Wan S, et al. Microglia activation and polarization after intracerebral hemorrhage in mice: the role of protease-activated receptor-1. Transl Stroke Res. 2016;7(6):478–87.

15. Zhao H, et al. Microglia/macrophage polarization after experimental intracerebral hemorrhage. Transl Stroke Res. 2015;6(6):407–9.

16. Ishida Y, et al. Induced expression of PD-1, a novel member of the immunoglobulin gene superfamily, upon programmed cell death. EMBO J. 1992;11(11):3887–95.

17. Parry RV, et al. CTLA-4 and PD-1 receptors inhibit T-cell activation by distinct mechanisms. Mol Cell Biol. 2005;25(21):9543–53.

18. Nguyen H, et al. Roles of phosphatidylinositol 3-kinase in interferon-gamma-dependent phosphorylation of STAT1 on serine 727 and activation of gene expression. J Biol Chem. 2001;276(36):33361–8.

19. Qin H, et al. SOCS3 deficiency promotes M1 macrophage polarization and inflammation. J Immunol. 2012;189(7):3439–48.

20. Butte MJ, et al. Programmed death-1 ligand 1 interacts specifically with the B7-1 costimulatory molecule to inhibit T cell responses. Immunity. 2007;27(1):111–22.

21. Kroner A, et al. A PD-1 polymorphism is associated with disease progression in multiple sclerosis. Ann Neurol. 2005;58(1):50–7.

22. Ren X, et al. Programmed death-1 pathway limits central nervous system inflammation and neurologic deficits in murine experimental stroke. Stroke. 2011;42(9):2578–83.

23. Saresella M, et al. A potential role for the PD1/PD-L1 pathway in the neuroinflammation of Alzheimer's disease. Neurobiol Aging. 2012;33(3):624 e11–22.

24. Deinsberger W, et al. Experimental intracerebral hemorrhage: description of a double injection model in rats. Neurol Res. 1996;18(5):475–7.

25. David S, Kroner A. Repertoire of microglial and macrophage responses after spinal cord injury. Nat Rev Neurosci. 2011;12(7):388–99.

26. Gao C, et al. Role of red blood cell lysis and iron in hydrocephalus after intraventricular hemorrhage. J Cereb Blood Flow Metab. 2014;34(6):1070–5.

27. Gao F, et al. Hydrocephalus after intraventricular hemorrhage: the role of thrombin. J Cereb Blood Flow Metab. 2014;34(3):489–94.

28. Hu X, et al. Macrophage antigen complex-1 mediates reactive microgliosis and progressive dopaminergic neurodegeneration in the MPTP model of Parkinson's disease. J Immunol. 2008;181(10):7194–204.

29. Murray PJ, et al. Macrophage activation and polarization: nomenclature and experimental guidelines. Immunity. 2014;41(1):14–20.

30. Carter LL, et al. PD-1/PD-L1, but not PD-1/PD-L2, interactions regulate the severity of experimental autoimmune encephalomyelitis. J Neuroimmunol. 2007;182(1-2):124–34.

31. Hanisch UK, Kettenmann H. Microglia: active sensor and versatile effector cells in the normal and pathologic brain. Nat Neurosci. 2007;10(11):1387–94.

32. Mosser DM, Edwards JP. Exploring the full spectrum of macrophage activation. Nat Rev Immunol. 2008;8(12):958–69.

33. Sica A, Bronte V. Altered macrophage differentiation and immune dysfunction in tumor development. J Clin Invest. 2007;117(5):1155–66.

34. Sheldon KE, et al. Shaping the murine macrophage phenotype: IL-4 and cyclic AMP synergistically activate the arginase I promoter. J Immunol. 2013;191(5):2290–8.

35. Ohmori Y, Hamilton TA. Interleukin-4/STAT6 represses STAT1 and NF-kappa B-dependent transcription through distinct mechanisms. J Biol Chem. 2000;275(48):38095–103.

36. Yao A, et al. Programmed death 1 deficiency induces the polarization of macrophages/microglia to the M1 phenotype after spinal cord injury in mice. Neurotherapeutics. 2014;11(3):636–50.

37. Bodhankar S, et al. PD-L1 enhances CNS inflammation and infarct volume following experimental stroke in mice in opposition to PD-1. J Neuroinflammation. 2013;10:111.

38. Riley JL. PD-1 signaling in primary T cells. Immunol Rev. 2009;229(1):114–25.

39. Gong AY, et al. MicroRNA-513 regulates B7-H1 translation and is involved in IFN-gamma-induced B7-H1 expression in cholangiocytes. J Immunol. 2009;182(3):1325–33.

Dimethylarginines in patients with intracerebral hemorrhage: association with outcome, hematoma enlargement, and edema

Hans Worthmann[1*†], Na Li[1,2†], Jens Martens-Lobenhoffer[3], Meike Dirks[1], Ramona Schuppner[1], Ralf Lichtinghagen[4], Jan T. Kielstein[5,6], Peter Raab[7], Heinrich Lanfermann[7], Stefanie M. Bode-Böger[3†] and Karin Weissenborn[1†]

Abstract

Background: Asymmetric dimethylarginine (ADMA)––the most potent endogenous NO-synthase inhibitor, has been regarded as mediator of endothelial dysfunction and oxidative stress. Considering experimental data, levels of ADMA and its structural isomer symmetric dimethylarginine (SDMA) might be elevated after intracerebral hemorrhage (ICH) and associated with clinical outcome and secondary brain injury.

Methods: Blood samples from 20 patients with acute ICH were taken at $\leq$ 24 h and 3 and 7 days after the event. Nine patients had favorable (modified Rankin Scale (mRS) at 90 days 0–2) outcome, and 11 patients unfavorable outcome (mRS 3–6). Patients' serum ADMA, SDMA, and L-arginine levels were determined by high-performance liquid chromatography–tandem mass spectrometry. Levels were compared to those of 30 control subjects without ICH. For further analysis, patients were grouped according to outcome, hematoma and perihematomal edema volumes, occurrence of hematoma enlargement, and cytotoxic edema as measured by computed tomography and serial magnetic resonance imaging.

Results: Levels of ADMA––but not SDMA and L-arginine––were elevated in ICH patients compared to controls (binary logistic regression analysis: ADMA $\leq$ 24 h, $p = 0.003$; 3 days $p = 0.005$; 7 days $p = 0.004$). If patients were grouped according to outcome, dimethylarginines were increased in patients with unfavorable outcome. The binary logistic regression analysis confirmed an association of SDMA levels $\leq$ 24 h ($p = 0.048$) and at 3 days ($p = 0.028$) with unfavorable outcome. ADMA $\leq$ 24 h was increased in patients with hematoma enlargement ($p = 0.003$), while SDMA $\leq$ 24 h was increased in patients with large hematoma ($p = 0.029$) and perihematomal edema volume ($p = 0.023$).

Conclusions: Our data demonstrate an association between dimethylarginines and outcome of ICH. However, further studies are needed to confirm this relationship and elucidate the mechanisms behind.

Keywords: ADMA, SDMA, Intracerebral hemorrhage, Outcome, Hematoma enlargement, Edema

* Correspondence: worthmann.hans@mh-hannover.de
†Equal contributors
[1]Department of Neurology, Hannover Medical School, 30623 Hannover, Germany
Full list of author information is available at the end of the article

Background

Intracerebal hemorrhage (ICH) is a detrimental disease with high morbidity and mortality [1]. Deterioration by secondary hematoma enlargement and perihematomal edema occurs frequently during the first days leading to a high rate of poor outcome underlining the need for effective therapy. Knowledge about molecular mechanisms being involved in these important complications that could facilitate therapeutic approaches is still sparse.

After ICH, thrombin and hemin, a hemoglobin metabolite, enter the brain parenchyma. Experimental data from cell culture models of microglia and cortical astrocytes indicate that these components lead to overexpression of inducible nitric oxide synthase (iNOS) and increased production of superoxide [2, 3]. Importantly, in ICH patients, levels of NO or NO metabolites were correlated with outcome. Chiang et al. showed an association of increased NO levels in cerebrospinal fluid with poor outcome at 6 months [4]. In contrast to this, Rashid et al. detected lower serum levels of NO metabolites in patients with poor outcome at discharge [5]. NO levels are differently influenced by dimetyhlarginines asymmetric dimetyhlarginine (ADMA) and its structural isomer symmetric dimethylarginine (SDMA).

Mono and dimethylarginines L-NG-monomethylarginine (N-NMMA), ADMA, and SDMA are generated by proteolysis from proteins with methylated arginine residues as catalyzed by protein arginine methyltransferases (PRMTs) [6, 7]. The structure of ADMA resembles L-arginine, which acts as the substrate of NOS to synthesize NO. For this reason, ADMA represents the most potent endogenous NOS inhibitor as it competes with L-arginine for NOS binding [8]. In acute ischemic stroke, it has been regarded as mediator of oxidative stress by inhibition and uncoupling of NO-synthases (for a review see [9]). Its structural isomer symmetric dimethylarginine (SDMA) inhibits production of NO levels differently through impairment of intracellular L-arginine uptake since L-arginine acts as the substrate of NOS [10]. SDMA increases the production of reactive oxygen species (ROS) as shown in monocytes [11].

By these mechanisms, dimethylarginines and L-arginine may contribute to the NO metabolism and oxidative stress also after ICH and might be involved in clinical outcome and secondary complications such as hematoma enlargement or perihematomal edema.

So far, dimethylarginine levels have been measured in only one study of ICH patients ($n = 22$) and did not differ from levels in control subjects [12]. However, the study by Wanby and colleagues leaves several questions unanswered since neither the time point of blood sampling has been specified nor have any clinical or radiological outcomes been analyzed in the study. Dimethylarginine levels may vary during the first days after ICH--similar to patients with ischemic stroke [13]. We expected a delayed increase in ADMA levels in ICH patients comparable to the findings in subarachnoid hemorrhage (SAH) patients [14, 15].

We aimed to investigate the temporal pattern of ADMA, SDMA, and L-arginine after ICH in regard to clinical outcome. In addition, we intended to examine the association of dimethylarginines with hematoma and perihematomal volumes and occurrence of hematoma enlargement and cytotoxic edema.

Methods

Study population

Twenty patients with primary ICH who presented within 24 h of symptom onset and were treated either at the stroke unit or the intensive care unit in the Department of Neurology at Hannover Medical School were enrolled. The patient cohort derived from a cohort of a former study [16]. Intracerebral hemorrhage was diagnosed by computed tomography (CT) scan or magnetic resonance tomography (MRI). Exclusion criteria were surgical ICH procedures, contraindication to MRI or refusal of participation. Thirty healthy subjects adjusted for sex and age served as controls. Patients and controls were assessed for age, sex, arterial hypertension, diabetes mellitus, estimated glomerular filtration rate (evaluated by CKD-EPI equation), hyperlipidemia, status of smoking, and treatment with anticoagulants and antiplatelets. In addition, in patients, baseline stroke severity (according to National Institutes of Health Stroke Scale Score (NIHSS) on admission) and clinical outcome (modified Rankin Scale (mRS) at 90 days) were obtained (favorable outcome mRS 0–2, unfavorable outcome mRS 3–6). For the definition of outcome groups, moderately and severely disabled patients as used in other studies [17] were combined in the unfavorable outcome group since in our patient cohort, the most severely disabled patients could not be included due to surgical procedures and impossibility of performance of serial MRI investigation.

The study was approved by the ethics committee of Hannover Medical School. Patients or a relative gave written informed consent.

Blood collection and measurement of ADMA, SDMA, and L-arginine

Venous blood samples were taken at ≤ 24 h (median 12 h) and 3 and 7 days after the event. Serum was stored at − 80 °C until assayed. Serum ADMA, SDMA, and L-arginine were assessed blindly without knowledge of any of the clinical information using high-performance liquid chromatography–tandem mass spectrometry (HPLC–MS–MS) [18]. The lower limits of quantification for ADMA were 0.15 µmol/l, for SDMA were 0.20 µmol/l, and for L-arginine were 7.5 µmol/l. The inter-assay precision was 3.77%, and the intra-assay precision was 2.12% for

ADMA, 3.86, and 2.83% for SDMA and 4.01 and 0.82% for L-arginine.

Imaging protocol and analysis

On admission, CT was performed for clinical diagnosis. Magnetic resonance imaging (MRI) was conducted at $\leq$ 24 h ($n = 18$), 3 days ($n = 18$), and 7 days ($n = 16$) after the event, as feasible. For detection of hematoma and perihematomal edema volume by manual segmentation on 3D-fluid-attenuated-inversion recovery-data, ITK-SNAP analysis software was used. Cytotoxic edema was defined by area of elevated diffusion-weighted imaging (DWI)-b1000-signal and decreased apparent diffusion coefficient (ADC) value (by > 10% compared with mirror region of interest (ROI)) outside of hematoma on T2*- and DWIb0-sequences. The manually outlined area was confirmed by 3D-multiplanar localization using the image analysis software. Patients were grouped according to median hematoma volume considering the initial MRI. In two patients, no MRI was conducted at $\leq$ 24 h due to a severe clinical deficit on admission. In these patients, MRI at 3 days was used for categorization of hematoma volume. Hematoma enlargement was defined by increase of hematoma volume > 33% or 6.0 ml calculated from first imaging (CT or MRI) to follow-up MRIs. When hematoma volumes from CT and MRI were compared, MRI volumes were adapted as proposed by Burgess et al. (CT volume = 0.8* MRI volume) [19]. Patients without MRI at 3 or 7 days ($n = 2$) were excluded from this analysis. For analysis of patient groups according to perihematomal edema volume, the maximum values from MRI ($\leq$ 24 h and 3 or 7 days) were used. In addition, patients were grouped for occurrence of cytotoxic edema as detected by MRI ($\leq$ 24 h and 3 or 7 days).

Statistical analysis

Statistical analysis was performed with the IBM SPSS Statistics 23. The data are presented as numbers and portion for categorical variables and median with interquartile range for continuous variables. The data were tested for statistically significant differences between patients and controls by Mann-Whitney U test for continuous data and Pearson chi-square for categorical data. The binary logistic regression analysis included ADMA levels and adjusted for co-variables age and estimated glomerular filtration rate (eGFR) using the method of backward stepwise. Within group comparisons of ADMA, SDMA and L-arginine levels at different time points were analyzed by Wilcoxon test. For the outcome analysis, patients were grouped into those with favorable and unfavorable outcome. In addition, Spearman rank correlation was performed between molecular marker levels and mRS at 90 days. To analyze the association of ADMA, SDMA, and L-arginine with imaging outcomes, patients were grouped according to

hematoma and perihematomal edema volume and occurrence of hematoma enlargement and cytotoxic edema. For the analysis of clinical and imaging outcomes, the data were tested for statistically significant differences between patient groups by Mann-Whitney U test for continuous data and Pearson chi-square for categorical data. The binary logistic regression analysis tested ADMA and SDMA levels for association with clinical outcome including age and eGFR as co-variables (method of backward stepwise). A p value < 0.05 was considered to indicate statistical significance.

Results

The study population consisted of 20 patients with ICH with a median age of 77 years (interquartile range 72–84). Clinical and demographical characteristics in patients and controls are shown in Table 1. Patients and controls did not significantly differ in regard to these parameters.

Temporal pattern of dimethylarginines after acute ICH

In controls ADMA levels were 0.438 µmol/L (interquartile range 0.389–0.476), SDMA levels were 0.551 µmol/L (interquartile range 0.465–0.631), and L-arginine levels

Table 1 Clinical characteristics of patients and controls

	ICH ($n = 20$)	Controls ($n = 30$)	P
Female	11 (55.0)	17 (56.7)	0.907
Male	9 (45.0)	13 (43.3)	
Age (years)	77 (72; 84)	71 (63; 76)	0.106
Hypertension	15 (75.0)	24 (80.0)	0.676
Smoker	1 (5.0)	4 (13.3)	0.336
Hyperlipoproteinemia	6 (30.0)	15 (50.0)	0.160
Diabetes mellitus	1 (5.0)	4 (13.3)	0.336
History of CVD	0 (0.0)	3 (10.0)	0.145
History of CHD	1 (5.0)	5 (16.7)	0.214
History of antiplatelets	4 (20.0)	9 (30.0)	0.430
History of anticoagulants	1 (5.0)	0 (0.0)	0.216
eGFR (ml/min per 1.73 m^2)	86.9 (65.4; 98.2)	70.7 (61.7; 86.6)	0.104
NIHSS on admission	9 (6; 15)	n.a.	–
mRS 90 days	3 (2; 4)	n.a.	–
Deep location of ICH	15 (75.0)	n.a.	–
IVH extension	2 (10.0)	n.a.	–
Hematoma volume (ml)	10.3 (3.1; 24.4)	n.a.	–
Hematoma enlargement	5 (25.0)	n.a.	–
Perihematomal edema (ml)	23.0 (11.9; 61.5)	n.a.	–
Cytotoxic edema	9 (45.0)	n.a.	–

Data are presented as numbers (percentages) or median (interquartile range).
$P < 0.05$ was considered statistically significant
CHD coronary heart disease, CVD cerebrovascular disease, eGFR estimated glomerular filtration rate, IVH intraventricular hematoma, mRS modified Rankin Scale, NIHSS National Institutes of Health Stroke Scale

were 74.65 μmol/L (interquartile range 63.70–91.43). Levels of ADMA, SDMA, and L-arginine with interquartile range for ICH patients are shown in Fig. 1a–c. ADMA levels were significantly increased at any time point in ICH patients compared to controls (≤ 24 h, $p < 0.001$; 3 days $p = 0.001$; 7 days, $p > 0.001$), while SDMA and L-arginine levels were not (Fig. 1a–c). However, L-arginine showed a trend for lower levels at ≤ 24 h ($p = 0.060$) and 3 days ($p = 0.063$).

The binary logistic regression analysis with co-variables age, and eGFR showed a significant elevation of ADMA levels at days 1, 3, and 7 in ICH patients compared to levels in controls (ADMA ≤ 24 h, $p = 0.003$; ADMA 3 days, $p = 0.005$; ADMA 7 days $p = 0.004$).

ADMA levels increased after the initial time point (≤ 24 h) until day 7 ($p = 0.030$) (Fig. 1a). SDMA levels decreased between the initial time point (≤ 24 h) and day 3 ($p = 0.029$) (Fig. 1b). No significant differences were seen for L-arginine levels in regard to the temporal evolution (Fig. 1c).

Dimethylarginines in relation to outcome

Patients were grouped according to mRS at 90 days as favorable (mRS 0–2) and unfavorable (mRS 3–6) outcome. Nine patients had favorable outcome, and 11 patients had unfavorable outcome. Outcome groups did not differ in regard to baseline characteristics and cardiovascular risk factors.

ADMA levels ≤ 24 h were significantly higher in patients with unfavorable than in patients with favorable outcome

($p = 0.031$) (Fig. 2a). SDMA levels at any time point were significantly elevated in patients with unfavorable outcome compared to those with favorable outcome (SDMA ≤ 24 h, $p = 0.016$; SDMA at 3 days, $p = 0.004$; SDMA at 7 days, $p = 0.031$) (Fig. 2b). For L-arginine, no significant differences were detected in regard to outcome groups (Fig. 2c).

The binary logistic regression analysis did not confirm increased ADMA levels ≤ 24 h in patients with unfavorable outcome ($p = 0.059$). Increased SDMA levels ≤ 24 h ($p = 0.048$) and at 3 days ($p = 0.028$) but not at 7 days ($p = 0.122$) remained significantly associated with unfavorable outcome.

Correlation analysis revealed a significant correlation of SDMA levels at ≤ 24 h and 3 days with mRS at 90 days, whereas SDMA at 7 days and ADMA levels ≤ 24 h only tended to correlate with mRS at 90 days (ADMA ≤ 24 h, $p = 0.088$; SDMA ≤ 24 h, $p = 0.029$; SDMA at 3 days, $p = 0.005$; SDMA at 7 days, $p = 0.081$) (Fig. 3a, b). At other time points, no association between ADMA, SDMA, or L-arginine and mRS at 90 days was detected.

Dimethylarginines in relation to secondary brain injury in ICH

Hematoma enlargement occurred in five patients and cytotoxic edema in nine patients (Table 1). To test the hypothesis that early levels of dimethylarginines (≤ 24 h) are associated with secondary brain injury, patients were grouped according to the median of hematoma and perihematomal edema volume as well as according to the occurrence of hematoma enlargement and cytotoxic

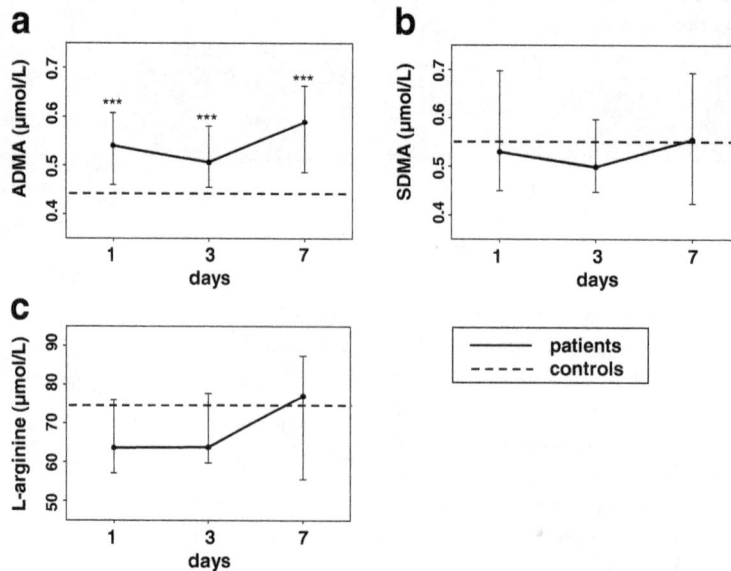

Fig. 1 a–c Time courses of ADMA, SDMA, and L-arginine in acute ICH. Data are presented as median (interquartile range). Values in controls are presented by dashed line. Differences between patients and controls: *** $p ≤ 0.001$. Within group comparisons of marker levels between initial (≤ 24 h) and follow-up time points: significant differences were detected for ADMA (≤ 24 h versus 7 days; $p = 0.030$) and SDMA (≤ 24 h versus 3 days; $p = 0.029$)

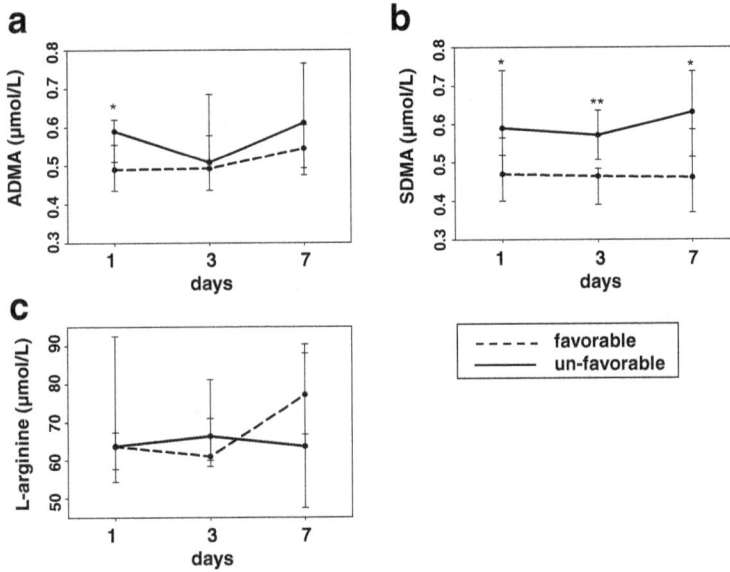

Fig. 2 a–c Comparison of time courses of ADMA, SDMA, and L-arginine after acute ICH in patients with favorable and unfavorable outcome. The data are presented as median (interquartile range). Differences between outcome groups: *$p \leq 0.05$; **$p \leq 0.01$

edema. Of note, these outcome groups did not differ in regard to baseline characteristics and cardiovascular risk factors.

In patients with higher hematoma volume (> median; $n = 10$), SDMA levels but not ADMA levels (≤ 24 h) were significantly higher compared to those with smaller hematoma volume (< median; $n = 10$) ($p = 0.029$). ADMA levels (≤ 24 h) were significantly higher in patients developing hematoma enlargement ($n = 5$) compared to patients without hematoma enlargement ($n = 13$) ($p = 0.003$). SDMA levels (≤ 24 h) were significantly higher in patients with larger perihematomal edema volume (> median; $n = 10$) compared to those with smaller perihematomal edema volume (< median; $n = 10$) ($p = 0.023$), while perihematomal edema mostly consists of vasogenic edema, in part of the patients cytotoxic edema, could be detected. In patients with occurrence of cytotoxic edema ($n = 9$), ADMA and SDMA levels (≤ 24 h) did not differ from those in patients without cytotoxic edema ($n = 11$).

Discussion

Our data show that (i) levels of ADMA are increased after acute ICH, (ii) higher levels of SDMA are associated with poor functional outcome, (iii) ADMA is associated with the occurrence of hematoma enlargement, and (iv) SDMA is associated with large hematoma and perihematomal edema volumes.

After ICH, inflammation, cellular damage, and proteolysis cause oxidative stress, which is known to increase protein arginine methyltransferase (PRMT) activity and decrease dimethylarginine dimethylaminohydrolase (DDAH) activity leading to elevated ADMA levels [20, 21]. In our study, ADMA levels but not SDMA levels were increased at each time point in ICH patients compared to controls. Of note,

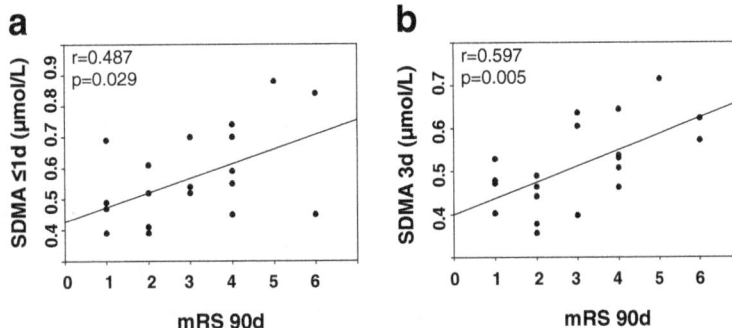

Fig. 3 a, b Correlation of SDMA $\leq$ 1 and 3 days with mRS at 90 days

Wanby et al. reported no increase of ADMA levels in 22 ICH patients [12]. But the design of both studies seems barely comparable. Wanby and colleagues took only one blood sample at an undefined time point during the first days after admission. However, in our study, ADMA levels were increased at each of the specified time points during the first week after the event. Therefore, differences in study results might not be related to the blood sampling schedule but to the patient cohort. We demonstrated an increase of ADMA in patients with poor outcome in the univariate analysis, while after adjustment for co-variables ADMA levels only tended to be associated with unfavorable outcome. Since Wanby et al. did not report clinical severity or outcome for their patients, it cannot be discussed if the difference between the study results might be due to differences in ICH severity. An association of ADMA levels with outcome might be explained by the larger extent of damage inducing more oxidative stress. Importantly, this hypothesis is supported by elevated ADMA levels in patients with hematoma enlargement. However, it remains unclear if ADMA is directly involved in the pathophysiology of hematoma enlargement. ADMA may trigger oxidative stress via uncoupling of endothelial NOS (eNOS) and iNOS resulting in production of the toxic compounds superoxide ($O_2{}^-$) and peroxynitrite ($ONOO{\cdot}^-$) [22, 23]. This may lead to further damage of the blood-brain barrier (BBB) facilitating hematoma enlargement. However, so far, direct evidence for ADMA-induced uncoupling of eNOS and iNOS is lacking for the cerebral circulation.

The continuous increase in ADMA levels between day 1 and day 7, as shown in our patient cohort, could possibly be explained by massive inflammation, proteolysis, and oxidative stress during the first days after ICH. Of note, follow-up data from a fraction of the patient cohort suggest that ADMA levels might be still elevated at day 90, although levels tended to decrease compared to those on day 7 (data not shown). However, so far, the length of and the reason for prolonged elevation of ADMA levels after ICH remain unclear.

Wanby et al. demonstrated lower levels of L-arginine in ICH patients than in controls [12]. In our study L-arginine––levels were also lower in the ICH patients than in the controls until day 3 after the event, but the level of significance was missed. Under conditions of L-arginine depletion, neuronal NOS (nNOS) synthesizes $O_2{}^-$ [24]. Therefore, it is suggested that lower levels of L-arginine in ICH patients result in increased $O_2{}^-$ production, potentially harming the zone of hypoperfusion surrounding the hematoma. Interestingly, addition of ADMA inhibited the nNOS-derived $O_2{}^-$ production [24]. This might indicate a beneficial effect of ADMA after ICH, potentially limiting the pathology of BBB damage. Another beneficial effect of ADMA might be reduction of perfusion by increase of vascular tone to lower the volume

of bleeding. In healthy subjects, infusion of ADMA with 0.10 mg/kg/min significantly decreased cerebral blood flow [25].

These ADMA effects might be pronounced in patients with poor outcome and hematoma enlargement since in these patients, ADMA production following cellular damage and proteolysis is particularly high. However, since these secondary complications are particularly detrimental and cause poor outcome, obviously any discussed beneficial ADMA effect might not be sufficient.

After ICH, elevated ADMA levels might also affect systemic blood pressure. Experimental data in rats showed that microinjection of ADMA in the rostral ventrolateral medulla reduced NO synthesis and increased blood pressure [26]. Importantly, high blood pressure after ICH has been associated with poor clinical outcome and secondary complications such as hematoma enlargement [27]. In addition, high blood pressure variability is associated with unfavorable outcome, possibly due to secondary injury of hypoperfused tissue affected by perihematomal edema [28]. However, optimized clinical management such as early intensive blood pressure-lowering is still discussed [29]. In particular, any treatment directly influencing NO levels cannot be recommended due to insufficient evidence. Recently, a systematic review has investigated safety and efficacy of the NO donor transdermal glyceryl trinitrate when applied after stroke. Patients showed blood pressure lowering, but outcome was not ameliorated [30]. Of note, the analyzed studies included both ischemic and hemorrhagic stroke patients.

SDMA levels were not different between ICH patients and controls in the current study and in the study of Wanby and colleagues [12]. Importantly, the current study showed a significant association of SDMA levels with outcome at 90 days. Giving a hint that SDMA is involved in the pathophysiology after acute ICH, SDMA levels measured in blood samples from the first day after the event were significantly higher in patients with larger compared to those with smaller hematoma and perihematomal edema volume. However, studies explaining these associations are so far missing in acute ICH patients and only data from other pathologies can be discussed. Recently, Feliers et al. demonstrated in glomerular endothelial cells, that SDMA causes eNOS uncoupling [31], a mechanism resulting in increased ROS production. It remains unclear, whether SDMA leads to eNOS uncoupling also in acute ICH. In another study, SDMA triggered ROS synthesis of monocytes by modulation of store-operated calcium channels [11]. Another mechanism, by which SDMA may add to poor outcome after ICH could be via pro-inflammatory effects.

Inflammation during the acute stage of ICH is of particular importance. Recently, leukocyte counts and the neutrophil-to-lymphocyte ratio on admission have been shown to be associated with functional outcome in ICH patients potentially contributing to neurological deterioration via edema formation [32]. Interestingly, also in ischemic stroke patients who developed parenchymal hematoma or in patients with symptomatic ICH after thrombolytic treatment, the neutrophil-to-lymphocyte ratio is increased [33]. SDMA might be involved in increased inflammation after ICH since in monocytes, it triggers nuclear factor kappa-light-chain-enhancer of activated B cell (NF-kappaB) activation and tumor necrosis factor-alpha (TNF-alpha) and interleukin-6 (IL-6) expression [34]. However, to our knowledge the association between dimethylarginines and inflammation in ICH patients has not been studied so far.

Limitations

This study was the first to investigate the temporal pattern of dimethylarginine levels after ICH and their association with clinical outcomes. Due to the small number of patients included, it is necessary to confirm the results in a larger study. In addition, there is no evidence that the demonstrated association of dimethylarginines with functional and radiological outcome reflects a causative effect of these mediators in the pathophysiology of ICH. However, in the current study, elaborated serial MRI imaging provided detection of radiological outcome markers which cannot be achieved in routine clinical care. Thereby, the association of dimethylarginine levels with hematoma enlargement and perihematomal edema could be investigated. To confirm these data, a step from bedside to bench to elucidate the underlying mechanisms in experimental studies is warranted.

Conclusions

ADMA and SDMA levels are increased after the acute event of ICH in relation to outcome and might be––though differentially––involved in secondary brain injury such as hematoma enlargement and perihematomal edema. However, further studies are needed to elucidate the mechanisms behind to investigate if there is any causal relationship between dimethylarginine levels, inflammatory response to, and outcome of intracerebral hemorrhage.

Abbreviations
ADC: Apparent diffusion coefficient; ADMA: Asymmetric dimethylarginine; BBB: Blood-brain barrier; CHD: Coronary heart disease; CT: Computed tomography; CVD: Cerebrovascular disease; DDAH: Dimethylarginine dimethylaminohydrolase; DWI: Diffusion weighted imaging; eGFR: Estimated glomerular filtration rate; eNOS: Endothelial nitric oxide synthase; HE: Hematoma enlargement; HPLC–MS–MS: High-performance liquid chromatography–tandem mass spectrometry; ICH: Intracerebral hemorrhage; IL-6: Interleukin-6; iNOS: Inducible nitric oxide synthase; IVH: Intraventricular hematoma; MRI: Magnetic resonance imaging; mRS: Modified Rankin Scale; NF-kappaB: Nuclear factor kappa-light-chain-enhancer of activated B cells; NIHSS: National Institutes of Health Stroke Scale Score; nNOS: Neuronal nitric oxide synthase; NOS: Nitric oxide synthase inhibitor; ONOO⁻: Peroxynitrite; $O_2 .^-$: Superoxide; PRMT: Protein arginine methyltransferase; ROI: Region of interest; ROS: Reactive oxygen species; SAH: Subarachnoid hemorrhage; SDMA: Symmetric dimethylarginine; TNF-alpha: Tumor necrosis factor-alpha

Acknowledgements
The authors thank Frank Dsiosa, Klaus Burfeind, and Bernadette Lüns for excellent technical assistance.

Funding
None

Authors' contributions
HW contributed to the conception and design of the study, the data acquisition, analysis, and interpretation, and the drafting and revision of the manuscript. NL contributed to the conception and design of the study, the data acquisition, analysis, and interpretation, and the revision of the manuscript. JM, MD, RS, and RL contributed to the data acquisition, analysis and interpretation, and to the revision of the manuscript. JTK and HL contributed to the data analysis and interpretation and to the revision of the manuscript. PR and SMB contributed to the design of the study, the data acquisition, analysis and interpretation and to the revision of the manuscript. KW contributed to the conception and design of the study, the data analysis and interpretation, and the revision of the manuscript. All authors read and approved the final manuscript.

Competing interests
The other authors declare that they have no competing interests.

Author details
[1]Department of Neurology, Hannover Medical School, 30623 Hannover, Germany. [2]Department of Neurology, Beijing Tiantan Hospital, Capital Medical University, Beijing, China. [3]Department of Clinical Pharmacology, Otto-von-Guericke-University of Magdeburg, University Hospital, Magdeburg, Germany. [4]Department of Clinical Chemistry, Hannover Medical School, Hannover, Germany. [5]Department of Nephrology and Hypertension, Hannover Medical School, Hannover, Germany. [6]Medical Clinic V, Academic Teaching Hospital Braunschweig, Braunschweig, Germany. [7]Institute of Diagnostic and Interventional Neuroradiology, Hannover Medical School, Hannover, Germany.

References
1. Van Asch CJ, Luitse MJ, Rinkel GJ, van der Tweel I, Algra A, Klijn CJ. Incidence, case fatality, and functional outcome of intracerebral haemorrhage over time, according to age, sex, and ethnic origin: a systematic review and meta-analysis. Lancet Neurol. 2010 Feb;9(2):167–76.
2. Ryu J, Pyo H, Jou I, Joe E. Thrombin induces NO release from cultured rat microglia via protein kinase C, mitogen-activated protein kinase, and NF-kappa B. J Biol Chem. 2000 Sep 29;275(39):29955–9.
3. Laird MD, Wakade C, Alleyne CH Jr, Dhandapani KM. Hemin-induced necroptosis involves glutathione depletion in mouse astrocytes. Free Radic Biol Med. 2008;45:1103–14.
4. Chiang MF, Chiu WT, Lin FJ, Thajeb P, Huang CJ, Tsai SH. Multiparametric analysis of cerebral substrates and nitric oxide delivery in cerebrospinal fluid

in patients with intracerebral haemorrhage: correlation with hemodynamics and outcome. Acta Neurochir. 2006;148:615–21.

5. Rashid PA, Whitehurst A, Lawson N, Bath PM. Plasma nitric oxide (nitrate/nitrite) levels in acute stroke and their relationship with severity and outcome. J Stroke Cerebrovasc Dis. 2003;12:82–7.

6. Nakajima T, Matsuoka Y, Kakimoto Y. Isolation and identification of N-G-monomethyl, N-G, N-G-dimethyl- and N-G, N' G-dimethylarginine from the hydrolysate of proteins of bovine brain. Biochim Biophys Acta. 1971 Feb 23; 230(2):212–22.

7. Lee DY, Teyssier C, Strahl BD, Stallcup MR. Role of protein methylation in regulation of transcription. Endocr Rev. 2005 Apr;26(2):147–70.

8. Vallance P, Leone A, Calver A, Collier J, Moncada S. Endogenous dimethylarginine as an inhibitor of nitric oxide synthesis. J Cardiovasc Pharmacol. 1992;20(Suppl 12):S60–2.

9. Chen S, Li N, Deb-Chatterji M, Dong Q, Kielstein JT, Weissenborn K, Worthmann H. Asymmetric dimethyarginine as marker and mediator in ischemic stroke. Int J Mol Sci 2012 Nov 28;13(12):15983-6004. Review.

10. Closs EI, Basha FZ, Habermeier A, Forstermann U. Interference of L-arginine analogues with L-arginine transport mediated by the y+ carrier hCAT-2B. Nitric Oxide. 1997;1:65–73.

11. Schepers E, Glorieux G, Dhondt A, Leybaert L, Vanholder R. Role of symmetric dimethylarginine in vascular damage by increasing ROS via store-operated calcium influx in monocytes. Nephrol Dial Transplant. 2009;24:1429–35.

12. Wanby P, Teerlink T, Brudin L, Brattstrom L, Nilsson I, Palmqvist P, et al. Asymmetric dimethylarginine (ADMA) as a risk marker for stroke and TIA in a Swedish population. Atherosclerosis. 2006;185:271–7.

13. Worthmann H, Chen S, Martens-Lobenhoffer J, Li N, Deb M, Tryc AB, Goldbecker A, Dong Q, Kielstein JT, Bode-Böger SM, Weissenborn K. High plasma dimethylarginine levels are associated with adverse clinical outcome after stroke. J Atheroscler Thromb. 2011;18(9):753–61.

14. Jung CS, Oldfield EH, Harvey-White J, Espey MG, Zimmermann M, Seifert V, et al. Association of an endogenous inhibitor of nitric oxide synthase with cerebral vasospasm in patients with aneurysmal subarachnoid hemorrhage. J Neurosurg. 2007;107:945–50.

15. Martens-Lobenhoffer J, Sulyok E, Czeiter E, Büki A, Kohl J, Firsching R, Tröger U, Bode-Böger SM. Determination of cerebrospinal fluid concentrations of arginine and dimethylarginines in patients with subarachnoid haemorrhage. J Neurosci Methods. 2007 Aug 15;164(1):155–60.

16. Li N, Worthmann H, Heeren M, Schuppner R, Deb M, Tryc AB, Bueltmann E, Lanfermann H, Donnerstag F, Weissenborn K, Raab P. Temporal pattern of cytotoxic edema in the perihematomal region after intracerebral hemorrhage: a serial magnetic resonance imaging study. Stroke. 2013 Apr;44(4):1144–6.

17. Phan TG, Chen J, Beare R, Ma H, Clissold B, Van Ly J, Srikanth V, VISTA-ICH Collaboration. Classification of different degrees of disability following intracerebral hemorrhage: a decision tree analysis from VISTA-ICH collaboration. Front Neurol. 2017 Feb 28;8:64.

18. Martens-Lobenhoffer J, Bode-Böger SM. Quantification of l-arginine, asymmetric dimethylarginine and symmetric dimethylarginine: a step improvement in precision by stable isotope dilution mass spectrometry. J Chromatogr B. 2012;904:140–3.

19. Burgess RE, Warach S, Schaewe TJ, Copenhaver BR, Alger JR, Vespa P, Martin N, Saver JL, Kidwell CS. Development and validation of a simple conversion model for comparison of intracerebral hemorrhage volumes measured on CT and gradient recalled echo MRI. Stroke. 2008 Jul;39(7):2017–20.

20. Leiper J, Murray-Rust J, McDonald N, Vallance P. S-nitrosylation of dimethylarginine dimethylaminohydrolase regulates enzyme activity: further interactions between nitric oxide synthase and dimethylarginine dimethylaminohydrolase. Proc Natl Acad Sci U S A. 2002 Oct 15;99(21):13527–32.

21. Sydow K, Münzel T. ADMA and oxidative stress. Atheroscler Suppl. 2003 Dec;4(4):41–51.

22. Wells SM, Holian A. Asymmetric dimethylarginine induces oxidative and nitrosative stress in murine lung epithelial cells. Am J Respir Cell Mol Biol. 2007 May;36(5):520–8.

23. Wadham C, Mangoni AA. Dimethylarginine dimethylaminohydrolase regulation: a novel therapeutic target in cardiovascular disease. Expert Opin Drug Metab Toxicol. 2009 Mar;5(3):303–19.

24. Cardounel AJ, Xia Y, Zweier JL. Endogenous methylarginines modulate superoxide as well as nitric oxide generation from neuronal nitric-oxide synthase: differences in the effects of monomethyl- and dimethylarginines in the presence and absence of tetrahydrobiopterin. J Biol Chem. 2005;280:7540–9.

25. Kielstein JT, Donnerstag F, Gasper S, Menne J, Kielstein A, Martens-Lobenhoffer J, Scalera F, Cooke JP, Fliser D, Bode-Böger SM. ADMA increases arterial stiffness and decreases cerebral blood flow in humans. Stroke. 2006 Aug;37(8):2024–9.

26. Tan X, Li JK, Sun JC, Jiao PL, Wang YK, Wu ZT, Liu B, Wang WZ. The asymmetric dimethylarginine-mediated inhibition of nitric oxide in the rostral ventrolateral medulla contributes to regulation of blood pressure in hypertensive rats. Nitric Oxide. 2017 Jul 1;67:58–67.

27. Rodriguez-Luna D, Piñeiro S, Rubiera M, Ribo M, Coscojuela P, Pagola J, Flores A, Muchada M, Ibarra B, Meler P, Sanjuan E, Hernandez-Guillamon M, Alvarez-Sabin J, Montaner J, Molina CA. Impact of blood pressure changes and course on hematoma growth in acute intracerebral hemorrhage. Eur J Neurol. 2013 Sep;20(9):1277–83.

28. Lattanzi S, Cagnetti C, Provinciali L, Silvestrini M. Blood pressure variability and clinical outcome in patients with acute Intracerebral hemorrhage. J Stroke Cerebrovasc Dis. 2015 Jul;24(7):1493–9.

29. Lattanzi S, Cagnetti C, Provinciali L, Silvestrini M. How should we lower blood pressure after cerebral hemorrhage? A systematic review and meta-analysis. Cerebrovasc Dis. 2017;43(5–6):207–13.

30. Bath PM, Krishnan K, Appleton JP. Nitric oxide donors (nitrates), L-arginine, or nitric oxide synthase inhibitors for acute stroke. Cochrane Database Syst Rev. 2017 Apr 21;4:CD000398.

31. Feliers D, Lee DY, Gorin Y, Kasinath BS. Symmetric dimethylarginine alters endothelial nitric oxide activity in glomerular endothelial cells. Cell Signal. 2015 Jan;27(1):1–5.

32. Lattanzi S, Cagnetti C, Provinciali L, Silvestrini M. Neutrophil-to-lymphocyte ratio predicts the outcome of acute intracerebral hemorrhage. Stroke. 2016 Jun;47(6):1654–7.

33. Guo Z, Yu S, Xiao L, Chen X, Ye R, Zheng P, Dai Q, Sun W, Zhou C, Wang S, Zhu W, Liu X. Dynamic change of neutrophil to lymphocyte ratio and hemorrhagic transformation after thrombolysis in stroke. J Neuroinflammation. 2016 Aug 26;13(1):199.

34. Schepers E, Barreto DV, Liabeuf S, Glorieux G, Eloot S, Barreto FC, Massy Z, Vanholder R, European Uremic Toxin Work Group (EUTox). Symmetric dimethylarginine as a proinflammatory agent in chronic kidney disease. Clin J Am Soc Nephrol. 2011 Oct;6(10):2374–83.

Isoliquiritigenin alleviates early brain injury after experimental intracerebral hemorrhage via suppressing ROS- and/or NF-κB-mediated NLRP3 inflammasome activation by promoting Nrf2 antioxidant pathway

Jun Zeng[1], Yizhao Chen[1]*(iD), Rui Ding[2], Liang Feng[3], Zhenghao Fu[4], Shuo Yang[5], Xinqing Deng[6], Zhichong Xie[1] and Shizhong Zheng[1]

Abstract

Background: Intracerebral hemorrhage (ICH) induces potently oxidative stress responses and inflammatory processes. Isoliquiritigenin (ILG) is a flavonoid with a chalcone structure and can activate nuclear factor erythroid-2 related factor 2 (Nrf2)-mediated antioxidant system, negatively regulate nuclear factor-κB (NF-κB) and nod-like receptor family, pyrin domain-containing 3 (NLRP3) inflammasome pathways, but its role and potential molecular mechanisms in the pathology following ICH remain unclear. The present study aimed to explore the effects of ILG after ICH and underlying mechanisms.

Methods: ICH model was induced by collagenase IV (0.2 U in 1 μl sterile normal saline) in male Sprague-Dawley rats weighing 280–320 g. Different doses of ILG (10, 20, or 40 mg/kg) was administrated intraperitoneally at 30 min, 12 h, 24 h, and 48 h after modeling, respectively. Rats were intracerebroventricularly administrated with control scramble small interfering RNA (siRNA) or Nrf2 siRNA at 24 h before ICH induction, and after 24 h, ICH model was established with or without ILG (20 mg/kg) treatment. All rats were dedicated at 24 or 72 h after ICH. Neurological deficits, histological damages, brain water content (BWC), blood-brain barrier (BBB) disruption, and neuronal degeneration were evaluated; quantitative real-time RT-PCR (qRT-PCR), immunohistochemistry/immunofluorescence, western blot, and enzyme-linked immunosorbent assay (ELISA) were carried out; catalase, superoxide dismutase activities and reactive oxygen species (ROS), and glutathione/oxidized glutathione contents were measured.

(Continued on next page)

---

* Correspondence: yizhao_chen@hotmail.com
[1]Department of Neurosurgery, Zhujiang Hospital, The National Key Clinical Specialty, The Neurosurgery Institute of Guangdong Province, Guangdong Provincial Key Laboratory on Brain Function Repair and Regeneration, The Engineering Technology Research Center of Education Ministry of China, Southern Medical University, Guangzhou 510282, China
Full list of author information is available at the end of the article

(Continued from previous page)

Results: ILG (20 and 40 mg/kg) markedly alleviated neurological deficits, histological damages, BBB disruption, brain edema, and neuronal degeneration, but there was no significant difference between two dosages. ILG (20 mg/kg) significantly suppressed the NF-κB and NLRP3 inflammasome pathways and activated Nrf2-mediated antioxidant system. Gene silencing of Nrf2 aggravated the neurological deficits, brain edema, and neuronal degeneration and increased the protein levels of NF-κB p65, NLRP3 inflammasome components, and IL-1β. ILG delivery significantly attenuated the effects of Nrf2 siRNA interference mentioned above.

Conclusions: Intraperitoneal administration of ILG after ICH reduced early brain impairments and neurological deficits, and the mechanisms were involved in the regulation of ROS and/or NF-κB on the activation of NLRP3 inflammasome pathway by the triggering of Nrf2 activity and Nrf2-induced antioxidant system. In addition, our experimental results may make ILG a potential candidate for a novel therapeutical strategy for ICH.

Keywords: ICH, Early brain injury, ILG, Nrf2, ROS, NF-κB, NLRP3 inflammasome

Background

Spontaneous intracerebral hemorrhage (ICH) belongs to a fatal cerebrovascular disorder, accounting for 15 to 20% in all stroke types, commonly accompanied with high morbidity and mortality [1, 2]. Brain injury after ICH is broadly classified as primary brain injury and secondary brain injury [3, 4]. Primary brain injury occurring within first several hours post ICH is caused by the hemorrhage and growth of hematoma which lead to the mechanical impairments and compression of adjacent cerebrovascular architecture [1, 3–5]. Hematoma size is a powerful and easy-to-use predictor of 30-day mortality and morbidity in patients with ICH, and large hemorrhage often indicates a poor prognosis [4, 6]. Blood components extravasated from the ruptured blood vessels and degradation products of blood cells can induce severe secondary brain injury including neurobehavioral deterioration, brain cell death, cerebral edema, and blood-brain barrier (BBB) disruption [1, 3–5]. Though the understanding of pathophysiological mechanisms to brain injury after ICH has been well improved in recent decades, there are still no effective therapies being available for the prevention of ICH-induced brain impairments [3–5, 7]. Furthermore, increasing evidences have shown that inflammatory response and oxidative stress which occur following ICH play a key role in pathophysiological processes of ICH-induced early brain dysfunctions [3–5, 7, 8].

Nuclear factor erythroid-2 related factor 2 (Nrf2) is a key transcription factor and master regulator of the cellular response of oxidative stress, which can induce the expression of antioxidant and detoxification enzymes and downstream proteins such as NAD(P)H: quinone oxidoreductase-1 (NQO1), catalase (CAT), superoxide dismutase (SOD), heme oxygenase-1 (HO-1), glutathione peroxidase (GPX), and glutathione-S-transferase (GST) [9, 10]. Recent study report showed that the expression of Nrf2 was gradually increased following ICH at 2 h, peaked at 24 h, and then slightly decreased with time until 10 days [11]. In addition, Nrf2 has been

identified to hold the neuroprotective effects against the early brain injury after ICH by translocating into nucleus after being activated, binding to the antioxidant response element (ARE), then initiating the expression of a series of antioxidant and detoxification enzymes and proteins, as a result, improving neurological deficits, alleviating brain edema, and decreasing the infiltration of inflammatory cells [11–15].

The NLRP3 (NALP3, cryopyrin) inflammasome [NLR (Nod-like receptor) family, pyrin domain-containing 3 inflammasome], a best characterized member of NLR family and one of the key components of innate immune system, has been reported by others [8, 16] and us [17] to take part in the processes of early brain injury after ICH via facilitating caspase-1 and interleukin-1beta (IL-1β) processing, which amplifies the inflammatory response and blockade or knockdown of NLRP3 inflammasome can alleviate the brain damages [8, 16, 17]. Recently, reports have indicated that Nrf2 could negatively regulate NLRP3 inflammasome activity by inhibiting reactive oxygen species (ROS)-induced NLRP3 inflammasome activation [18, 19]. However, the relationship between Nrf2 antioxidant pathway and NLRP3 inflammasome activation and whether Nrf2 reduces the early brain injury via the suppression of NLRP3 inflammasome and whether the above-mentioned inhibitory effect is involved in Nrf2 mediated ROS and/or nuclear factor-κB (NF-κB) suppression have not been explored in the experimental rat ICH model.

Isoliquiritigenin (ILG), a component of *Glycyrrhiza uralensis* (*G. uralensis*), is a flavonoid with a chalcone structure and it holds multiple biological activities [20]. Recent papers have shown that ILG was a potent inhibitor of NLRP3 inflammasome [21, 22] and NF-κB [23–25], thus exerting a protective effect. Also, there were reports showing that ILG could activate Nrf2-mediated antioxidant pathway via promoting Nrf2 translocation into the nucleus and then initiating a series of genes to express [9, 26–29]. However, it remains unclear whether ILG has a protective effect against the early brain injury following ICH, and the detailed molecular mechanisms have not been elucidated. Thus, in this study, we are attempting to explore the effects of ILG on the early brain injury after an experimental rat intracerebral hemorrhage model and the potential molecular mechanisms.

Methods

Animals

Adult male Sprague-Dawley rats (SD rats) weighing between 280 and 320 g (8–10 weeks) were obtained from the Animal Experiment Center of Southern Medical University. All experimental procedures and animal care were approved by the Southern Medical University Ethics Committee and were conducted in accordance with the guidelines of the National Institutes of Health on the care and use of animals. All rats were housed in a light-, temperature-, and humidity-controlled specific pathogen-free (SPF) environment (under a 12-h light/dark cycle with constant temperature about 25 °C and relative humidity approximating 55%). All rats had free access to standard food and water during the experiments.

Experimental design and groups

Experiments were conducted in a rat model of collagenase type IV-induced ICH. In the first experiment, 180 rats were used (183 rats suffered to the surgery, 180 rats survived) to evaluate the effects of ILG on the early brain injury post ICH. The rats were randomly and evenly assigned to five groups of 36 rats each, namely, sham group, ICH + vehicle-1 [dimethylsulfoxide (DMSO)] group, ICH + ILG 10 mg/kg group, ICH + ILG 20 mg/kg group, and ICH + ILG 40 mg/kg group. All rats in this experiment were evaluated with a Modified Neurological Severity Score (mNSS) ($n = 12$) scale at 24 or 72 h after ICH, except for the rats that perform extravasation detection of Evans blue (EB) dyes ($n = 6$) at the same time points. Then, the rats were killed, and brain tissue samples were taken to perform brain water content (BWC) measurements ($n = 6$), hematoxylin and eosin (H&E) staining ($n = 6$), and Fluoro-Jade® C (FJC) staining ($n = 6$).

In the second experiment, 120 rats were used (122 rats experienced the operation, 120 rats survived) to explore the underlying molecular mechanisms of ILG's effects on the early brain injury after ICH. The rats were randomized into four groups (30 rats per group): sham group, ICH group, ICH + vehicle-1 (DMSO) group, and ICH + ILG 20 mg/kg group. All rats in the experiment were sacrificed at 24 h after ICH for real-time reverse transcription-quantitative polymerase chain reaction (RT-qPCR) ($n = 6$), western blot (WB) ($n = 6$), immunohistochemistry (IHC)/immunofluorescence (IF) ($n = 6$), enzyme-linked immunosorbent assay (ELISA) ($n = 6$), and glutathione/oxidized glutathione (GSH/GSSG) contents, ROS content, CAT activity, and SOD activity analyses ($n = 6$).

In the third experiment, 132 rats were used (132 of 137 rats after the surgery survived) to execute the study on effects of Nrf2 small interfering RNA (siRNA) interference and Nrf2 siRNA together with ILG co-administration on early brain injury following ICH. The rats were randomly divided into six groups (sham group, ICH + vehicle-2 [mixtures of Entranster™ in vivo transfection reagent and siRNA diluent (RNase-free H_2O)] group, ICH + control scramble siRNA group, ICH + Nrf2 siRNA group, ICH + Nrf2 siRNA + vehicle-1 group, ICH + Nrf2 siRNA + ILG 20 mg/kg group). All rats were decapitated to perform related RT-qPCR ($n = 6$), WB ($n = 6$), mNSS scoring ($n = 6$), BWC ($n = 6$), FJC staining analyses ($n = 6$).

ICH model

The procedure for ICH model in rats has been described in previous publications with some small modifications [17, 30]. In brief, the rats were anesthetized by intraperitoneal injection (i.p.) of pentobarbital sodium (45 mg/kg). Then, the animals were placed in a rat brain stereotaxic apparatus and under aseptic condition. Rectal temperature was maintained at 37 °C throughout the surgical procedure using an insulation board connected with water bath circulation system. Next, a midline incision on the scalp to expose the skull and bregma and a cranial burr hole (1 mm in diameter) was drilled in the right part of the brain, a 5-μl microsyringe with a needle tip (Shanghai high pigeon industry & trade co., LTD, Shanghai, China) was inserted stereotactically through the burr hole and into the right striatum which coordinates were 0.1 mm anterior, 3.5 mm lateral, and 6.0 mm ventral to the bregma. Collagenase type IV (0.2 U in 1 μl sterile normal saline) was administrated over a period of 10 min via stereotaxic intrastriatal injection. The needle was kept in situ for an additional 10 min to prevent back-flow. Then, the microsyringe was slowly removed and the craniotomy was sealed with bone wax. Finally, the wound was sutured. The sham-operated rats were treated via the same way except that they were administrated 1 μl sterile normal saline into the right striatum. The rats were allowed to recover in separate cages with free access to food and water.

In vivo siRNA transfection and drug delivery

The transfection of Nrf2 siRNA for rat brains in vivo were conducted according to the method described formerly [17, 31, 32]. Briefly, the rats were placed under anesthesia, then a cranial burr hole (1 mm in diameter) was drilled, following a 25-μl microsyringe with a needle tip (Shanghai high pigeon industry & trade co., LTD, Shanghai, China) was inserted stereotaxically into the right lateral ventricle. The stereotaxic coordinates were 1.5 mm posterior, 1.0 mm lateral, and 3.2 mm below the horizontal plane of the bregma [32]. Nrf2 siRNA (sc-156128, Santa Cruz biotechnology, USA) and control scramble siRNA (sc-37007, Santa Cruz Biotechnology, USA) were applied with in vivo transfection reagent (Entranster™-in vivo, 18668-11-1, Engreen Biosystem Co., Ltd., Beijing, China) at 24 h before modeling by intracerebroventricular injection [31, 32]. The microsyringe was left in place for an additional 10 min after administration and then slowly withdrawn. At last, the incision was closed with sutures. The sham-operated rats received a cranial burr hole, but only a needle was inserted.

ILG (1811912, Shanghai Macklin Biochemical Co., Ltd., Shanghai, China) was dissolved into DMSO (D5879, Sigma-Aldrich) solution (20 mg/ml). The rats were administered intraperitoneally with either ILG at 10, 20, and 40 mg/kg or the same volume of DMSO at 30 min, 12 h, 24 h, and 48 h after ICH induction.

Behavioral assessment

We used a mNSS scale [33, 34] to assess the behavioral deficits at 24 h and 72 h after ICH, which was performed by two trained investigators and both of whom had been blinded to animal grouping. The mNSS is consisted of motor, sensory, balance, and reflex tests. Neurological function is graded via the scale of 0–18 points (1–6, mild injury; 7–12, moderate injury; 13–18, severe injury; the scores of 0 and 18 represent normal performance and severe neurological deficit, respectively). In the severity scores of neurological function injury, 1 score point is obtained for the incapacity to complete the test or the absence of a tested reflex. Thus, a higher score indicates a more severe neurological injury [33–35].

Measurement of BWC

BWC was evaluated via a wet/dry weight method, as previously described [36, 37]. Briefly, at 24 or 72 h after ICH, the rats were deeply anesthetized with an i.p. of pentobarbital sodium and then were decapitated. The brain of the rats were immediately removed and separated into five parts, namely ipsilateral and contralateral cortex, ipsilateral and contralateral basal ganglia, and cerebellum. The cerebellum was used as an internal control. Each part was placed on a pre-weighed piece of aluminum foil and obtained the wet weight by an electric analytic balance, and then was dried at 100 °C for 24 h in an electric oven to get the dry weight. BWC was assessed using the following formula: [(wet weight – dry weight)]/(wet weight) × 100%.

Evaluation of BBB permeability

Quantitative analysis of BBB permeability was evaluated via EB dye (Wako Pure Chemical Industries, Ltd., Japan) extravasation, as described previously with minor modifications [38–40]. Briefly, the rats were anesthetized and administered intravenously 2% EB solution in normal saline (4 ml/kg) by the femoral vein. After a circulation of 2 h, intracardiac perfusion was performed under deep anesthesia with 0.01 M phosphate buffer solution (PBS) (pH 7.4) of 250 ml to clear EB dyes in cerebral circulation. Subsequently, the brains were removed and the brain samples were immediately separated into the left hemisphere and right hemisphere. Tissue samples were then incubated in 50% trichloroacetic acid solution (2 ml). Following homogenization and centrifugation (15,000 rpm for 20 min), the supernatant (1 ml) was diluted with ethanol (1: 3), and its fluorescence intensity was measured at an excitation wavelength of 620 nm and an emission wavelength of 680 nm with an automatic microplate reader. The EB dye leakage was expressed as micrograms per gram brain weight.

Preparation of paraffin-embedded sections

Paraffin-embedded sections were made as previously described [17, 35, 40] with some modifications. After deep anesthetization with pentobarbital sodium, the rats were transcardially perfused with 250 ml of 0.01 M PBS (pH 7.4) followed by 500 ml 4% paraformaldehyde solution. And then, the brains were removed and post-fixed by immersion in the same fixative solution at 4 °C for 24–48 h. After dehydration and vitrification, tissue samples were embedded in paraffin, and 4-μm sections were prepared. The sections were then dewaxed in xylene, rehydrated in graded ethanol and deionized water, and then processed for H&E, IHC, IF, and FJC staining.

H&E staining

The coronal brain sections (4-μm thickness, paraffin-embedded) were prepared as mentioned above, then were stained with eosin for 10 s followed by hematoxylin re-staining for 5 min. After dehydrated in graded ethanol and cleared in xylene, slides were mounted by neutral balsam. Images were obtained using a microscope (Leica-DM2500, Germany).

IHC staining

IHC staining was conducted as described previously [35, 36] with a few modifications. Coronal paraffin-embedded brain sections (4-μm thickness) were prepared as before-mentioned and antigen retrieval was performed by heat treatment in a microwave oven for 21 min in Tris–ethylene diamine tetraacetic acid (EDTA) buffer solution (0.05 mol/l Tris, 0.001 mol/l EDTA; pH 8.5). Endogenous peroxidase activity was inactivated using 0.3% H_2O_2 for 10 min followed by washing with PBS. After blocking by 5% bovine serum albumin (BSA) for 20 min, the slides were incubated overnight at 4 °C with the following primary antibodies used: rabbit monoclonal anti-NF-κB p65 (D14E12) XP® antibody (1:800, #8242, Cell Signaling Technology); rabbit polyclonal anti-Nrf2 (L593) antibody (1:200, BS1258, Bioworld); rabbit polyclonal anti-HO-1 antibody (1:200, BS6626, Bioworld); goat polyclonal anti-NQO1 antibody (1:200, ab2346, Abcam); mouse monoclonal anti-Cryopyrin (NLRP3) (6F12) antibody (1:100, sc-134306, Santa Cruz Biotechnology); mouse monoclonal anti-3-Nitrotyrosine (3-NT) antibody [39B6] (1:200, ab61392, Abcam); mouse monoclonal anti-8-Hydroxyguanosine (8-OHdG) antibody [N45.1] (1:200, ab48508, Abcam); rabbit polyclonal anti-Iba-1 antibody (1:600, WAKO, Osaka, Japan); and mouse monoclonal anti-CD68 antibody [ED1] (1:200, ab31630, Abcam). After washing with PBS, the sections were incubated with biotinylated goat anti-mouse IgG, goat anti-rabbit IgG, and donkey anti-goat IgG secondary antibodies for 20 min and then incubated with horseradish peroxidase (HRP)-streptavidin reagent for 20 min. Finally, immunoreactivity was detected using 3,3-diaminobenzidine (DAB), followed by re-staining with hematoxylin. Images were obtained by using a microscope (Leica-DM2500, Germany). The number of immunopositive cells in the perihematomal region was counted in a blinded manner and was expressed as number/0.1 mm^2 areas.

IF staining

IF staining was performed as described previously [17, 35] with a few modifications. Coronal paraffin-embedded 4-μm thickness brain sections were prepared as mentioned above. Antigen retrieval was conducted as IHC staining. After blocking by 5% BSA for 40 min, sections were incubated overnight at 4 °C with the following primary antibody used: rabbit polyclonal anti-myeloperoxidase (MPO) antibody (1:50, ab9535, Abcam). After washing with PBS, sections were then incubated with the secondary antibody: Alexa Fluor 594 goat anti-rabbit IgG (H + L) (1:100, A-11012, Invitrogen) for 1 h at room temperature. Following washing three times with PBS, the sections were re-stained by 4′6-diamidino-2-phenylindole (DAPI) for 10 min. Then, images were obtained with a fluorescence microscope (ZEISS-AXIO Scope. Al, Germany).

FJC staining

For the detection of degenerating neuron, FJC staining was conducted as described previously with some modifications [41]. Briefly, rat brain sections were prepared as mentioned above, then sections were rinsed with distilled water and immersed into 0.06% potassium permanganate solution for 10 min followed by transferred into a 0.0001% solution of FJC (AG325, Merck millipore) dissolved in 0.1% acetic acid vehicle for 30 min. After washing with distilled water, the slides were put into an oven at 50 °C for 20 min. The dried slides were then

cleared in xylene for 5 min and then coverslipped with DPX mountant for histology (06522-100 ml, Sigma). Four high-power images (×400 magnification) were taken around hematoma using a fluorescence microscope (ZEISS-AXIO Scope, Al, Germany) in each slide. FJC staining positive cells were counted on these four areas.

Real-time RT-qPCR

Quantitative real-time RT-PCR assessment for the messenger RNA (mRNA) levels was conducted via using Prime Script RT-PCR kits (RR047A and RR820A, Takara) according to the manufacturer's instructions. The mRNA level of β-actin was used as an internal control. The real-time PCR program steps were 95 °C for 30 s, 40 cycles of 95 °C for 3 s, 60 °C for 34 s. The mRNA level of each target gene was normalized to that of β-actin mRNA. Fold-induction was calculated using the $2^{-\Delta\Delta CT}$ method, as previously described [42, 43]. The specific sequences of primers used were shown as Table 1.

WB

WB was performed according to our previous study method [17, 35]. We used the following primary antibodies to perform the WB analyses: rabbit monoclonal anti-NF-κB p65 (D14E12) XP® antibody (1:1000, #8242, Cell Signaling Technology); rabbit polyclonal anti-Nrf2 (L593) antibody (1:500, BS1258, Bioworld); mouse monoclonal anti-Cryopyrin (NLRP3) (6F12) antibody (1:1000, sc-134306, Santa Cruz Biotechnology); rabbit polyclonal anti-PYCARD (ASC) antibody (1:500, A1170, Abclonal); goat polyclonal anti-caspase-1 p20 (M-19) antibody(1:1000, sc-1218, Santa Cruz Biotechnology); rabbit polyclonal anti-IL-1β (H-153) antibody (1: 1000, sc-7884, Santa Cruz Biotechnology); and rabbit polyclonal anti-IL-18 (H-173) antibody (1:1000, sc-7954, Santa Cruz Biotechnology), and glyceraldehyde 3-phosphate dehydrogenase (GAPDH) (1:1000, Cell Signaling Technology) was used as an internal reference. Blot bands were quantified via densitometry with ImageJ software (National Institutes of Health, Baltimore, MD, USA), and protein levels were expressed as the ratio of values of the detected protein bands to that of GAPDH bands.

Table 1 Primers used in real-time qRT-PCR reactions

Gene	Forward primer (5'-3')	Reverse primer (5'-3')
NLRP3	CGGTGACCTTGTGTGTGCTT	TCATGTCCTGAGCCATGGAAG
ASC	GACAGTACCAGGCAGTTCGT	AGTAGGGCTGTGTTTGCCTC
Caspase-1	GAACAAAGAAGGTGGCGCAT	AGACGTGTACGAGTGGGTGT
IL-1beta	CCTATGTCTTGCCCGTGGAG	CACACACTAGCAGGTCGTCA
IL-18	ACCACTTTGGCAGACTTCACT	ACACAGGCGGGTTTCTTTTG
Nqo1	GTTTGCCTGGCTTGCTTTCA	ACAGCCGTGGCAGAACTATC
HO-1	GGTGATGGCCTCCTTGTACC	GTGGGGCATAGACTGGGTTC
Actin	TCAGCAAGCAGGAGTACGATG	GTGTAAAACGCAGCTCAGTAACA

Cytokine ELISA assay

At 24 h after ICH, the rats were deeply anesthetized. The serum samples from intracardiac puncture blood and the supernatant samples from perihematomal brain tissue homogenate were obtained and stored at −80 °C until use. Measurements of IL-1β and IL-18 levels were conducted by a double-antibody sandwich ELISA Array Kit according to the reagent manufacturer's instructions. Briefly, prepared tissue supernatant or serum samples were added to monoclonal antibody enzyme well which is pre-coated with rats IL-1β or IL-18 antibodies labeled with biotin and combined with Streptavidin-HRP to form immune complex, then incubated for 1.5 h in a 37 °C condition and washed three times with PBS to remove the uncombined enzyme. After adding the chromogen solution A and B, the samples were detected using an automatic microplate reader at 450 nm.

Measurements of CAT activity, SOD activity and ROS content, GSH/GSSG contents

CAT assay kit (visible light) (A007-1), total SOD assay kit (Hydroxylamine method) (A001-1), ROS assay kit (E004), and total GSH/GSSG assay kit (A061-1) were all purchased from Nanjing Jiancheng Bioengineering Institute (Nanjing, China) and were used to measure the CAT activity, SOD activity and ROS content, GSH/GSSG contents according to the instructions of reagent manufacturers, respectively.

Statistical analysis

All data were presented as means ± standard deviation (SD). Statistical analyses were performed with SPSS version 19.0 software (SPSS, Inc., Chicago, IL, USA), and plots were drawn by GraphPad Prism 5 software (GraphPad Software, Inc., San Diego, CA). If data are equal variances, one-way analysis of variance (ANOVA) followed by least significant difference (LSD) tests were used to compare differences among multiple groups; for the results being unequal, Dunnett's T3 tests were taken into account. Differences with a $p < 0.05$ were considered statistically significant.

Results

ILG improved behavioral deficits and reduced histological damages at 24 and 72 h after ICH by intraperitoneal administration

Figure 1a shows the representative macrographs (left, sham, 24 h; right, ICH, 24 h). The rats subject to ICH induction showed obvious behavioral deficits at 24 and 72 h after ICH graded by a mNSS score scale ($p < 0.01$ vs. sham, 24 h and 72 h). Administration of ILG at the dosage of 10 mg/kg was not significantly effective for the improvement of behavioral deficits (vehicle-DMSO vs. 10 mg/kg: 10.33 ± 1.07 vs. 10.25 ± 1.14, $p > 0.05$, 24 h;

8.92 ± 0.79 vs. 9.00 ± 0.95, $p > 0.05$, 72 h). However, ILG obviously reduced the mNSS scores at 20 mg/kg (vehicle-DMSO vs. 20 mg/kg: vs. 8.25 ± 0.87, $p < 0.01$, 24 h; vs. 6.25 ± 1.06, $p < 0.01$, 72 h) and 40 mg/kg (vehicle-DMSO vs. 40 mg/kg: vs. 8.17 ± 0.94, $p < 0.01$, 24 h; vs. 6.83 ± 1.03, $p < 0.01$, 72 h), but the effects between two dosages were no significant difference (20 vs. 40 mg/kg, $p > 0.05$, 24 and 72 h) (Fig. 1b). Consistent with the behavioral results, H&E staining of brain tissues surrounding the hematoma showed that ILG treatment obviously improved histological impairments at the dosages of 20 and 40 mg/kg, but 10 mg/kg were not (Fig. 1c). Besides, we also evaluated the effect of ILG (20 mg/kg) on hematoma volume at 24 and 72 h after ICH induction (Additional file 1D). Typical magnetic resonance imaging (MRI) T2-weighted images (T2WI) were obtained (Additional file 2A). The hematoma volume of ICH + DMSO group at 24 and 72 h after ICH were 24.81 ± 1.64, 29.11 ± 2.06 mm^3, respectively. ILG administration significantly reduced hematoma volume to 22.95 ± 3.26 mm^3 at 72 h after ICH but not 24 h (23.10 ± 2.02 mm^3) ($p < 0.05$ vs. ICH + DMSO, 72 h; $p > 0.05$ vs. ICH + DMSO, 24 h) (Additional file 2B). Consequently, the results indicated that ILG treatment (20 mg/kg) had no notably effect on bleeding but possibly promoted hematoma clearance after ICH induction.

Intraperitoneal administration of ILG alleviated brain edema and disruption of BBB at 24 and 72 h after ICH

After induction of ICH at 24 and 72 h, BWC increased clearly ($p < 0.01$ vs. sham, 24 and 72 h) and Evans blue dyes significantly extravasated through disrupted BBB ($p < 0.01$ vs. sham, 24 and 72 h). The effects of ILG treatment on the brain edema and BBB disruption were in keeping with that on the behavioral deficits and brain tissue damages. Assessment of BWC using a wet/dry weight method showed that ILG treatment at the dosage of 10 mg/kg (vehicle-DMSO vs. 10 mg/kg: $81.96 \pm 0.68\%$ vs. $81.57 \pm 0.64\%$, $p > 0.05$, 24 h; $81.40 \pm 0.73\%$ vs. $81.05 \pm 0.90\%$, $p > 0.05$, 72 h) was unable to improve brain edema, but the dosages at 20 mg/kg (vehicle-DMSO vs. 20 mg/kg: vs. $80.40 \pm 0.87\%$, $p < 0.01$, 24 h; vs. $79.65 \pm 1.01\%$, $p < 0.01$, 72 h) and 40 mg/kg (vehicle-DMSO vs. 40 mg/kg: vs. $80.07 \pm 0.43\%$, $p < 0.01$, 24 h; vs. $79.53 \pm 0.85\%$, $p < 0.01$, 72 h) did play a positive role on the reduction of brain edema. However, there was no clear difference on the extent of protective effects about the ILG dosages of 20 and 40 mg/kg (20 vs. 40 mg/kg: $p > 0.05$, 24 and 72 h) (Fig. 1d, e). Quantitative measurements of EB dyes after extravasation in the ipsilateral hemisphere indicated that ILG treatment significantly alleviated the extravasation of EB dyes at the dosages of 20 mg/kg ($p < 0.01$ vs. vehicle-DMSO, 24 and 72 h) and 40 mg/kg ($p < 0.01$ vs. vehicle-DMSO, 24

Isoliquiritigenin alleviates early brain injury after experimental intracerebral hemorrhage via suppressing...

85

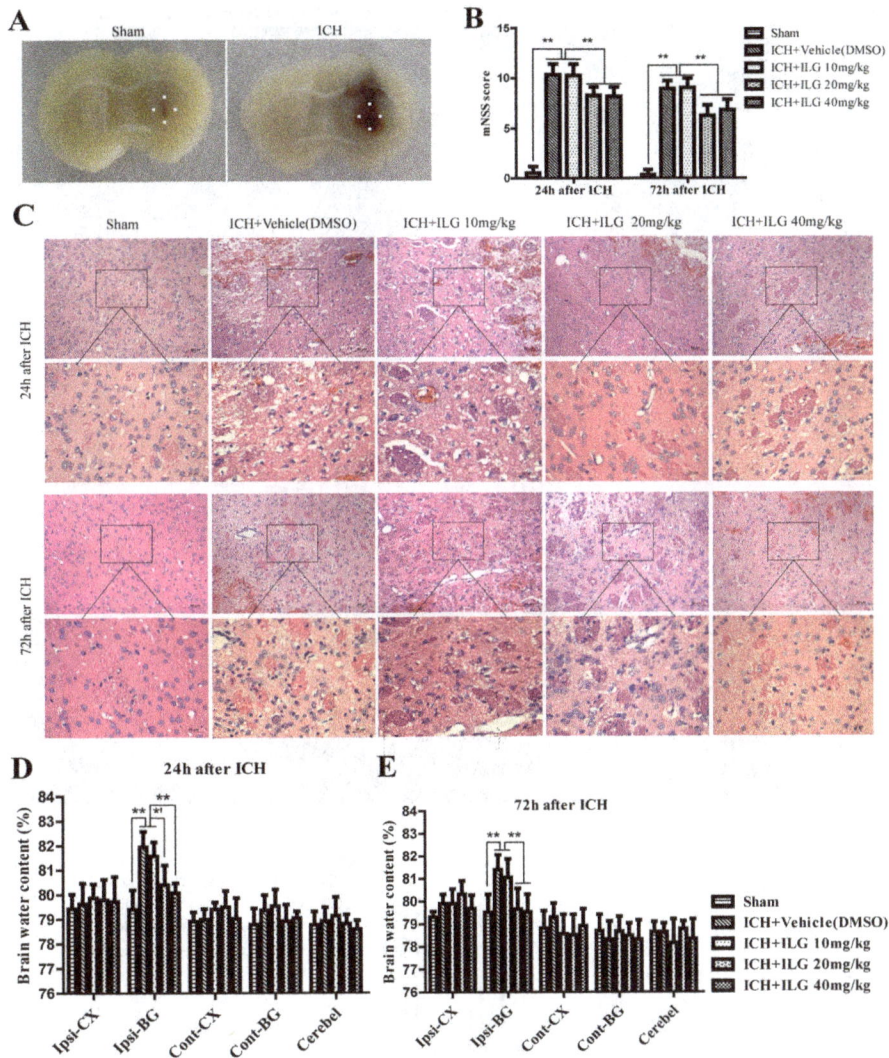

Fig. 1 Representative macrographs and the effects of ILG treatment on ICH-induced brain impairments (**a–e**). Typical macrographs (*left*: sham, 24 h after operation; *right*: 24 h after ICH induction) (**a**). ILG administration at the doses of 20 and 40 mg/kg at 24 and 72 h after ICH induction significantly reduced the neurological deficits assessed by a mNSS score scale (**b**) ($n = 12$ rats/group). Similarly, ILG treatment at doses of 20 and 40 mg/kg markedly alleviated the histological changes evaluated via H&E staining (**c**) ($n = 6$ rats/group) and BWC (**d, e**) ($n = 6$ rats/group) measured by the dry/wet weight method at 24 and 72 h after ICH. *Scale bar* = 50 and 20 μm. Values are shown as means ± SD. ***p < 0.01*; *: ICH + vehicle (DMSO) vs. ICH + ILG 20 mg/kg, $p < 0.01$; ICH + ILG 10 mg/kg vs. ICH + ILG 20 mg/kg, $p < 0.05$

and 72 h), but not 10 mg/kg ($p > 0.05$ vs. vehicle-DMSO, 24 and 72 h) after ICH modeling (Fig. 2a, b).

ILG administration decreased the number of degenerating neurons in the brain tissue surrounding the hematoma after ICH induction

To further estimate the effects of ILG treatment on brain damages in a rat ICH model, we assessed the neuronal degeneration in brain tissue of perihematomal region. FJC$^+$ neurons were significantly increased in the brain tissue surrounding hematoma after ICH ($p < 0.01$ vs. sham, 24 and 72 h) and administration of ILG at the dosages of 20 mg/kg ($p < 0.01$ vs. vehicle-DMSO, 24 and

72 h) and 40 mg/kg ($p < 0.01$ vs. vehicle-DMSO, 24 and 72 h) markedly dropped the number of FJC$^+$ cells. Additionally, a 10 mg/kg dosage of ILG treatment had no distinct effect on the reduction of degenerating neurons ($p > 0.05$ vs. vehicle-DMSO, 24 and 72 h) and treatment results of ILG between 20 and 40 mg/kg were similar (20 vs. 40 mg/kg: $p > 0.05$, 24 and 72 h) (Fig. 2c, d).

In conclusion, experimental results displayed above clearly suggested that ILG treatment by intraperitoneal delivery significantly reduced the behavioral deficits, histological impairments, BBB disruption, brain edema and degenerating neurons of perihematomal brain tissue at the doses of 20 and 40 mg/kg, but there were no

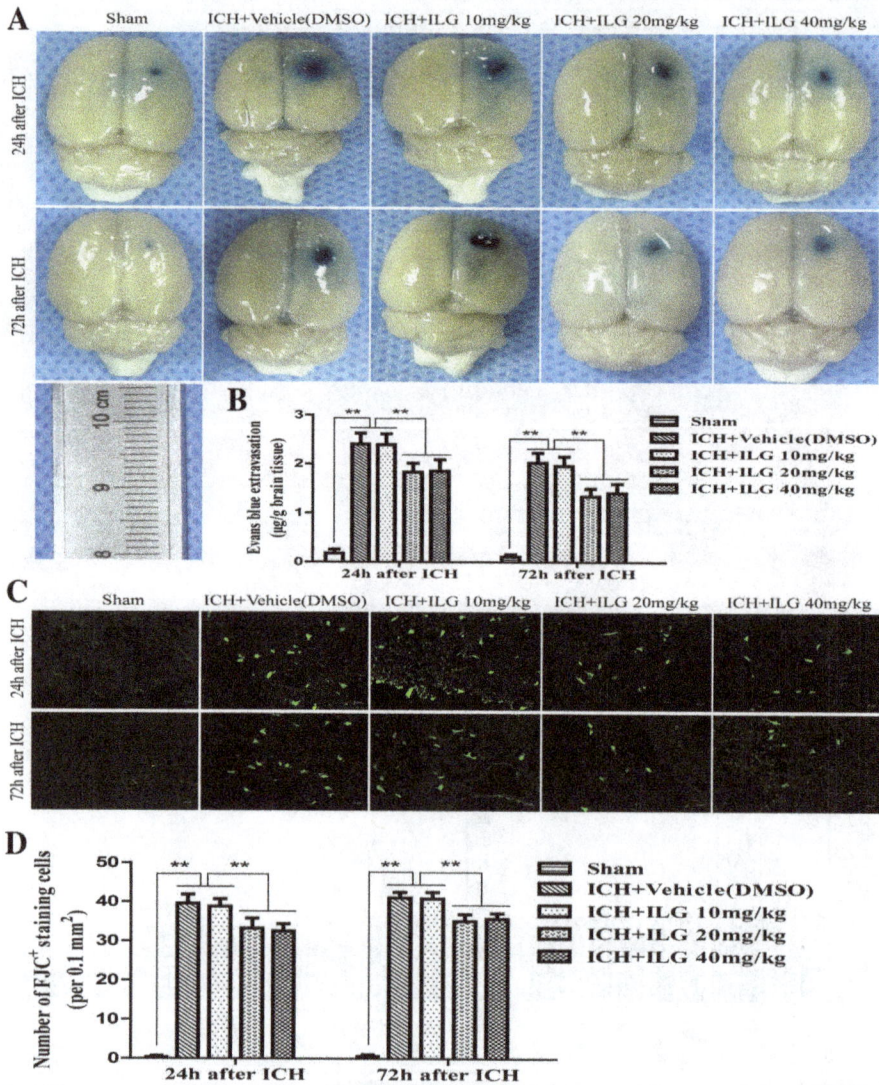

Fig. 2 Effects of ILG on BBB disruption and the number of degenerating neuron following ICH (**a-d**). ILG administration at the dosages of 20 and 40 mg/kg significantly alleviated the extravasation of EB dyes and the number of FJC+ staining cells. Macroscopic images of brains with extravasated EB dyes (**a**) and corresponding quantitative analyses (**b**) ($n = 6$ rats/group). Typical microscopic images for FJC+ staining cells from injury brain tissues (**c**) and quantitative analyses of the number of FJC+ staining cells (**d**) ($n = 6$ rats/group). Scale bar = 20 μm. Values are reported as means ± SD. **$p < 0.01$

obvious difference on the extent between them. Thus, we selected the dosage of 20 mg/kg to further explore the potential molecular mechanisms of ILG's protective effects on early brain injury after ICH induction.

The expression and nuclear translocation of Nrf2 was promoted by ILG treatment at 24 h after ICH induction and that of NF-κB p65 was suppressed

ILG was reported to hold capacity to activate the Nrf2-mediated antioxidant system and inhibit the activation of NF-κB. Thus, we guessed that whether ILG alleviated early brain injury post ICH involved in Nrf2 and NF-κB pathways. In order to verify our supposition, we performed WB analyses and IHC staining using the perihematomal brain

tissue at 24 h after ICH and the results suggested that ILG 20 mg/kg treatment significantly increased the expression of total Nrf2 protein ($p < 0.01$ vs. ICH) (Fig. 3a, d) and decreased that of total NF-κB p65 protein ($p < 0.01$ vs. ICH) (Fig. 3a, b). Typical IHC images were obtained from the injury brain tissue (Fig. 4). Meanwhile, Nrf2 protein level in the cytoplasm was significantly dropped ($p < 0.01$ vs. ICH) (Fig. 3a, e) and notably increased in the nucleus ($p < 0.01$ vs. ICH) (Fig. 3a, g); cytoplasmic level of NF-κB p65 was significantly increased ($p < 0.01$ vs. ICH) (Fig. 3a, c) and the nuclear level was notably deceased ($p < 0.01$ vs. ICH) (Fig. 3a, f). Consequently, experimental results indicated that ILG promoted the expression and nuclear translocation of Nrf2 and suppressed that of NF-κB p65.

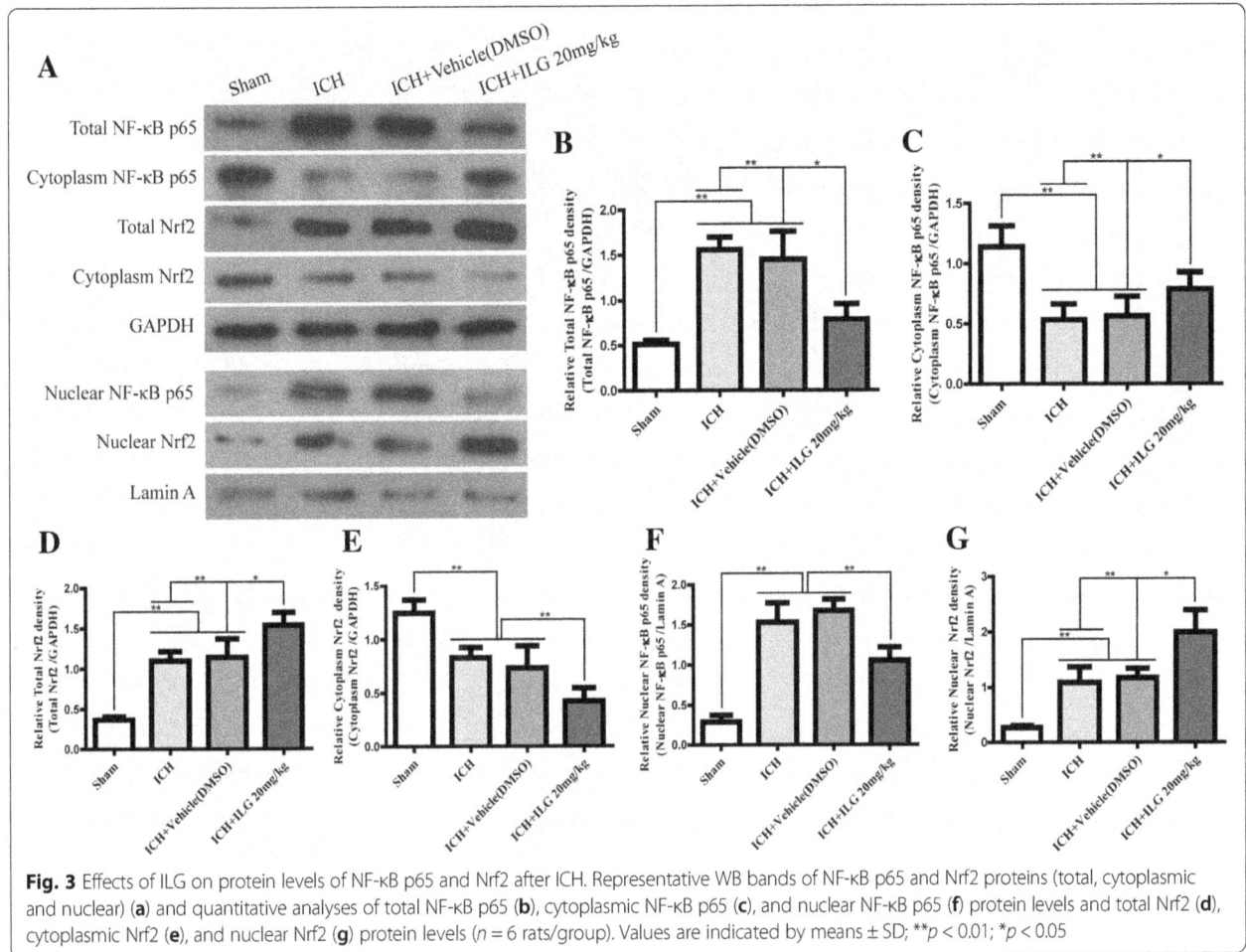

Fig. 3 Effects of ILG on protein levels of NF-κB p65 and Nrf2 after ICH. Representative WB bands of NF-κB p65 and Nrf2 proteins (total, cytoplasmic and nuclear) (**a**) and quantitative analyses of total NF-κB p65 (**b**), cytoplasmic NF-κB p65 (**c**), and nuclear NF-κB p65 (**f**) protein levels and total Nrf2 (**d**), cytoplasmic Nrf2 (**e**), and nuclear Nrf2 (**g**) protein levels ($n = 6$ rats/group). Values are indicated by means ± SD; **$p < 0.01$; *$p < 0.05$

The components of NLRP3 inflammasome pathway and subsequent IL-1β/IL-18 release were suppressed by ILG treatment

Activation of NLRP3 inflammasome and induction of its components aggravated the early brain injury after ICH, and blockades were protective reported by our [17] and other studies [8, 16]. In addition, a recent study showed that Nrf2 negatively regulates NLRP3 inflammasome activity by inhibiting ROS [18]. Therefore, we investigated that whether ILG decreased the activation and induction of NLRP3 inflammasome pathway components or not. The results showed that ILG at the dosage of 20 mg/kg significantly suppressed the expression of NLRP3 inflammasome components: NLRP3, ASC, caspase-1 ($p < 0.01$ vs. ICH) (Fig. 5a, b, c, e), and blocked the activation of NLRP3 inflammasome as indicated by the reduction of cleaved IL-1β and IL-18 ($p < 0.01$ vs. ICH) (Fig. 5a, g, i). Representative IHC images of NLRP3 protein were shown (Fig. 4). Consistent with the above results, ILG treatment obviously reduced the protein levels of pro-IL-1β ($p < 0.01$ vs. ICH) (Fig. 5a, f) and pro-IL-18 ($p < 0.01$ vs. ICH) (Fig. 5a, h) and increased the expression of pro-caspase-1 ($p < 0.05$ vs. ICH) (Fig. 5a, d).

ILG delivery reduced the markers of oxidative stress injury, infiltration of MPO⁺, CD68⁺, Iba-1⁺ cells, and expression of MPO in the brain tissue surrounding the hematoma

Excessive production of ROS mediates seriously oxidative injury and is a key promoting factor for the activation of NLRP3 inflammasome, and the antioxidant responses initiated through nuclear translocation of Nrf2 could alleviate the ROS-induced brain injury and inflammatory cell infiltration. Therefore, we probed that if ILG treatment at 20 mg/kg dropped the production of oxidative stress markers 3-NT and 8-OHdG by IHC staining and infiltration of neutrophils (indicated by MPO, a neutrophil marker) using IF staining and WB analyses. The results suggested that ILG (20 mg/kg) could significantly decrease the amounts of 3-NT⁺ cells ($p < 0.01$ vs. ICH) (Fig. 6a, b), 8-OHdG⁺ cells ($p < 0.05$ vs. ICH) (Fig. 6a, c) in perihematomal brain tissues. Also, the expression level of MPO was notably decreased in the injury brain tissue ($p < 0.01$ vs. ICH) (Fig. 7c), and representative IF images and WB band of MPO protein were shown, respectively (Fig. 7a, b). Meanwhile, ILG (20 mg/kg) could significantly drop the amounts of CD68⁺, Iba-1⁺ (CD68

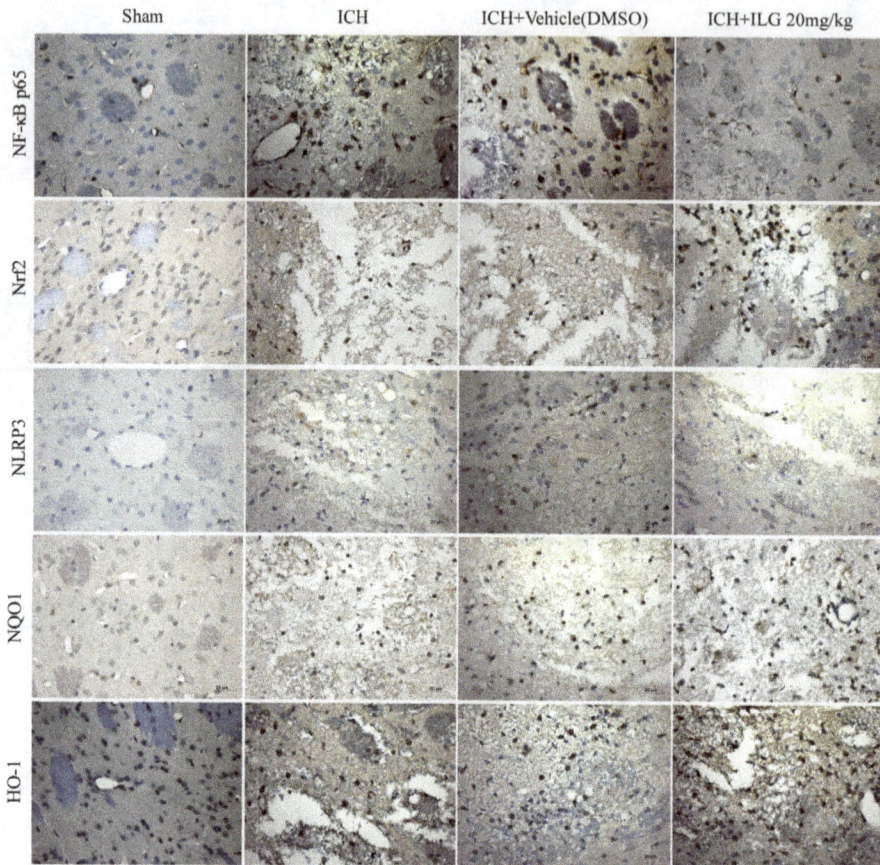

Fig. 4 Effects of ILG on protein levels of NF-κB and Nrf2 pathways evaluated by IHC staining. Typical IHC images of NF-κB p65, Nrf2, NLRP3, NQO1, and HO-1 (*n* = 6 rats/group). *Scale bar* = 20 μm

and Iba-1, the microglia/macrophage markers) cell recruitments in injury brain tissue after ICH as well ($p < 0.05$ vs. ICH) (Additional file 2C, D, E).

ILG treatment lowered the mRNA levels of NLRP3 inflammasome, NF-κB, and Nrf2 pathway components

To further explore the effects of ILG treatment on the mRNA levels of NLRP3 inflammasome, NF-κB, and Nrf2 pathway components at 24 h after ICH induction, we performed relative real-time RT-qPCR study. The results showed that 24 h after ICH induction, the mRNA levels of NLRP3, ASC, caspase-1, IL-1β, IL-18, NQO1, and HO-1 were obviously increased ($p < 0.01$ vs. sham) (Fig. 8) and ILG (20 mg/kg) significantly weakened the increases of NLRP3, caspase-1, IL-18 ($p < 0.05$ vs. ICH) (Fig. 8a, c, e), ASC, and IL-1β mRNA levels ($p < 0.01$ vs. ICH) (Fig. 8b, d). Meanwhile, NQO1 ($p < 0.01$ vs. ICH) (Fig. 8f) and HO-1 ($p < 0.05$ vs. ICH) (Fig. 8g) were further distinctly upregulated at the mRNA levels by ILG treatment. In addition, representative IHC images of NQO1 and HO-1 proteins were shown (Fig. 4).

Inflammatory cytokine levels in the brain tissue and serum from the blood of cardiac puncture were both significantly reduced by ILG treatment

We measured the levels of inflammatory cytokines IL-1β and IL-18 both in perihematomal brain tissues and the serum, respectively. The results were similar to the previous experimental findings, namely, ILG treatment significantly dropped the levels of IL-1β in damaged brain tissues and the serum ($p < 0.01$ vs. ICH) (Fig. 8h, i). The contents of IL-18 in the damaged brain tissue and serum were significantly decreased as well ($p < 0.01$ vs. ICH) (Fig. 8j, k).

ILG reduced the contents of ROS and GSSG, increased the level of GSH and upregulated the enzyme activities of SOD and CAT

We also detected the activities of SOD and CAT enzymes and the contents of GSH/GSSG and ROS after ILG treatment at 24 h post ICH. Experimental results indicated that after ICH induction, enzyme activities of CAT and SOD and the content of GSH were significantly decreased ($p < 0.01$ vs. sham) (Fig. 8l, m, o), the levels of GSSG and ROS were evidently increased ($p < 0.01$ vs. sham) (Fig. 8o, n).

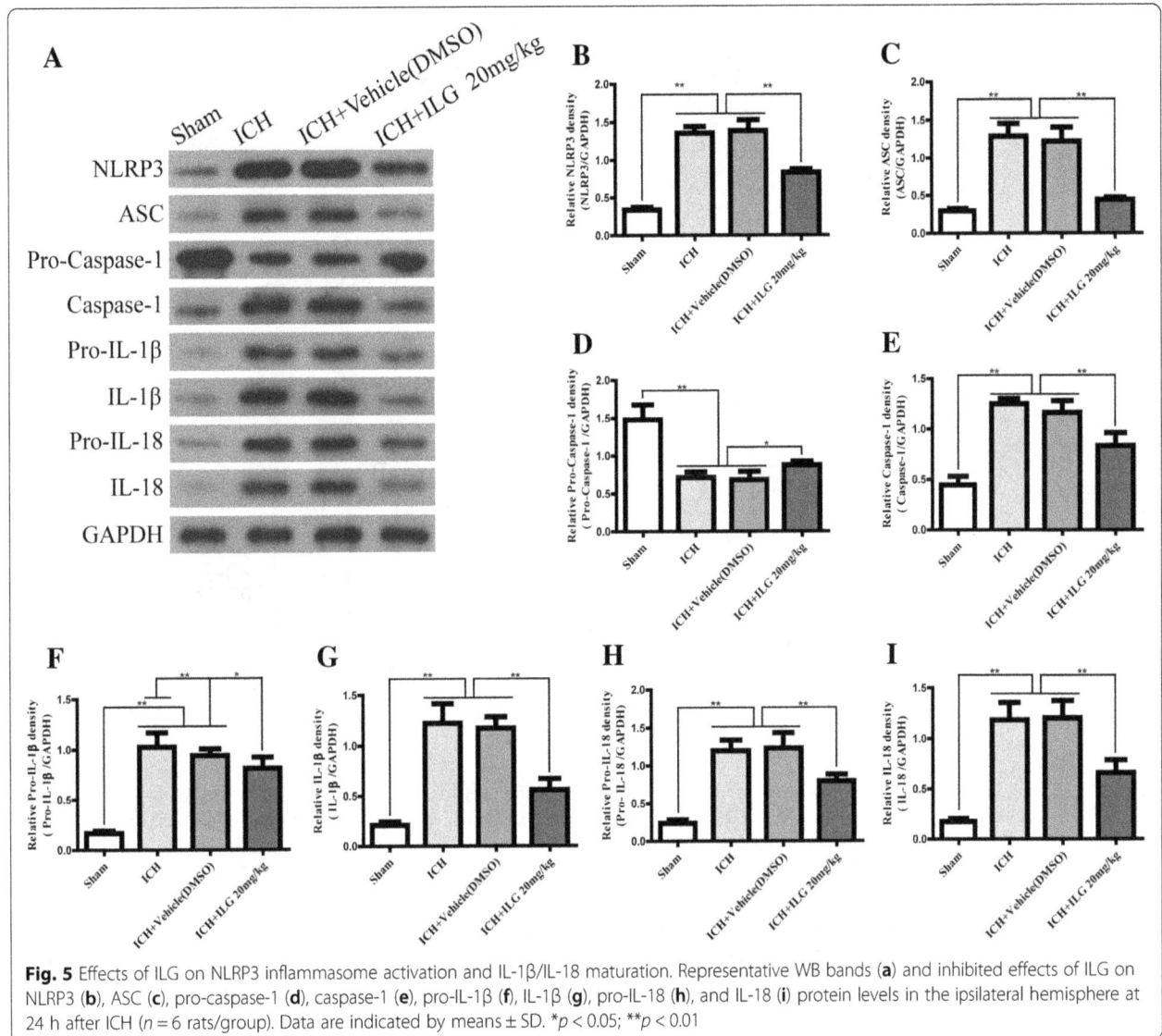

Fig. 5 Effects of ILG on NLRP3 inflammasome activation and IL-1β/IL-18 maturation. Representative WB bands (**a**) and inhibited effects of ILG on NLRP3 (**b**), ASC (**c**), pro-caspase-1 (**d**), caspase-1 (**e**), pro-IL-1β (**f**), IL-1β (**g**), pro-IL-18 (**h**), and IL-18 (**i**) protein levels in the ipsilateral hemisphere at 24 h after ICH ($n = 6$ rats/group). Data are indicated by means ± SD. *$p < 0.05$; **$p < 0.01$

ILG treatment at 20 mg/kg could strikingly reverse the decreases of CAT and SOD enzyme activities, increases of GSSG and ROS levels, and reduction of GSH content ($p < 0.01$ vs. ICH) (Fig. 8l–o).

Nrf2 siRNA interference aggravated the behavioral deficits and brain edema and raised the number of FJC⁺ cells and administration of ILG lowered those uncomfortable effects

In our studies mentioned above, some preliminary conclusions were obtained that ILG could effectively reduce the early brain injury after ICH induction and the protective effects of ILG might be involved in the regulation of Nrf2, ROS, NF-κB, and NLPR3 inflammasome pathways. We wondered if ILG treatment reduced the brain injury mediated by NLRP3 inflammasome pathway via Nrf2 activation-induced ROS and/or NF-κB inhibition.

We conducted the Nrf2 siRNA interfering and Nrf2 siRNA together with ILG 20 mg/kg co-treatment research by intraventricular injection and intraperitoneal delivery, respectively. Interfering effects of Nrf2 siRNA were identified using real-time RT-qPCR and WB analyses. The results showed that Nrf2 siRNA significantly dropped the mRNA and protein expression ($p < 0.01$ vs. vehicle-2) levels of Nrf2 (Fig. 9a–c). In the study, we found that Nrf2 siRNA interference markedly exacerbated the function deficits (Nrf2 siRNA vs. vehicle-2: 13.67 ± 0.91 vs. 10.89 ± 0.96, $p < 0.01$) (Fig. 9d) and brain edema (Nrf2 siRNA vs. vehicle-2: $83.57 \pm 0.80\%$ vs. $82.35 \pm 0.98\%$, $p < 0.05$) (Fig. 9f) and increased the amounts of degenerating neuronal cells ($p < 0.01$ vs. vehicle-2) (Fig. 9e, g) at 24 h after ICH induction. However, ILG administration (20 mg/kg) distinctly reversed those uncomfortable results: function deficits (Nrf2

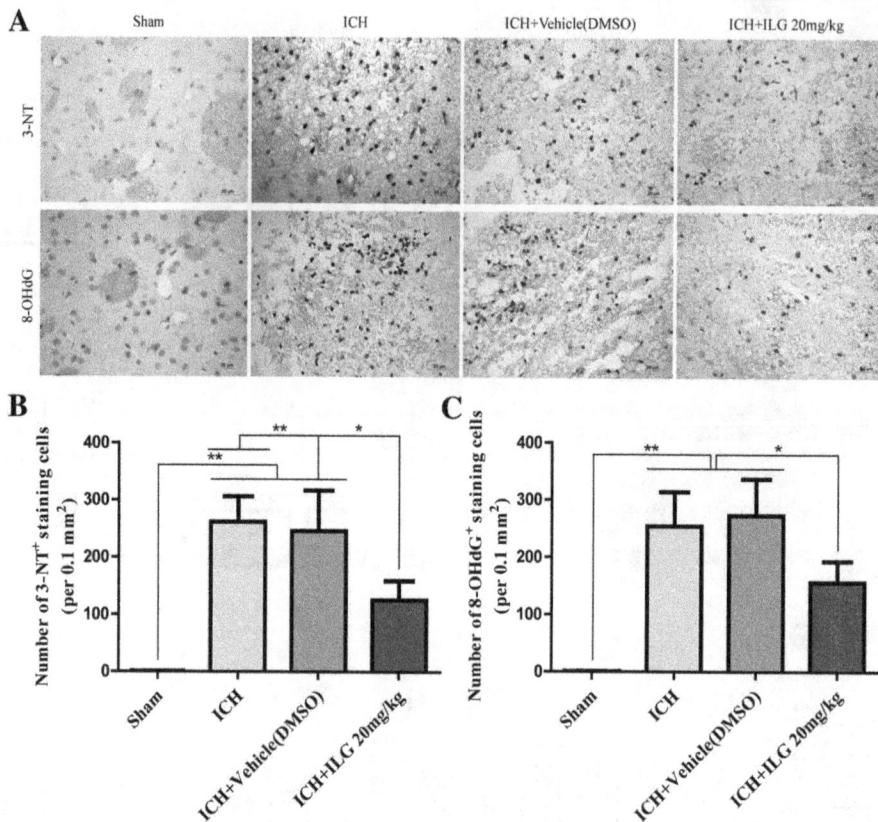

Fig. 6 Effects of ILG on oxidative stress marker levels in the injury brain tissue after ICH. ILG significantly decreased the oxidative stress marker levels (3-NT and 8-OHdG) after ICH. Typical oxidative stress markers 3-NT and 8-OHdG IHC images (**a**) and quantitative analyses (**b**, **c**) ($n = 6$ rats/group). *Scale bar* = 20 μm. Values are reported as means ± SD. **$p < 0.01$; *$p < 0.05$

siRNA vs. Nrf2 siRNA + ILG 20 mg/kg: vs. 11.89 ± 0.90, $p < 0.01$), brain edema (Nrf2 siRNA vs. Nrf2 siRNA + ILG 20 mg/kg: vs. 82.27 ± 0.57%, $p < 0.05$), and FJC$^+$ cells ($p < 0.01$ vs. Nrf2 siRNA) (Fig. 9d–g).

Nrf2 siRNA interference increased the expression of NF-κB p65 and NLRP3 inflammasome components and triggered the activation of NLRP3 inflammasome pathway and ILG reduced these effects

We further evaluated the effects of Nrf2 siRNA on the expression of NF-κB p65 and induction and activation of NLRP3 inflammasome pathway components. We found that Nrf2 siRNA interfering could significantly increase the expression of NF-κB p65 ($p < 0.05$ vs. vehicle-2) (Fig. 10a, b); NLRP3 inflammasome components: NLRP3, ASC, caspase-1, and downstream molecule, IL-1β ($p < 0.01$ vs. vehicle-2) (Fig. 10a, c, d, e, f). ILG at the dosage of 20 mg/kg and Nrf2 siRNA co-administration obviously alleviated the enhancement of protein expression levels of NF-κB p65, caspase-1, IL-1β ($p < 0.05$ vs. Nrf2 siRNA) (Fig. 10a, b, e, f), NLRP3, and ASC ($p < 0.01$ vs. Nrf2 siRNA) (Fig. 10a, c, d) after Nrf2 siRNA treatment at 24 h following ICH.

Discussion

Accumulating studies have displayed that oxidative stress and inflammation played key roles in the pathophysiological processes of early brain injury after ICH induction and inhibition of them were beneficial [5, 7, 44–46]. In our first experiment, we found that ILG administration at the dosages of 20 and 40 mg/kg ameliorated the early brain tissue impairments and behavioral defects as indicated by the reduction of mNSS scores and FJC$^+$ neuronal cells, the improvement of histological damages, BBB disruption, and brain edema at 24 and 72 h post ICH modeling and obtained the ideal dose of ILG at 20 mg/kg for the following experiments. In the second experiment, the results showed that ILG delivery at 20 mg/kg activated the Nrf2-mediated antioxidative signaling pathway and suppressed the activation of NF-κB and NLRP3 inflammasome pathways as indicated by the increasing of nuclear translocation and decreasing of the cytoplasmic level of Nrf2, the reduction of nuclear translocation and upregulation of cytoplasmic level of NF-κB p65, and the induction and activation of NLRP3 inflammasome (components) and its downstream molecules. In the third experiment, we found that Nrf2 siRNA notably

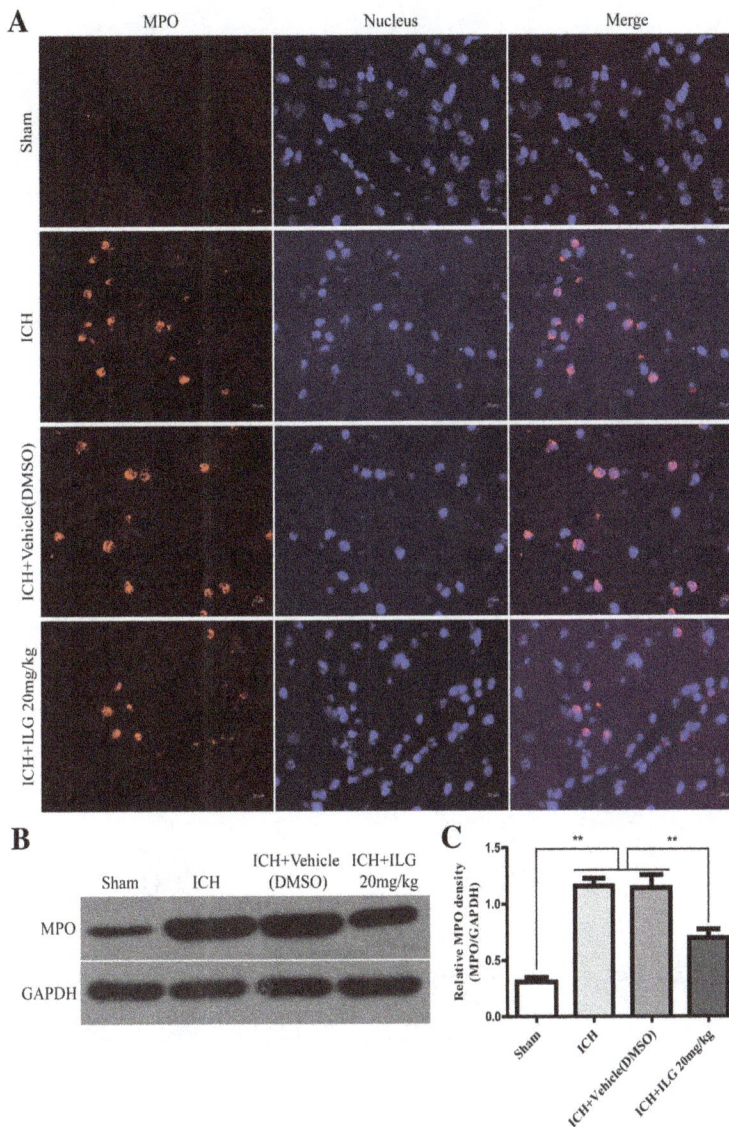

Fig. 7 Effects of ILG on the number of MPO$^+$ cells in perihematomal brain tissues (**a–c**). Representative microscopic images (**a**), WB bands (**b**), and quantitative analysis of the bands (**c**) ($n = 6$ rats/group). *Scale bar* = 20 μm. Values are reported as means ± SD. ***p* < 0.01

exacerbated the early brain injury post ICH as supported by aggravated behavioral deficits, brain edema, and degeneration of neuronal cells, and ILG treatment visibly alleviated the effects. Based on the results above, we hypothesized here that ILG alleviates early brain injury after ICH induction by activating Nrf2 antioxidant pathway, inhibiting the activation and induction of NLRP3 inflammasome (components), and this process may be involved in the suppression of ROS and/or NF-κB signaling pathways. Potential molecular mechanisms of ILG's effects on the early brain injury after ICH induction is shown in Additional file 3.

Results from our study have powerful evidence showing that ILG possesses a brain cell-protective function, and this was in line with previous studies in vivo [47–50] and

in vitro [26, 51, 52]. Pretreatment of ILG significantly alleviated neurological deficits, cerebral infarct, and brain edema, and these neuroprotective effects are involved in the increases of brain ATP content, energy charge (EC) and total adenine nucleotides (TAN) and preservation of brain Na$^+$ K$^+$ ATPase activity, SOD, CAT, and GSH-Px, and inhibition of the increase of brain MDA content in a rat cerebral ischemia-reperfusion model [50]. Toxicity of brain cells induced by cocaine and methamphetamine delivery was also able to be attenuated by ILG treatment [47–49]. Consistently, in in vitro studies, ILG protected neuronal cells from glutamate and 6-hydroxydopamine (6-OHDA)-induced neurotoxicity by reducing the production of ROS [51, 52]. Meanwhile, a recent report also showed that ILG treatment could notably alleviate

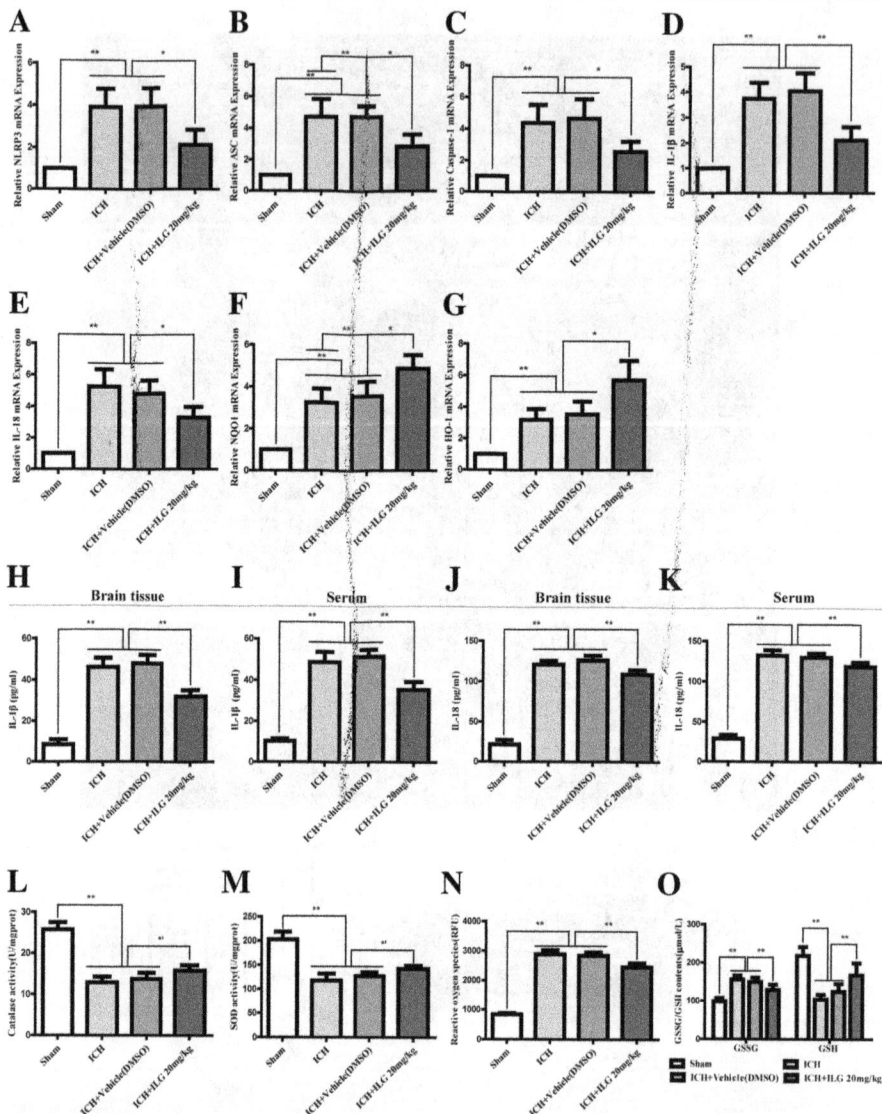

Fig. 8 Effects of ILG on the mRNA levels of NLRP3 inflammasome pathway components and downstream molecules of Nrf2-mediated antioxidant system, contents of inflammatory cytokines and antioxidants, and activity of antioxidative enzymes. ILG treatment at 20 mg/kg notably decreased the mRNA levels of NLRP3 (**a**), ASC (**b**), caspase-1 (**c**), IL-1β (**d**), IL-18 (**e**), and further increased the NQO1 (**f**), HO-1 (**g**) mRNA levels (n = 6 rats/group). Similarly, ILG administration at 20 mg/kg obviously reduced the levels of IL-1β (**h**, **i**) and IL-18 (**j**, **k**) in the perihematomal brain tissue and serum measured by ELISA (n = 6 rats/group). Besides, ILG delivery also markedly reversed the reduction of CAT and SOD activities (**l**, **m**), increasing of ROS (**n**) and GSSG (**o**) contents and decreasing of GSH level (**o**) (n = 6 rats/group). Values are reported as means ± SD. $**p < 0.01$; $*p < 0.05$; $*$: ICH vs. ICH + ILG 20 mg/kg, $p < 0.01$; ICH + vehicle (DMSO) vs. ICH + ILG 20 mg/kg, $p < 0.05$

rotenone and sodium nitroprusside (SNP)-induced oxidative stress and nitrosative stress by improving MMP, ATP levels, and neural cell viability [26].

ILG, one of the active extracts isolated from *G. uralensis*, is a flavonoid with chalcone structure and is brain-permeable after administration [53], which showed various biological activities including anti-inflammatory, antioxidative stress [9]. Increasing studies suggested that ILG exerts biological effects by activating Nrf2-mediated antioxidative system and eliminating ROS [9] and was the most potent inducer to stimulate the expression of Nrf2

and its downstream genes [28]. The activation mechanisms of Nrf2 by ILG might be involved in the alkylation of kelchlike ECH-associated protein 1 (Keap1) at specific cysteine residues, especially at the site of C151, a most reactive cysteine residue site of human Keap1 [54]. At the same time, there were reports showing that ILG upregulated the expression of HO-1 in RAW264.7 macrophages through the extracellular signal-regulated kinase1/2 (ERK1/2) pathway post lipopolysaccharide (LPS) treatment [55] and had inhibitory effects on LPS-induced inflammatory responses of mouse macrophages by suppressing NF-κB signaling

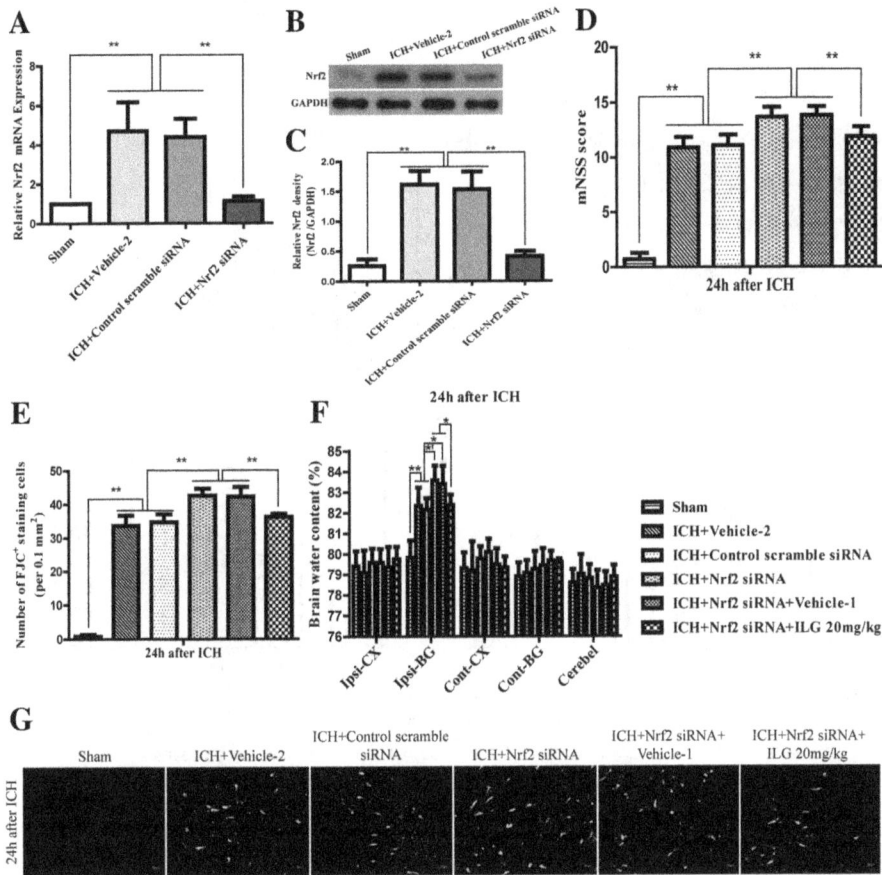

Fig. 9 Effects of Nrf2 siRNA delivery and Nrf2 siRNA with ILG 20 mg/kg co-administration in ICH rats. Real-time RT-qPCR assay of Nrf2 after siRNA delivery 24 h following ICH ($n = 6$ rats/group) (**a**). WB assay (**b**) and quantification (**c**) of Nrf2 protein after siRNA treatment 24 h following ICH ($n = 6$ rats/group); mNSS score (**d**) at 24 h post ICH ($n = 18$ rats/group). BWC (**f**) at 24 h after ICH ($n = 6$ rats/group). FJC staining (**g**) and quantification (**e**) of FJC$^+$ staining cells ($n = 6$ rats/group). Data represent means ± SD. *Scale bar* = 20 μm. **$p < 0.01$; *$p < 0.05$. *: ICH + vehicle-2 vs. ICH + Nrf2 siRNA, $p < 0.05$; ICH + control scramble siRNA vs. ICH + Nrf2 siRNA, $p < 0.01$

involved in the blockade of inhibitor of κBα (IκBα) degradation and phosphorylation [56]. In addition, recent reports also indicated that ILG induced the activation of Nrf2 as indicated by an increase in its nuclear translocation and the expression of Nrf2-targeted phase II enzymes, such as HO-1 and NQO1 [29]. In addition to the regulation of ILG on Nrf2 pathway, increasing evidences have suggested that ILG notably inhibited the activation of NF-κB pathway by suppressing LPS-induced TLR4/MD-2 homodimerization [57], blocking IκBα phosphorylation and degradation, reducing NF-κB p65 nuclear translocation [58], downregulating mRNA and protein levels of NF-κB and its activation [25, 59], and inhibiting RANKL-stimulated NF-κB expression and nuclear translocation [23].

The NLRP3 inflammasome, a best characterized pattern recognition receptor (PRR) in innate immune response, played a crucial component in the early brain injury post ICH [8, 16, 17] and was composed by a sensor (NLRP3 protein), an adaptor (ASC protein), and an effector (zymogen pro-caspase-1) [60, 61]. Production

of ROS, mitochondrial DNA or the mitochondrial phospholipid cardiolipin, potassium efflux, changes in cell volume, calcium, and lysosomal impairments have all been proposed as critical active signals to trigger the activation of NLRP3 inflammasome [60, 61]. Activation of NLRP3 inflammasome demands two signals. One is the stimulus of NF-kB pathway that after NF-κB activation, NF-κB translocates into the nucleus, after binding with DNA and initiating the transcription and translation of IL-1β precursor protein and NLRP3 protein; another one is to trigger the assembly of NLRP3 inflammasome and lead to its stimulus such as production of ROS. Following triggered, active NLRP3 inflammasome recruits precursor caspase-1 and cleaves it into active caspase-1, and then the cleaved caspase-1 processes IL-1β and IL-18 precursors into mature IL-1β and IL-18, eventually augmenting the inflammatory responses and impairments [60, 61].

Recently, several studies have demonstrated that NLRP3 inflammasome pathway was activated after ICH

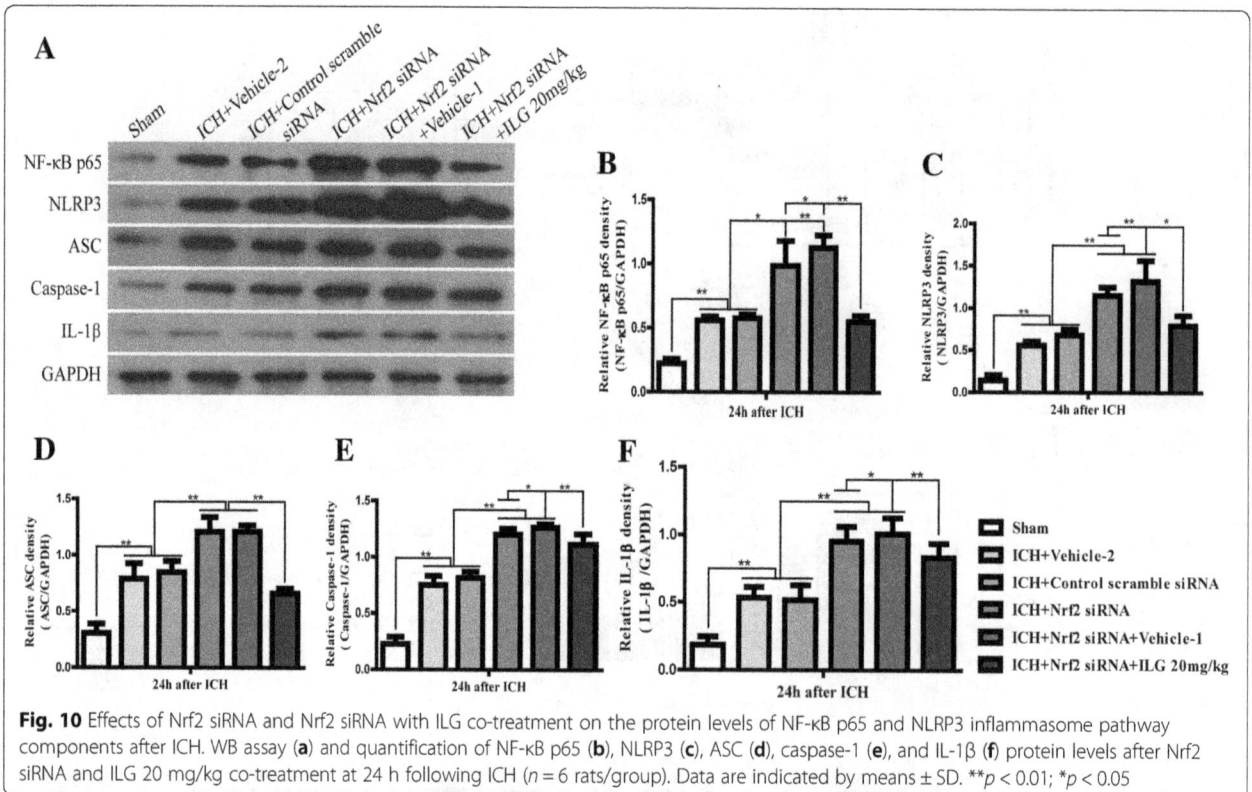

Fig. 10 Effects of Nrf2 siRNA and Nrf2 siRNA with ILG co-treatment on the protein levels of NF-κB p65 and NLRP3 inflammasome pathway components after ICH. WB assay (**a**) and quantification of NF-κB p65 (**b**), NLRP3 (**c**), ASC (**d**), caspase-1 (**e**), and IL-1β (**f**) protein levels after Nrf2 siRNA and ILG 20 mg/kg co-treatment at 24 h following ICH ($n = 6$ rats/group). Data are indicated by means ± SD. **$p < 0.01$; *$p < 0.05$

induction, and the inhibiting of NLRP3 using siRNA or recombinant adenovirus encoding NLRP3 RNAi could attenuate the brain injury including improving behavioral deficits and reducing brain edema and MPO level. Hence, ROS and the activation of NF-κB pathway were the crucial upstream signals, and blocking them can reduce the activation of NLRP3 inflammasome. In our study, we have verified that Nrf2 triggering via ILG administration significantly decreased the production of oxidative stress markers 3-NT and 8-OHdG and suppressed the activation of NF-κB; meanwhile, the NLRP3 inflammasome was restrained. The results suggested that Nrf2 could downregulate the activity and expression of NLRP3 inflammasome (components) and were in keeping with previous reports [18, 22]. To further proved our assumption, we conducted Nrf2 siRNA interfering and Nrf2 siRNA + ILG 20 mg/kg co-administration study in a rat ICH model. The results showed that after Nrf2 siRNA treatment, the brain injuries were more severe and ILG (20 mg/kg) obviously attenuated the impairments. These also were consistent with the studies of other groups, namely, Nrf2 was involved in the regulation of ILG-mediated NLRP3 inflammasome activation [18, 22] and the activation of Nrf2 pathway was neuroprotective [9, 12, 13, 31].

Microglia are the key immune cells existing in the central nervous system (CNS) and are commonly referred to as the macrophage of the brain. Microglia

are considered to be the first non-neuronal cells to react to various pathological processes after ICH and thus once the condition ictus, microglia are immediately activated by a various of blood components and then activated microglia release multiple cytokines and chemokines, following peripheral inflammatory cells (including neutrophils, macrophages) infiltrating into the hemorrhagic brain and are activated, next producing a mass of cytokines, chemokines, and cytotoxicity substance [4, 62]. Thus, both the activation and infiltration of neutrophils and microglia/macrophages synergistically contribute to the inflammatory brain injury post ICH and play crucial role on the pathological mechanisms [4, 62]. Our experimental results have shown that ILG administration could notably reduce the number of perihematomal neutrophils and microglia/macrophages as well.

Also, iron, one key component of hemoglobin (Hb) metabolites, was reported to be involved in the secondary brain injury. Excessive production of iron could lead to oxidative brain impairments by Fenton reaction, which yields massive ROS. Furthermore, HO-1 promotes the level of iron by participating in the degradation of heme [63, 64]. Besides, ILG was also reported to counteract iron-catalyzed oxidative stress damages in HepG2 cells by AMPK-mediated GSK3β inhibition which was involved in mitochondrial dysfunction and superoxide generation [65]. Meanwhile, in our experiments, we found that ILG administration could significantly inhibit the level of ROS and promote the expression of HO-1 in the injury brain tissue. Thus, the relationship of iron metabolism and neuroprotective effects of ILG needs to be further explored.

Thrombin, a serine protease produced immediately in brain after ICH to prevent the bleeding. It may be a central injury mechanism of ICH and was shown to mediate the secondary brain injury by multiple pathways including complement cascade and protease-activated receptors (PAR) [63, 64]. Recently, thrombin was also reported to be involved in the activation of NLRP3 inflammasome and microglia and induced severe brain injury including brain edema, BBB disruption, and brain cell loss [66, 67]. In our study, we found that ILG 20 mg/kg could efficaciously block-ade the activation of NLRP3 inflammasome and infiltration of neutrophils and microglia/macrophages into the injury brain tissue. Thus, whether ILG exerts its protective effects involved in the thrombin-mediated brain injury pathway remains to be further investigated.

There are several potential limitations deserving attention in our experiments. Firstly, ILG was reported to perform a variety of biological functions by regulating multiple signaling pathways, and we mainly concentrated on the Nrf2, ROS, NF-κB, and NLRP3 inflammasome pathways. However, ILG may exert its effects on other signaling pathways. Secondly, we just carried out our study on a kind of ICH model (sterile-filtered collagenase type IV-induced), not concurrently on other ICH models such as autologous blood-imitated model of ICH. The results derived from our experiments should be more convincing by more than one model to be verified. Finally, collagenase itself is a kind of foreign matter and is unavoidable to trigger extra inflammatory responses. Consequently, further experiments are needed to settle these issues.

Conclusions

Taken together, our experiments have identified that ILG administration notably attenuated the early brain injury after ICH induction and the underlying molecular mechanisms of these beneficial effects are involved in the regulation of ROS and/or NF-κB on the activation of NLRP3 inflammasome pathway by the triggering of Nrf2 activity and Nrf2-induced anti-oxidant system. In addition, our experimental results might provide a novel therapeutical strategy for ICH.

Additional files

Additional file 1: Experimental design and groups (a-c). MRI and Hematoma Volume Evaluation (d). The captions of Additional file 2 and 3 (e). (PDF 235 kb)

Additional file 2: Effects of ILG on the hematoma volume and expansion at 24 h and 72 h after ICH (a, b) and effects of ILG on the number of CD68$^+$, Iba-1$^+$ cells in the perihematomal brain tissue at 24 h after ICH (c-e). Representative MRI T2WI images (a) and quantitative analyses of hematoma volume (b) (n = 6 rats / group). Representative microscopic images (c) and quantitative analyses of CD68$^+$, Iba-1$^+$ cells (d, e) (n = 6 rats /group). Scale bar = 20 μm. Values are reported as means ± SD. ** p < 0.01, * p < 0.05. (TIF 7318 kb)

Additional file 3: Mechanism diagram. Underlying molecular mechanisms of ILG's neuroprotective effects on the early brain injury after ICH induction. ILG alleviated the early brain injury following ICH may be involved in the regulation of ROS and / or NF-κB on the activation of NLRP3 inflammasome pathway by the triggering of Nrf2 activity and the induction of Nrf2-mediated antioxidant system. (TIF 232 kb)

Abbreviations

3-NT: 3-Nitrotyrosine; 6-OHDA: 6-Hydroxydopamine; 8-OHdG: 8-Hydroxyguanosine; ANOVA: Analysis of variance; ARE: Antioxidant response element; BBB: Blood-brain barrier; BSA: Bovine serum albumin; BWC: Brain water content; CAT: Catalase; CNS: Central nervous system; DAB: 3,3-Diaminobenzidine; DAPI: 4'6-Diamidino-2-phenylindole; DMSO: Dimethylsulfoxide; EB: Evans blue; EC: Energy charge; EDTA: Ethylene diamine tetraacetic acid; ELISA: Enzyme-linked immunosorbent assay; ERK1/2: Extracellular signal-regulated kinase1/2; FJC: Fluoro-Jade® C; G. uralensis: Glycyrrhiza uralensis; GAPDH: Glyceraldehyde 3-phosphate dehydro-genase; GPX: Glutathione peroxidase; GSH/GSSG: Glutathione/oxidized glutathione; GST: Glutathione-S-transferase; H&E: Hematoxylin and eosin; Hb: Hemoglobin; HO-1: Heme oxygenase-1; HRP: Horseradish peroxidase; i.p.: Intraperitoneal injection; ICH: Intracerebral hemorrhage; IF: Immunofluorescence; IHC: Immunohistochemistry; IL-1β: Interleukin-1 beta; ILG: Isoliquiritigenin; IκBα: Inhibitor of κBα; Keap1: Kelchlike ECH-associated protein 1; LPS: Lipopolysaccharide; LSD: Least significant difference; mNSS: Modified Neurological Severity Score; MPO: Myeloperoxidase; MRI: Magnetic resonance imaging; NF-κB: Nuclear factor-κB; NLRP3: Nod-like receptor family, pyrin domain-containing 3; NO: Nitric oxide; NQO1: NAD(P)H: quinone oxidoreductase-1; Nrf2: Nuclear factor erythroid-2 related factor 2; PAR: Protease-activated receptor; PBS: Phosphate buffer solution; PRR: Pattern recognition receptor; ROS: Reactive oxygen species; RT-qPCR: Real-time reverse transcription-quantitative polymerase chain reaction; SD: Standard deviation; SD rats: Sprague-Dawley rats; siRNA: Small interfering RNA; SNP: Sodium nitroprusside; SOD: Superoxide dismutase; SPF: Specific pathogen-free; T2WI: T2-weighted images; TAN: Total adenine nucleotides; WB: Western blot

Acknowledgements
It has been shown as Funding.

Funding
This work was supported by the National Natural Science Foundation of China (Nos. 81671125, 81271314, and 30500526), Special Project on the Integration of Industry, Education and Research of Guangdong Province and Ministry of Education (No. 2012B091100154), Natural Science Foundation of Guangdong (No. 2014A030313346 and 5300468), and the Guangdong Provincial Clinical Medical Centre for Neurosurgery (No. 2013B020400005).

Authors' contributions
YZC and JZ conceived and designed the experiments. JZ performed the experiments. YZC and JZ analyzed the data. JZ wrote the paper. YZC, RD, LF, SY, XQD, ZHF, ZCX, and SZZ contributed to the paper revision, provided experimental technical support, and assisted in completing the study at different stages. All authors read and approved the final manuscript.

Competing interests
The authors declare that they have no competing interests.

Author details

[1]Department of Neurosurgery, Zhujiang Hospital, The National Key Clinical Specialty, The Neurosurgery Institute of Guangdong Province, Guangdong Provincial Key Laboratory on Brain Function Repair and Regeneration, The Engineering Technology Research Center of Education Ministry of China, Southern Medical University, Guangzhou 510282, China. [2]Department of Neurosurgery, Jingmen No. 1 People's Hospital, Jingmen 448000, Hubei, China. [3]Department of Neurosurgery, Affiliated Hospital of Xiangnan University, Chenzhou 423000, Hunan, China. [4]Department of Neurosurgery, The Fifth Affiliated Hospital of Southern Medical University, Guangzhou 510900, Guangdong, China. [5]Department of Neurosurgery, Gaoqing Campus of Central Hospital of Zibo, Gaoqing People's Hospital, Gaoqing, Zibo 256300, Shandong, China. [6]Department of Neurosurgery, 999 Brain Hospital, Jinan University, Guangzhou 510510, Guangdong, China.

References

1. Keep RF, Hua Y, Xi G. Intracerebral haemorrhage: mechanisms of injury and therapeutic targets. Lancet Neurol. 2012;11:720–31.

2. Adeoye O, Broderick JP. Advances in the management of intracerebral hemorrhage. Nat Rev Neurol. 2010;6:593–601.

3. Chen S, Yang Q, Chen G, Zhang JH. An update on inflammation in the acute phase of intracerebral hemorrhage. Transl Stroke Res. 2015;6:4–8.

4. Zhou Y, Wang Y, Wang J, Anne SR, Yang QW. Inflammation in intracerebral hemorrhage: from mechanisms to clinical translation. Prog Neurobiol. 2014; 115:25–44.

5. Hu X, Tao C, Gan Q, Zheng J, Li H, You C. Oxidative stress in intracerebral hemorrhage: sources, mechanisms, and therapeutic targets. Oxid Med Cell Longev. 2016;2016:3215391.

6. Broderick JP, Brott TG, Duldner JE, Tomsick T, Huster G. Volume of intracerebral hemorrhage. A powerful and easy-to-use predictor of 30-day mortality. Stroke. 1993;24:987–93.

7. Duan X, Wen Z, Shen H, Shen M, Chen G. Intracerebral hemorrhage, oxidative stress, and antioxidant therapy. Oxid Med Cell Longev. 2016;2016: 1203285.

8. Ma Q, Chen S, Hu Q, Feng H, Zhang JH, Tang J. NLRP3 inflammasome contributes to inflammation after intracerebral hemorrhage. Ann Neurol. 2014;75:209–19.

9. Denzer I, Munch G, Friedland K. Modulation of mitochondrial dysfunction in neurodegenerative diseases via activation of nuclear factor erythroid-2-related factor 2 by food-derived compounds. Pharmacol Res. 2016;103:80–94.

10. Calkins MJ, Johnson DA, Townsend JA, Vargas MR, Dowell JA, Williamson TP, Kraft AD, Lee JM, Li J, Johnson JA. The Nrf2/ARE pathway as a potential therapeutic target in neurodegenerative disease. Antioxid Redox Signal. 2009;11:497–508.

11. Shang H, Yang D, Zhang W, Li T, Ren X, Wang X, Zhao W. Time course of Keap1-Nrf2 pathway expression after experimental intracerebral haemorrhage: correlation with brain oedema and neurological deficit. Free Radic Res. 2013;47:368–75.

12. Iniaghe LO, Krafft PR, Klebe DW, Omogbai EK, Zhang JH, Tang J. Dimethyl fumarate confers neuroprotection by casein kinase 2 phosphorylation of Nrf2 in murine intracerebral hemorrhage. Neurobiol Dis. 2015;82:349–58.

13. Zhao X, Sun G, Zhang J, Ting SM, Gonzales N, Aronowski J. Dimethyl fumarate protects brain from damage produced by intracerebral hemorrhage by mechanism involving Nrf2. Stroke. 2015;46:1923–8.

14. Wang J, Fields J, Zhao C, Langer J, Thimmulappa RK, Kensler TW, Yamamoto M, Biswal S, Dore S. Role of Nrf2 in protection against intracerebral hemorrhage injury in mice. Free Radic Biol Med. 2007;43:408–14.

15. Zhao X, Sun G, Zhang J, Strong R, Dash PK, Kan YW, Grotta JC, Aronowski J. Transcription factor Nrf2 protects the brain from damage produced by intracerebral hemorrhage. Stroke. 2007;38:3280–6.

16. Yuan B, Shen H, Lin L, Su T, Zhong S, Yang Z. Recombinant adenovirus encoding NLRP3 RNAi attenuate inflammation and brain injury after intracerebral hemorrhage. J Neuroimmunol. 2015;287:71–5.

17. Feng L, Chen Y, Ding R, Fu Z, Yang S, Deng X, Zeng J. P2X7R blockade prevents NLRP3 inflammasome activation and brain injury in a rat model of intracerebral hemorrhage: involvement of peroxynitrite. J Neuroinflammation. 2015;12:190.

18. Liu X, Zhang X, Ding Y, Zhou W, Tao L, Hu R. Nuclear factor E2-related factor-2 (Nrf2) negatively regulates NLRP3 inflammasome activity by inhibiting reactive oxygen species (ROS)-induced NLRP3 priming. Antioxid Redox Signal. 2017;26(1):28–43.

19. Rzepecka J, Pineda MA, Al-Riyami L, Rodgers DT, Huggan JK, Lumb FE, Khalaf AI, Meakin PJ, Corbet M, Ashford ML, et al. Prophylactic and therapeutic treatment with a synthetic analogue of a parasitic worm product prevents experimental arthritis and inhibits IL-1beta production via NRF2-mediated counter-regulation of the inflammasome. J Autoimmun. 2015;60:59–73.

20. Peng F, Du Q, Peng C, Wang N, Tang H, Xie X, Shen J, Chen J. A review: the pharmacology of isoliquiritigenin. Phytother Res. 2015;29:969–77.

21. Gnanaguru G, Choi AR, Amarnani D, D'Amore PA. Oxidized lipoprotein uptake through the CD36 receptor activates the NLRP3 inflammasome in human retinal pigment epithelial cells. Invest Ophthalmol Vis Sci. 2016;57:4704–12.

22. Honda H, Nagai Y, Matsunaga T, Okamoto N, Watanabe Y, Tsuneyama K, Hayashi H, Fujii I, Ikutani M, Hirai Y, et al. Isoliquiritigenin is a potent inhibitor of NLRP3 inflammasome activation and diet-induced adipose tissue inflammation. J Leukoc Biol. 2014;96:1087–100.

23. Liu S, Zhu L, Zhang J, Yu J, Cheng X, Peng B. Anti-osteoclastogenic activity of isoliquiritigenin via inhibition of NF-kappaB-dependent autophagic pathway. Biochem Pharmacol. 2016;106:82–93.

24. Kwon HM, Choi YJ, Choi JS, Kang SW, Bae JY, Kang IJ, Jun JG, Lee SS, Lim SS, Kang YH. Blockade of cytokine-induced endothelial cell adhesion molecule expression by licorice isoliquiritigenin through NF-kappaB signal disruption. Exp Biol Med (Maywood). 2007;232:235–45.

25. Wu Y, Chen X, Ge X, Xia H, Wang Y, Su S, Li W, Yang T, Wei M, Zhang H, et al. Isoliquiritigenin prevents the progression of psoriasis-like symptoms by inhibiting NF-kappaB and proinflammatory cytokines. J Mol Med (Berl). 2016;94:195–206.

26. Denzer I, Munch G, Pischetsrieder M, Friedland K. S-allyl-L-cysteine and isoliquiritigenin improve mitochondrial function in cellular models of oxidative and nitrosative stress. Food Chem. 2016;194:843–8.

27. Foresti R, Bains SK, Pitchumony TS, de Castro BL, Drago F, Dubois-Rande JL, Bucolo C, Motterlini R. Small molecule activators of the Nrf2-HO-1 antioxidant axis modulate heme metabolism and inflammation in BV2 microglia cells. Pharmacol Res. 2013;76:132–48.

28. Gong H, Zhang BK, Yan M, Fang PF, Li HD, Hu CP, Yang Y, Cao P, Jiang P, Fan XR. A protective mechanism of licorice (Glycyrrhiza uralensis): isoliquiritigenin stimulates detoxification system via Nrf2 activation. J Ethnopharmacol. 2015;162:134–9.

29. Park SM, Lee JR, Ku SK, Cho IJ, Byun SH, Kim SC, Park SJ, Kim YW. Isoliquiritigenin in licorice functions as a hepatic protectant by induction of antioxidant genes through extracellular signal-regulated kinase-mediated NF-E2-related factor-2 signaling pathway. Eur J Nutr. 2016;55(8):2431–44.

30. Rosenberg GA, Mun-Bryce S, Wesley M, Kornfeld M. Collagenase-induced intracerebral hemorrhage in rats. Stroke. 1990;21:801–7.

31. Xue F, Huang JW, Ding PY, Zang HG, Kou ZJ, Li T, Fan J, Peng ZW, Yan WJ. Nrf2/antioxidant defense pathway is involved in the neuroprotective effects of Sirt1 against focal cerebral ischemia in rats after hyperbaric oxygen preconditioning. Behav Brain Res. 2016;309:1–8.

32. Dang B, Li H, Xu X, Shen H, Wang Y, Gao A, He W, Wang Z, Chen G. Cyclophilin A/cluster of differentiation 147 interactions participate in early brain injury after subarachnoid hemorrhage in rats. Crit Care Med. 2015;43:e369–81.

33. Chen J, Li Y, Wang L, Zhang Z, Lu D, Lu M, Chopp M. Therapeutic benefit of intravenous administration of bone marrow stromal cells after cerebral ischemia in rats. Stroke. 2001;32:1005–11.

34. Chen J, Sanberg PR, Li Y, Wang L, Lu M, Willing AE, Sanchez-Ramos J, Chopp M. Intravenous administration of human umbilical cord blood reduces behavioral deficits after stroke in rats. Stroke. 2001;32:2682–8.

35. Ding R, Feng L, He L, Chen Y, Wen P, Fu Z, Lin C, Yang S, Deng X, Zeng J, Sun G. Peroxynitrite decomposition catalyst prevents matrix metalloproteinase-9 activation and neurovascular injury after hemoglobin injection into the caudate nucleus of rats. Neuroscience. 2015;297:182–93.

36. Ding R, Chen Y, Yang S, Deng X, Fu Z, Feng L, Cai Y, Du M, Zhou Y, Tang Y. Blood-brain barrier disruption induced by hemoglobin in vivo: Involvement of up-regulation of nitric oxide synthase and peroxynitrite formation. Brain Res. 2014;1571:25–38.

37. Yang F, Wang Z, Zhang JH, Tang J, Liu X, Tan L, Huang QY, Feng H. Receptor for advanced glycation end-product antagonist reduces blood-brain barrier damage after intracerebral hemorrhage. Stroke. 2015;46:1328–36.

38. Belayev L, Busto R, Zhao W, Ginsberg MD. Quantitative evaluation of blood-brain barrier permeability following middle cerebral artery occlusion in rats. Brain Res. 1996;739:88–96.

39. Uyama O, Okamura N, Yanase M, Narita M, Kawabata K, Sugita M. Quantitative evaluation of vascular permeability in the gerbil brain after transient ischemia using Evans blue fluorescence. J Cereb Blood Flow Metab. 1988;8:282–4.

40. Yang S, Chen Y, Deng X, Jiang W, Li B, Fu Z, Du M, Ding R. Hemoglobin-induced nitric oxide synthase overexpression and nitric oxide production contribute to blood-brain barrier disruption in the rat. J Mol Neurosci. 2013;51:352–63.

41. Schmued LC, Stowers CC, Scallet AC, Xu L. Fluoro-Jade C results in ultra high resolution and contrast labeling of degenerating neurons. Brain Res. 2005;1035:24–31.

42. Min H, Jang YH, Cho IH, Yu SW, Lee SJ. Alternatively activated brain-infiltrating macrophages facilitate recovery from collagenase-induced intracerebral hemorrhage. Mol Brain. 2016;9:42.

43. Livak KJ, Schmittgen TD. Analysis of relative gene expression data using real-time quantitative PCR and the 2(-Delta Delta C(T)) Method. Methods. 2001;25:402–8.

44. Mracsko E, Veltkamp R. Neuroinflammation after intracerebral hemorrhage. Front Cell Neurosci. 2014;8:388.

45. Qu J, Chen W, Hu R, Feng H. The injury and therapy of reactive oxygen species in intracerebral hemorrhage looking at mitochondria. Oxid Med Cell Longev. 2016;2016:2592935.

46. Ziai WC. Hematology and inflammatory signaling of intracerebral hemorrhage. Stroke. 2013;44:S74–8.

47. Jang EY, Choe ES, Hwang M, Kim SC, Lee JR, Kim SG, Jeon JP, Buono RJ, Yang CH. Isoliquiritigenin suppresses cocaine-induced extracellular dopamine release in rat brain through GABA(B) receptor. Eur J Pharmacol. 2008;587:124–8.

48. Jeon JP, Buono RJ, Han BG, Jang EY, Kim SC, Yang CH, Hwang M. Proteomic and behavioral analysis of response to isoliquiritigenin in brains of acute cocaine treated rats. J Proteome Res. 2008;7:5094–102.

49. Lee MJ, Yang CH, Jeon JP, Hwang M. Protective effects of isoliquiritigenin against methamphetamine-induced neurotoxicity in mice. J Pharmacol Sci. 2009;111:216–20.

50. Zhan C, Yang J. Protective effects of isoliquiritigenin in transient middle cerebral artery occlusion-induced focal cerebral ischemia in rats. Pharmacol Res. 2006;53:303–9.

51. Hwang CK, Chun HS. Isoliquiritigenin isolated from licorice Glycyrrhiza uralensis prevents 6-hydroxydopamine-induced apoptosis in dopaminergic neurons. Biosci Biotechnol Biochem. 2012;76:536–43.

52. Yang EJ, Min JS, Ku HY, Choi HS, Park MK, Kim MK, Song KS, Lee DS. Isoliquiritigenin isolated from Glycyrrhiza uralensis protects neuronal cells against glutamate-induced mitochondrial dysfunction. Biochem Biophys Res Commun. 2012;421:658–64.

53. Mogami S, Sadakane C, Nahata M, Mizuhara Y, Yamada C, Hattori T, Takeda H. CRF receptor 1 antagonism and brain distribution of active components contribute to the ameliorative effect of rikkunshito on stress-induced anorexia. Sci Rep. 2016;6:27516.

54. Luo Y, Eggler AL, Liu D, Liu G, Mesecar AD, van Breemen RB. Sites of alkylation of human Keap1 by natural chemoprevention agents. J Am Soc Mass Spectrom. 2007;18:2226–32.

55. Lee SH, Kim JY, Seo GS, Kim YC, Sohn DH. Isoliquiritigenin, from Dalbergia odorifera, up-regulates anti-inflammatory heme oxygenase-1 expression in RAW264.7 macrophages. Inflamm Res. 2009;58:257–62.

56. Wang R, Zhang CY, Bai LP, Pan HD, Shu LM, Kong AN, Leung EL, Liu L, Li T. Flavonoids derived from liquorice suppress murine macrophage activation by up-regulating heme oxygenase-1 independent of Nrf2 activation. Int Immunopharmacol. 2015;28:917–24.

57. Honda H, Nagai Y, Matsunaga T, Saitoh S, Akashi-Takamura S, Hayashi H, Fujii I, Miyake K, Muraguchi A, Takatsu K. Glycyrrhizin and isoliquiritigenin suppress the LPS sensor toll-like receptor 4/MD-2 complex signaling in a different manner. J Leukoc Biol. 2012;91:967–76.

58. Zhu L, Wei H, Wu Y, Yang S, Xiao L, Zhang J, Peng B. Licorice isoliquiritigenin suppresses RANKL-induced osteoclastogenesis in vitro and prevents inflammatory bone loss in vivo. Int J Biochem Cell Biol. 2012;44:1139–52.

59. Watanabe Y, Nagai Y, Honda H, Okamoto N, Yamamoto S, Hamashima T, Ishii Y, Tanaka M, Suganami T, Sasahara M, et al. Isoliquiritigenin attenuates adipose tissue inflammation in vitro and adipose tissue fibrosis through inhibition of innate immune responses in mice. Sci Rep. 2016;6:23097.

60. Sharma D, Kanneganti TD. The cell biology of inflammasomes: mechanisms of inflammasome activation and regulation. J Cell Biol. 2016;213:617–29.

61. Lamkanfi M, Dixit VM. Mechanisms and functions of inflammasomes. Cell. 2014;157:1013–22.

62. Zhang Z, Zhang Z, Lu H, Yang Q, Wu H, Wang J. Microglial polarization and inflammatory mediators after intracerebral hemorrhage. Mol Neurobiol. 2017;54:1874–86.

63. Babu R, Bagley JH, Di C, Friedman AH, Adamson C. Thrombin and hemin as central factors in the mechanisms of intracerebral hemorrhage-induced secondary brain injury and as potential targets for intervention. Neurosurg Focus. 2012;32:E8.

64. Hua Y, Keep RF, Hoff JT, Xi G. Brain injury after intracerebral hemorrhage: the role of thrombin and iron. Stroke. 2007;38:759–62.

65. Choi SH, Kim YW, Kim SG. AMPK-mediated GSK3beta inhibition by isoliquiritigenin contributes to protecting mitochondria against iron-catalyzed oxidative stress. Biochem Pharmacol. 2010;79:1352–62.

66. Wan S, Cheng Y, Jin H, Guo D, Hua Y, Keep RF, Xi G. Microglia activation and polarization after intracerebral hemorrhage in mice: the role of protease-activated receptor-1. Transl Stroke Res. 2016;7(6):478–87.

67. Zuo D, Ye X, Yu L, Zhang L, Tang J, Cui C, Bao L, Zan K, Zhang Z, Yang X, et al. ROS/TXNIP pathway contributes to thrombin induced NLRP3 inflammasome activation and cell apoptosis in BV2 cells. Biochem Biophys Res Commun. 2017;485(2):499–505.

P2X7R blockade prevents NLRP3 inflammasome activation and brain injury in a rat model of intracerebral hemorrhage: involvement of peroxynitrite

Liang Feng[1], Yizhao Chen[1*], Rui Ding[2], Zhenghao Fu[3], Shuo Yang[4], Xinqing Deng[5] and Jun Zeng[1]

Abstract

Background: The NLR family, pyrin domain-containing 3 (NLRP3) inflammasome plays a key role in intracerebral hemorrhage (ICH)-induced inflammatory injury, and the purinergic 2X7 receptor (P2X7R) is upstream of NLRP3 activation. This study aimed to investigate how P2X7R functions in ICH-induced inflammatory injury and how the receptor interacts with the NLRP3 inflammasome.

Methods: Rats were treated with P2X7R small interfering RNA (siRNA) 24 h before undergoing collagenase-induced ICH. A selective P2X7R inhibitor (blue brilliant G, BBG) or a peroxynitrite ($ONOO^-$) decomposition catalyst (5,10,15,20-tetrakis(4-sulfonatophenyl)porphyrinato iron(III) [FeTPPS]) was injected 30 min after ICH. Brain water content, hemorrhagic lesion volume, and neurological deficits were evaluated, and western blot, immunofluorescence, and terminal deoxynucleotidyl transferase dUTP nick end labeling (TUNEL) were carried out.

Results: Striatal P2X7R and NLRP3 inflammasomes were activated after ICH. Gene silencing of P2X7R suppressed NLRP3 inflammasome activation and interleukin (IL)-1β/IL-18 release and significantly ameliorated brain edema and neurological deficits. Additionally, enhanced NADPH oxidase 2 (NOX2, gp91^{phox}) and inducible nitric oxide synthase (iNOS), as well as their cytotoxic product ($ONOO^-$) were markedly attenuated by BBG treatment following ICH. This was accompanied by downregulations of the inflammasome components, IL-1β/IL-18 and myeloperoxidase (MPO, a neutrophil marker). Most importantly, inflammasome activation and IL-1β/IL-18 release were significantly inhibited by $ONOO^-$ decomposition with FeTPPS.

Conclusions: Our findings implicate that P2X7R exacerbated inflammatory progression and brain damage in ICH rats possibly via NLRP3 inflammasome-dependent IL-1β/IL-18 release and neutrophil infiltration. $ONOO^-$, a potential downstream signaling molecule of P2X7R, may play a critical role in triggering NLRP3 inflammasome activation.

Keyword: P2X7R, NLRP3, Peroxynitrite, Intracerebral hemorrhage, NOX2, IL-1β

Background

Spontaneous intracerebral hemorrhage (ICH) is a devastating stroke subtype, with high morbidity and mortality [1]. Unfortunately, no satisfactory pharmacologic treatments have been found for clinical practice, mainly due to a lack of knowledge underlying the mechanisms of post-

ICH brain damage. There is an urgent need to clarify the pathophysiology of this disease to identify effective therapies.

Accumulating evidence suggests that innate immunity and inflammatory responses are involved in ICH-induced secondary brain injury [1–3]. The intracellular Nod-like receptors have recently been shown to play a critical role in the process of innate immunity and inflammatory responses [4]. The NLR family, pyrin domain-containing 3 (NLRP3) inflammasome, the best characterized member of Nod-like receptor family, is a multiprotein complex that

* Correspondence: yizhao_chen@hotmail.com
[1]The National Key Clinical Specialty, The Engineering Technology Research Center of Education Ministry of China, Guangdong Provincial Key Laboratory on Brain Function Repair and Regeneration, Department of Neurosurgery, Zhujiang Hospital, Southern Medical University, Guangzhou 510282, China
Full list of author information is available at the end of the article

contains the adaptor protein apoptosis-associated speck-like protein containing a CARD (ASC) and the effector caspase-1. Once activated, caspase-1 can cleave the pro forms of interleukin (IL)-1β and IL-18 into their mature and active forms, which leads to the recruitment and activation of other immune cells, such as neutrophils [5]. In this regard, evidence indicates that the NLRP3 inflammasome plays a pivotal role in ICH [2] and other central nervous system (CNS) conditions [6–11], but the precise mechanisms associated with inflammasome activation continue to be debated.

The role of ATP-gated transmembrane cation channel P2X7R in the signaling cascade has received particular attention due to its widespread involvement as a key regulatory element of NLRP3 inflammasome activation [12]. A growing number of studies have demonstrated the important pathophysiological functions of P2X7R in CNS disorders, including ischemic stroke, subarachnoid hemorrhage, neurotrauma, epilepsy, neuropathic pain, and neurodegenerative illnesses [13, 14]. However, the specific role of P2X7R in ICH has not yet been established, and the interaction between P2X7R and the NLRP3 inflammasome in the development of ICH-induced brain injury remains unclear.

In the case of ICH, both NADPH oxidase 2 (NOX2) and inducible nitric oxide synthase (iNOS) have been reported to contribute to brain injury; knockout mice exhibit less brain edema and cell death than wild-type controls following ICH [15, 16]. Superoxide anion (O_2^-) and nitric oxide (NO), released through NOX and iNOS in activated microglia, act as devastating pro-inflammatory mediators in CNS diseases [17]. More importantly, peroxynitrite ($ONOO^-$), the product of a diffusion-controlled reaction of NO with O_2^-, is a more potent oxidant species and is involved in the pathologies of ischemic stroke, neurotrauma, and neurodegenerative diseases [18–20]. We previously demonstrated that abundant $ONOO^-$ formed in a hemoglobin (Hb)-induced ICH rat model [21], but the exact mechanisms of $ONOO^-$ in brain injury after ICH have not been fully characterized. Besides its ability to oxidize or nitrate proteins, lipids, and DNA, $ONOO^-$ can also lead to destructive pathological consequences by triggering the activation of several biochemical pathways engaged in the development of neuroinflammation and IL-1β production [22–24]. However, the precise link between $ONOO^-$ formation and IL-1β secretion in ICH is unclear.

The P2X7R acts as an upstream molecule of NOX2 activation signaling in many in vivo and in vitro disease

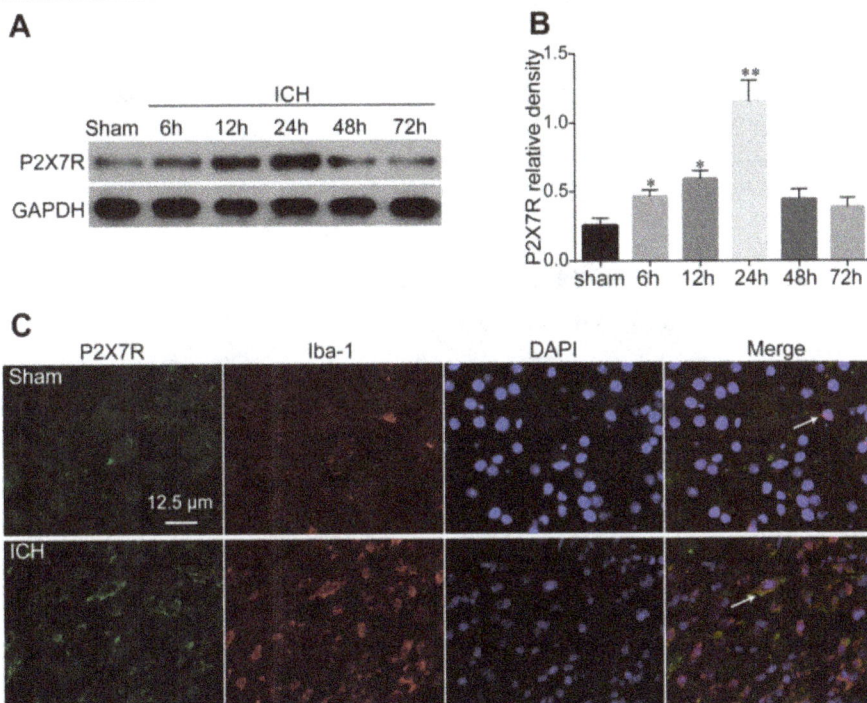

Fig. 1 Expression profile of P2X7R and its cellular location after collagenase-induced intracerebral hemorrhage (ICH). Western blot analysis (**a**) for the time course of P2X7R expression in the ipsilateral hemisphere of Sham and ICH rats within 72 h. Quantification of P2X7R (**b**) expression is shown, n = 4 rats per group and time point. Confocal images (**c**) of double immunofluorescence for P2X7R expression in Iba-1-positive microglia 24 h following ICH, n = 6 rats per group. Scale bar = 12.5 µm. Data represent means ± SD. *P < 0.05 vs. Sham, **P < 0.01 vs. Sham. *GAPDH* glyceraldehyde 3-phosphate dehydrogenase, *ICH* intracerebral hemorrhage

models [25–27]. NOX2-mediated oxidative stress was recently proposed to be responsible for activation of the NLRP3 inflammasome and subsequent neurovascular damage in ischemic stroke [7]. Notably, P2X7R-dependent NADPH oxidase activation and $ONOO^-$ formation play key roles in caspase-1 and IL-1β processing in endotoxin-primed human monocytes [28]. In an animal model of lipopolysaccharide (LPS)-induced striatum injury, activated P2X7R in microglia was associated with increased iNOS and 3-nitrotyrosine (3-NT, a reliable marker of $ONOO^-$), and this was reversed by the P2X7R antagonist oxidized ATP (oxATP) [29]. Despite this knowledge, the potential roles of P2X7R and NLRP3 inflammasomes and NOX2/iNOS-dependent $ONOO^-$ formation in the development of ICH-induced brain damage remain to be clarified.

We hypothesized that $ONOO^-$, formed from NOX2-derived O_2^- and iNOS-derived NO, may be involved in transducing P2X7R-mediated IL-1β/IL-18 production and brain injury via NLRP3 inflammasome activation after ICH. We first investigated the expression profiles of P2X7R and the NLRP3 inflammasome components. Next, a mixed small interfering (si) RNA was applied to knock down P2X7R in vivo, and alterations in NLRP3 inflammasome components and functional outcomes were measured. We then explored the therapeutic effect of the selective P2X7R antagonist, blue brilliant G (BBG). Additionally, we observed iNOS- and NOX2-dependent formation of $ONOO^-$ and their alterations in ICH rats following BBG treatment. Finally, to determine whether

$ONOO^-$ is involved in P2X7R-mediated NLRP3 inflammasome activation, we used an $ONOO^-$ decomposition catalyst in vivo and measured the expression levels of P2X7R and NLRP3 inflammasome components.

Materials and methods
Animals
Sprague–Dawley (SD) male rats weighing 280–320 g were purchased from the Animal Experiment Center of Southern Medical University (Guangzhou, China). All experimental procedures and animal care were approved by the Southern Medical University Ethics Committee.

ICH model
After anesthetization (0.3 ml/100 g, 10 % chloral hydrate, Sigma-Aldrich, St. Louis, MO, USA), an incision was made on the skin along the sagittal midline to expose the skull. A burr hole (1 mm) was drilled 3 mm lateral and 1 mm anterior to the bregma, then a 30-gauge needle was inserted through the burr hole into the striatum (6 mm ventral from the skull surface), and ICH was induced by stereotaxic infusion of bacterial collagenase VII-S (0.25U in 1.0 μl sterile saline, Sigma-Aldrich) over a 10-min period. In the Sham group, rats were subjected to only a needle insertion as described above. The needle was kept in situ for another 10 min to prevent backflow and then slowly removed. The craniotomies were sealed with bone wax. Rats were allowed to recover in separate cages with free access to food and water.

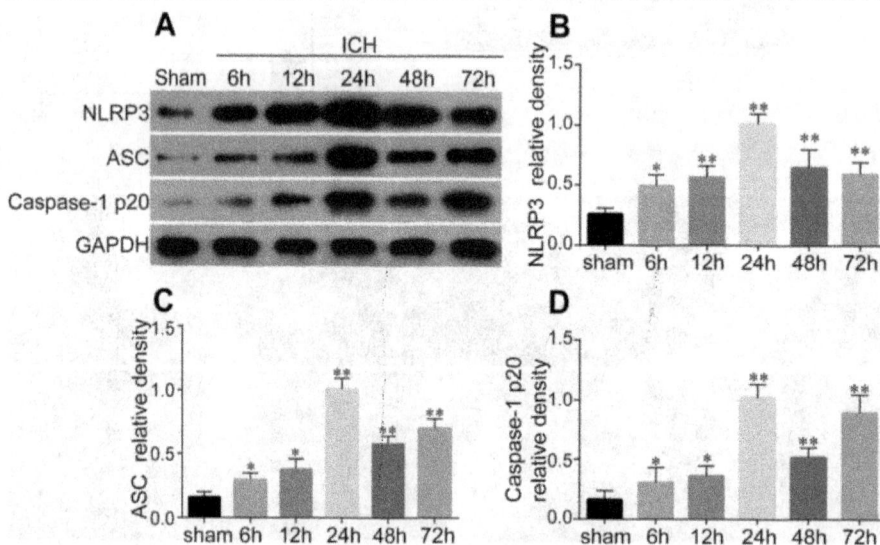

Fig. 2 Expression profiles of NLRP3, ASC, and caspase-1 p20 subunit after ICH. Western blot analysis (**a**) for the time course expressions of NLRP3 (**b**), ASC (**c**), and caspase-1 p20 subunit (**d**) in the ipsilateral hemisphere of Sham and ICH rats within 72 h. Quantification of NLRP3, ASC, and caspase-1 p20 subunit expression is shown, respectively, $n = 4$ rats per group and time point. Data represent means ± SD. $^*P < 0.05$ vs. Sham, $^{**}P < 0.01$ vs. Sham. *ASC* adaptor protein apoptosis-associated speck-like protein containing a CARD, *GAPDH* glyceraldehyde 3-phosphate dehydrogenase, *ICH* intracerebral hemorrhage, *NLRP3* pyrin domain-containing 3

Experimental protocol

Four separate experiments were conducted as shown in Additional file 1.

Experiment 1

Thirty-six rats were divided into six groups (Sham, and 6, 12, 24, 48, and 72 h after ICH). The expression levels of P2X7R, NLRP3, ASC, and caspase-1 were detected by western blot. The tissue for immunofluorescence (IF) was collected 24 h after ICH induction.

Experiment 2

Eighty-eight rats were randomized into four groups: Sham, Vehicle (ICH + saline, intracerebroventricular injection), Scramble small interfering RNA (siRNA) (1000 pmol, 2 μl, ICH + scramble siRNA), and P2X7R siRNA (1000 pmol, 2 μl, ICH + P2X7R siRNA). siRNA silencing efficacy was assessed by western blot. Brain water content and modified Neurological Severity Score (mNSS) were also measured.

Experiment 3

One hundred and thirty-two rats were randomized into four groups: Sham, Vehicle (ICH + saline, intraperitoneal injection), BBG (50 mg/kg), and BBG (100 mg/kg). For the 72-h study, BBG was administered daily by intraperitoneal injection. Western blot, hematoxylin and eosin (H&E) staining, immunofluorescence (IF), and terminal deoxynucleotidyl transferase dUTP nick end labeling (TUNEL) were measured 24 h after ICH induction; mNSS and brain water content were detected at both 24 and 72 h.

Experiment 4

Thirty-three rats were randomized into three groups: Sham, Vehicle (ICH + saline, intraperitoneal injection), and FeTPPS (30 mg/kg). Western blotting was performed 24 h after ICH induction.

siRNA and drug delivery

BBG (Sigma-Aldrich) was diluted at 50 and 100 mg/kg in Vehicle (saline) solution. Rats were treated intraperitoneally with either BBG or Vehicle immediately after ICH induction and at 12, 36, and 60 h.

For in vivo siRNA administration, P2X7R siRNA or non-silencing RNA (Sigma-Aldrich) was applied 24 h before ICH by intracerebroventricular injection as previously described [2]. A cranial burr hole (1 mm) was drilled, and a 30-gauge needle was inserted stereotaxically into the right lateral ventricle. To improve the gene

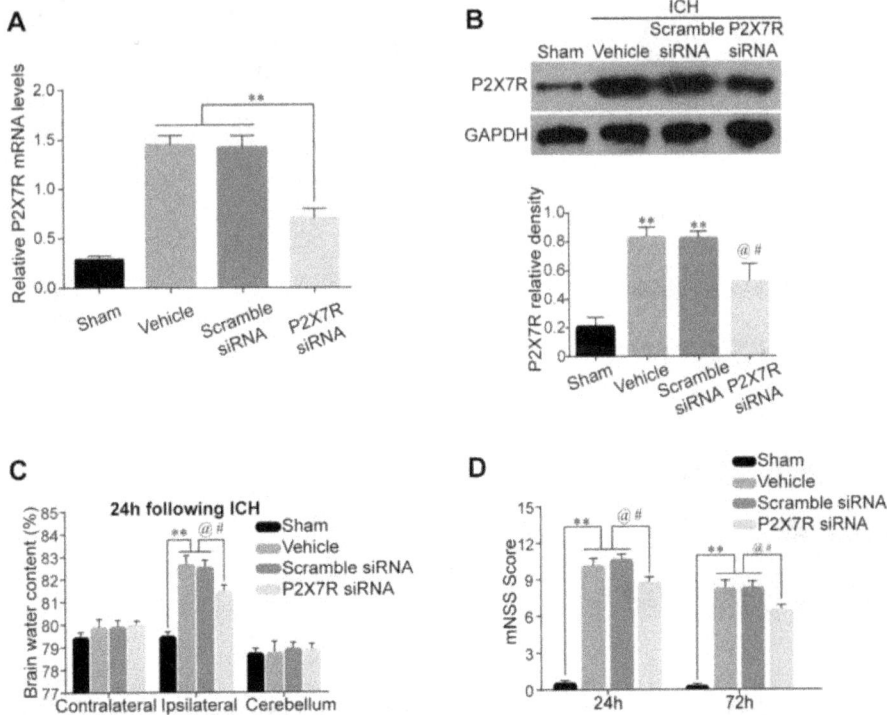

Fig. 3 Effects of P2X7R small interfering RNA (siRNA) treatment in ICH rats. RT-PCR of P2X7R after siRNA treatment 24 h following ICH, $n = 6$ rats per group (**a**). Western blot assay and quantification of P2X7R (**b**) after siRNA treatment 24 h following ICH, $n = 4$ rats per group. Brain edema (**c**) at 24 h after ICH, $n = 6$ rats per group. mNSS (**d**) at 24 and 72 h after ICH, $n = 6$ rats per group. Data represent means ± SD. $^{**}P < 0.01$ vs. Sham, $^{@}P < 0.05$ vs. Vehicle, $^{#}P < 0.05$ vs. ICH + Scramble siRNA. *GAPDH* glyceraldehyde 3-phosphate dehydrogenase, *mNSS* modified Neurological Severity Score, *siRNA* small interfering RNA

silence efficiency, two different sequences targeting P2X7R siRNA were combined (a)sense:5′-CAGUGAA UGAGUACUACUA-3′; antisense:5′-UAGUAGUACU CAUUCACUG-3′; (b)sense:5′-CUCUUGAGGAGCGC CGAAA-3′;antisense:5′-UUUCGGCGCUCCUCAAGA G-3′. siRNA was dissolved in RNA free water. Scrambled control siRNA (1000 pmol, 2 μl), P2X7R siRNA (1000 pmol, 2 μl), or RNA free water (2 μl) was delivered intracerebroventricularly for 2 min. The needle was left in place for an additional 10 min after injection and then slowly withdrawn.

FeTPPS (Millipore, Billerica, MA, USA) was diluted to 30 mg/kg in Vehicle (saline) solution. Rats were treated intraperitoneally with either FeTPPS or Vehicle immediately and at 12 h after ICH induction. The FeTPPS dose was selected based on our previous reports that showed that it is effectively protected against injury [30].

RT-PCR

Rats were anesthetized and decapitated. Lesioned tissues (about 40 mg) were obtained, and total RNA was extracted from the tissue with GeneJET™ RNA Purification Kit (Thermo Fisher Scientific Inc., Waltham, MA, USA). RNA (1 μg) was reverse-transcribed to cDNA with high capacity (Life Technologies, Carlsbad, CA, USA). RT-PCR was performed in an ABI Prism 7500 sequence detection system (Applied Biosystems, Foster City, CA, USA) using specific primers designed from known sequences. GAPDH was used as an endogenous control gene. Sequence-specific primers for P2X7R, NLRP3, and GADPH were as follows:

P2X7R, 5′-CTACTCTTCGGTGGGGGCTT-3′ (forward primer),
P2X7R, 5′-CTCTGGATCCGGGTGACTTT-3′ (reverse primer);
NLRP3, 5′-CTGCATGCCGTATCTGGTTG-3′

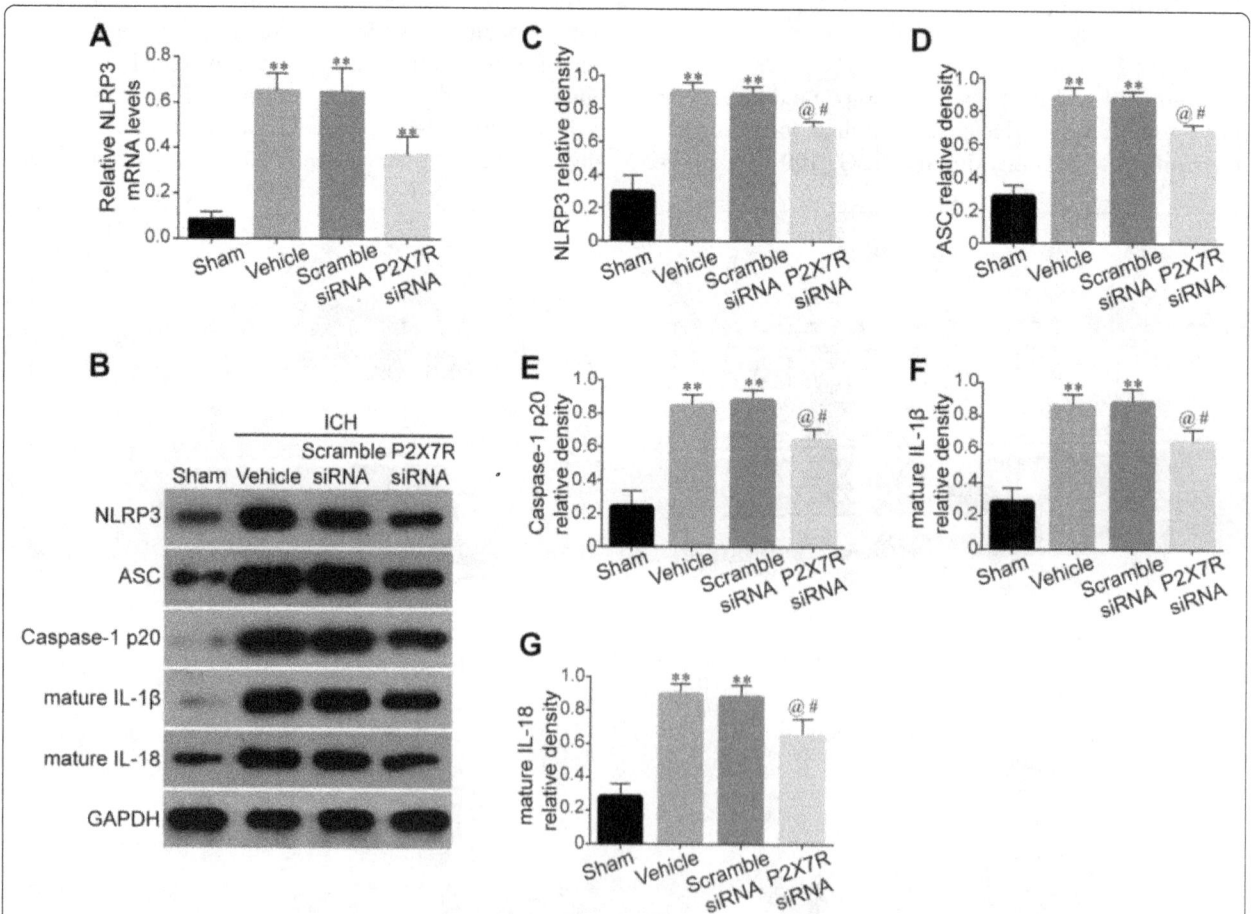

Fig. 4 Effects of P2X7R siRNA on NLRP3 inflammasome activation and IL-1β/IL-18 maturation after ICH. RT-PCR of NLRP3 after P2X7R siRNA treatment 24 h following ICH (**a**), $n = 6$ rats per group. Western blot assay (**b**) and quantification of NLRP3 (**c**), ASC (**d**), caspase-1 p20 subunit (**e**), IL-1β (**f**), and IL-18 (**g**) after P2X7R siRNA treatment 24 h following ICH, $n = 4$ rats per group. Data represent means ± SD. $**P < 0.01$ vs. Sham, $@P < 0.05$ vs. Vehicle, $\#P < 0.05$ vs. ICH + Scramble siRNA. *ASC* adaptor protein apoptosis-associated speck-like protein containing a CARD, *GAPDH* glyceraldehyde 3-phosphate dehydrogenase, *ICH* intracerebral hemorrhage, *IL* interleukin, *NLRP3* The NLR family, pyrin domain-containing 3

(forward primer),
NLRP3, 5′-GCTGAGCAAGCTAAAGGCTTC-3′
(reverse primer);
GAPDH, 5′-AGACAGCCGCATCTTCTTGT-3′
(forward primer),
GAPDH, 5′- TGATGGCAACAATGTCCACT-3'
(reverse primer);

Western blot

Western blotting was performed as described previously [30]. The following primary antibodies were used: rabbit polyclonal anti-P2X7R (1:1000, Alomone Labs, Jerusalem, Israel), rabbit polyclonal anti-NLRP3 antibody (1:1000, Santa Cruz, Biotechnology, Santa Cruz, CA, USA), rabbit polyclonal anti-ASC antibody (1:500, Abclonal, Cambridge,

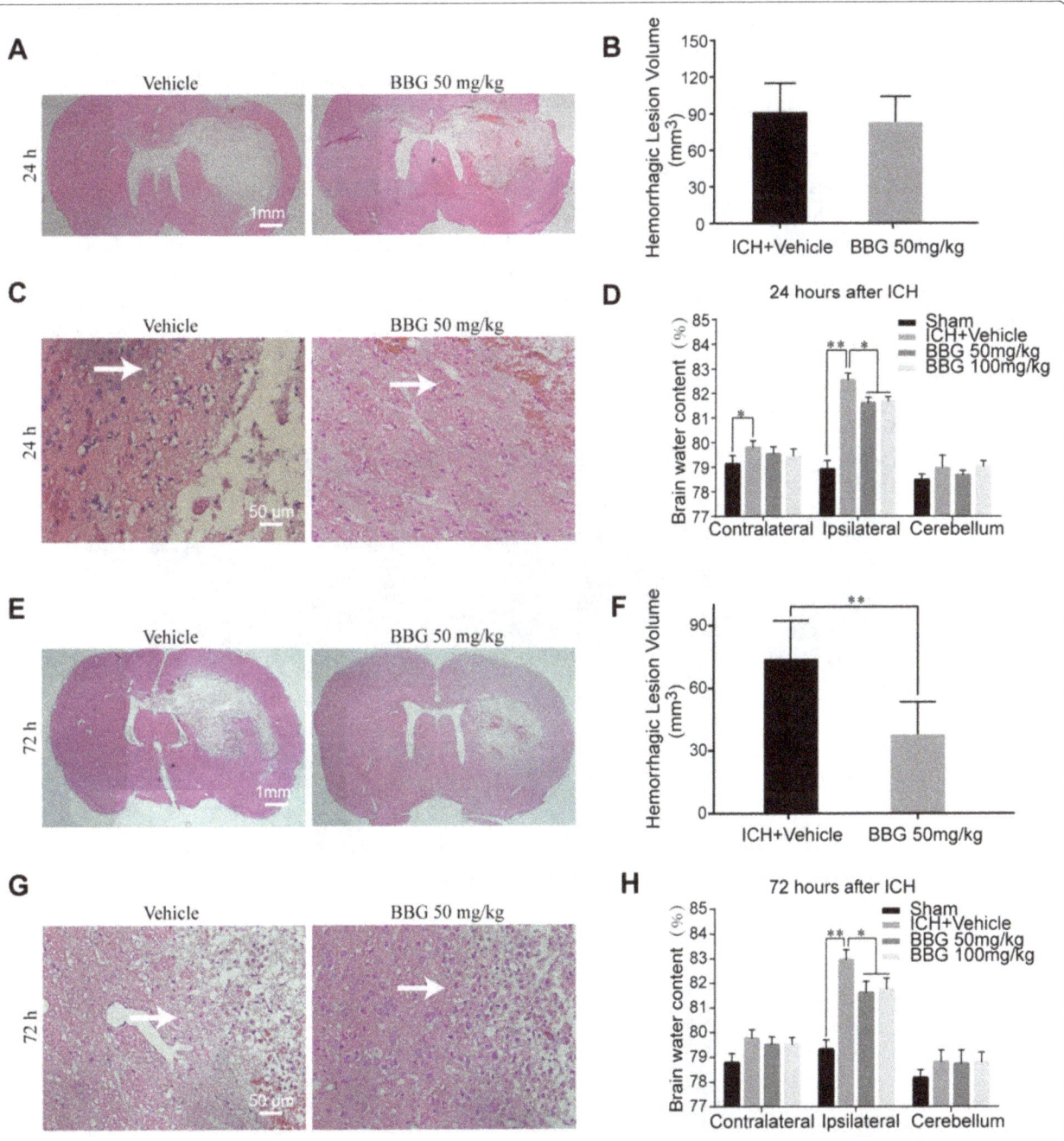

Fig. 5 Effects of BBG on brain edema in ICH rats. BBG treatment evidently reduced brain edema at 24 (**d**) and at 72 h (**h**) after ICH. Hematoxylin and eosin (H&E) showed the hemorrhagic lesion volume alteration after BBG treatment at 24 (**a**, **b**) and at 72 h (**e**, **f**) following ICH. Tissue damage after BBG treatment at 24 (**c**) and at 72 h (**g**) following ICH. $n = 6$ rats per group. Data represent means ± SD. $^{*}P < 0.05$, $^{**}P < 0.01$. *BBG* brilliant blue G, *ICH* intracerebral hemorrhage

MA, USA), mouse monoclonal anti-caspase-1 p20 antibody (1:1000, Santa Cruz Biotechnology), rabbit polyclonal anti-IL-1β antibody (1:1000, Millipore), rabbit monoclonal anti-IL-18 antibody (1:1000, Abcam, Cambridge, UK), mouse monoclonal anti-nitrotyrosine antibody (1:1000, Abcam), mouse monoclonal anti-iNOS antibody (1:200, Santa Cruz Biotechnology), mouse monoclonal anti-gp91[phox] antibody (1:2000, BD Transduction Laboratories, San Jose, CA, USA), and rabbit polyclonal anti-myeloperoxidase antibody (MPO, 1:500, Abcam). GAPDH (1:1000, Cell Signaling Technology, Danvers, MA, USA) was employed as the loading control. Blot bands were quantified by densitometry with ImageJ software (National Institutes of Health, Baltimore, MD, USA).

Paraffin section preparations
The sections were processed as previously described [30] with minor modifications. After anesthetization, rats were transcardially perfused with 200 ml saline followed by 400 ml 4 % paraformaldehyde solution. Brain tissues were then removed and fixed by immersion in the same solution at 4 °C for 24 h. After dehydration and

vitrification, they were embedded in paraffin, and 3-μm sections were prepared. Sections were dewaxed, rehydrated, and then processed for IF and TUNEL.

Histological examination
Coronal sections (1 mm apart) [31] were prepared accordingly and then stained with H&E. Hemorrhagic volumes were calculated using Image Pro Plus 6.0 software (Media Cybernetics, USA) to span the entire hematoma [32].

IF
Antigen retrieval was performed by heat treatment in a microwave oven for 21 min in Tris–EDTA buffer solution (0.05 mol/L Tris, 0.001 mol/L EDTA; pH 8.5). Sections were incubated for 30 min in 5 % bovine serum albumin (BSA) and then incubated at 4 °C overnight with primary antibodies (rabbit polyclonal anti-P2X7R, 1:500, Alomone labs; mouse monoclonal anti-3-Nitrotyrosine, 1:400, Abcam; rabbit polyclonal anti-nitrotyrosine antibody, 1:200, Millipore; rabbit polyclonal anti-MPO antibody, 1:50, Abcam; rabbit polyclonal anti-iNOS antibody, 1:40, Santa Cruz Biotechnology; rabbit

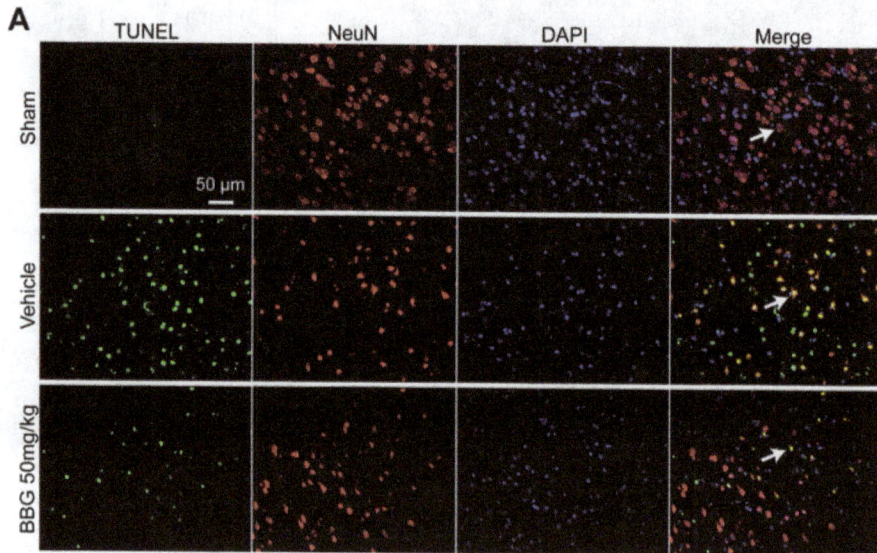

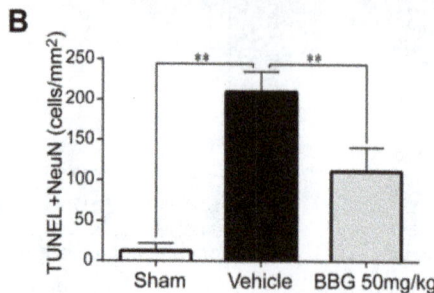

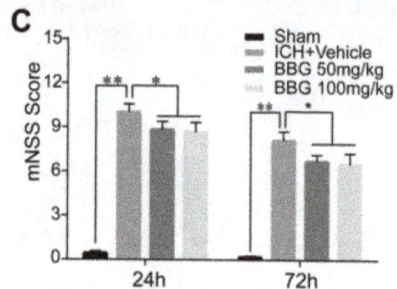

Fig. 6 Effects of BBG on neuronal apoptosis and neurological outcomes in ICH rats. BBG significantly reduced the number of apoptotic neurons (**a**, **b**) 24 h following ICH, $n = 6$ rats per group. BBG significantly improved neurological deficits (**c**) at 24 and at 72 h after ICH, $n = 6$ rats per group. Scale bar = 50 μm. Data represent means ± SD. $^{*}P < 0.05$, $^{**}P < 0.01$. *BBG* brilliant blue G

polyclonal anti-Iba-1 antibody, 1:600, WAKO, Osaka, Japan; goat polyclonal anti-Iba-1 antibody, 1:300, Abcam; mouse monoclonal gp91^{phox} antibody, 1:400, BD Transduction Laboratories). For double-staining experiments, primary antibodies were separately incubated overnight at 4 °C. After they were washed with phosphate-buffered saline (PBS), sections were then incubated with secondary antibodies. Images were obtained using confocal microscopes (FV10i-W, Olympus, Tokyo, Japan; LSM780, Zeiss, Oberkochen, Germany).

TUNEL

At 24 h after ICH, TUNEL staining was performed with an in situ apoptosis detection kit (Roche, Basel, Switzerland) according to the manufacturer's instruction. For NeuN and TUNEL co-staining, the sections were first labeled with a NeuN antibody (1:400, Abcam), followed by TUNEL. The slides were analyzed using a fluorescence microscope (Bx51, Olympus).

Brain water content measurement

Brain edema was evaluated by a common wet/dry method as previously described [33]. Briefly, at 24 or 72 h post-ICH, rats were anesthetized and decapitated. The brains were removed and immediately separated into contralateral and ipsilateral hemispheres and the cerebellum and wet weighed. The cerebellum was used as an internal control. Brain specimens were dried in an oven at 100 °C for 24 h to obtain the dry weight. The water content was expressed as a percentage of the wet weight: ([wet weight] − [dry weight]) / (wet weight) × 100 %.

Behavioral testing

Behavioral tests were assessed with mNSS at 24 and 72 h after ICH by an investigator who was blinded to the experimental groups [34].

Statistical analysis

Data are shown as mean ± SD. Statistical analysis was performed using SPSS 13.0 (SPSS Inc., Chicago, IL, USA).

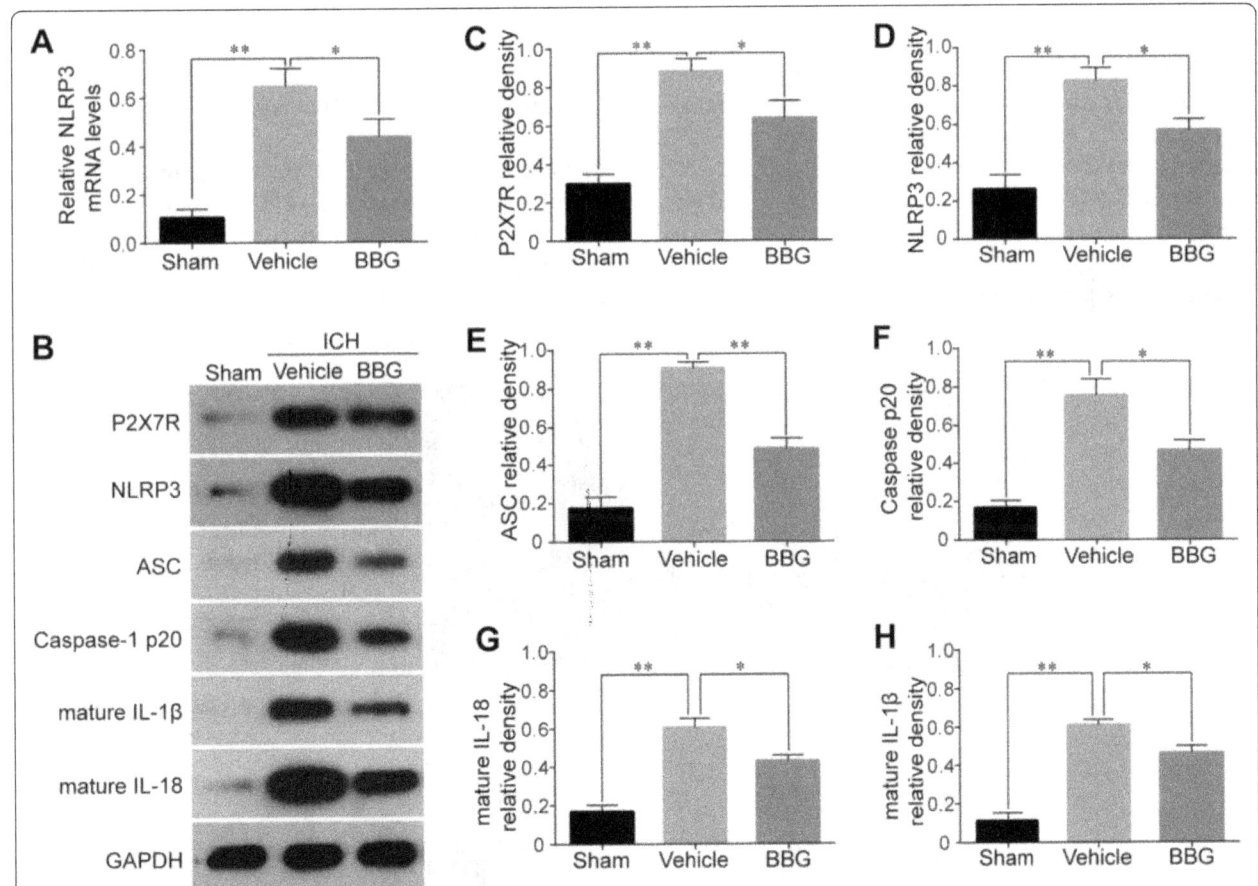

Fig. 7 Effects of BBG on NLRP3 inflammasome activation and IL-1β/IL-18 maturation. RT-PCR of NLRP3 after BBG treatment 24 h following ICH, n = 6 rats per group (**a**). Representative western blot (**b**) and therapeutic effects of BBG on P2X7R (**c**), NLRP3 (**d**), ASC (**e**), caspase-1 p20 subunit (**f**), mature IL-1β (**g**), and mature IL-18 (**h**) levels in the ipsilateral hemisphere 24 h after ICH, n = 4 rats per group. Data represent means ± SD. *P < 0.05, **P < 0.01. ASC adaptor protein apoptosis-associated speck-like protein containing a CARD, BBG brilliant blue G, GAPDH glyceraldehyde 3-phosphate dehydrogenase, ICH intracerebral hemorrhage, IL interleukin, NLRP3 pyrin domain-containing 3

Comparison between groups was determined by Student's t tests or one-way analysis of variance (ANOVA) followed by least significant difference (LSD) tests with multiple comparisons. The statistically significant level was $P < 0.05$.

Results

P2X7R was increased and mainly expressed in microglia cells following ICH

Protein content was analyzed at different time points after injection to investigate whether P2X7R would respond to collagenase-induced ICH. As shown by western blot (Fig. 1a, b), P2X7R levels were significantly elevated at 6 h after ICH ($P < 0.05$ vs. Sham) and peaked at around 24 h ($P < 0.01$ vs. Sham) when P2X7R levels were nearly 4.5 times more than those in the Sham group. Following the peak, P2X7R levels decreased, returning close to baseline levels at 72 h.

Double immunolabeling was performed to identify the cell type that expresses P2X7R. The results showed that P2X7R was predominantly expressed in microglia cells (Fig. 1c) and not in other cell types, such as astrocytes or neurons (Additional file 2).

NLRP3, ASC, and caspase-1 were upregulated after ICH

NLRP3 inflammasome has been proposed to be downstream of P2X7R [12]. We evaluated the expressions of NLRP3 inflammasome components by western blot (Fig. 2a). NLRP3 (Fig. 2b), ASC (Fig. 2c), and cleaved caspase-1 (Fig. 2d) were significantly upregulated at 6 h ($P < 0.05$ vs. Sham) and reached their peak at 24 h post-ICH ($P < 0.01$ vs. Sham). Following this peak, levels of all three proteins declined

but still remained higher than those in the Sham group at 48 h ($P < 0.05$ vs. Sham) and 72 h ($P < 0.05$ vs. Sham).

P2X7R RNA interference reduced brain water content and improved neurological outcomes

We next explored whether P2X7R is involved in brain injury following ICH. Two P2X7R siRNA mixtures were applied 24 h before ICH induction. Silencing efficacy by RT-PCR demonstrated a significant inhibitory effect of P2X7R siRNA on its mRNA levels ($P < 0.01$) (Fig. 3a). Western blot (Fig. 3b) showed 41.3 and 40.7 % reductions of P2X7R in the P2X7R siRNA group compared with the Vehicle and Scramble siRNA groups, respectively (both $P < 0.05$), at 24 h after ICH. Brain water content in the ipsilateral hemisphere was significantly increased in the Vehicle (82.56 ± 0.72 % vs. Sham, 79.40 ± 0.44 %, $P < 0.01$) and Scramble siRNA (82.44 ± 0.75 % vs. Sham, 79.40 ± 0.44 %, $P < 0.01$) groups at 24 h post-ICH, while that in P2X7R siRNA group was decreased to 81.39 ± 0.58 % ($P < 0.05$ vs. Vehicle or Scramble siRNA) (Fig. 3c). Consistent with the brain edema results, P2X7R siRNA administration significantly ameliorated neurological deficits at 24 h (8.66 ± 1.15 vs. Vehicle, 10.00 ± 1.95, $P < 0.05$; vs. Scramble siRNA, 10.50 ± 1.26, $P < 0.05$) and 72 h (6.33 ± 0.81 vs. Vehicle, 8.10 ± 1.96, $P < 0.05$; vs. Scramble siRNA, 8.16 ± 1.16, $P < 0.05$) post-ICH (Fig. 3d).

P2X7R RNA interference inhibited NLRP3 inflammasome activation and subsequent IL-1β/IL-18 release

NLRP3 inflammasome is actively involved in brain injury after ICH [2]. We further clarify the role of P2X7R in NLRP3/ASC/caspase-1 activation and the subsequent

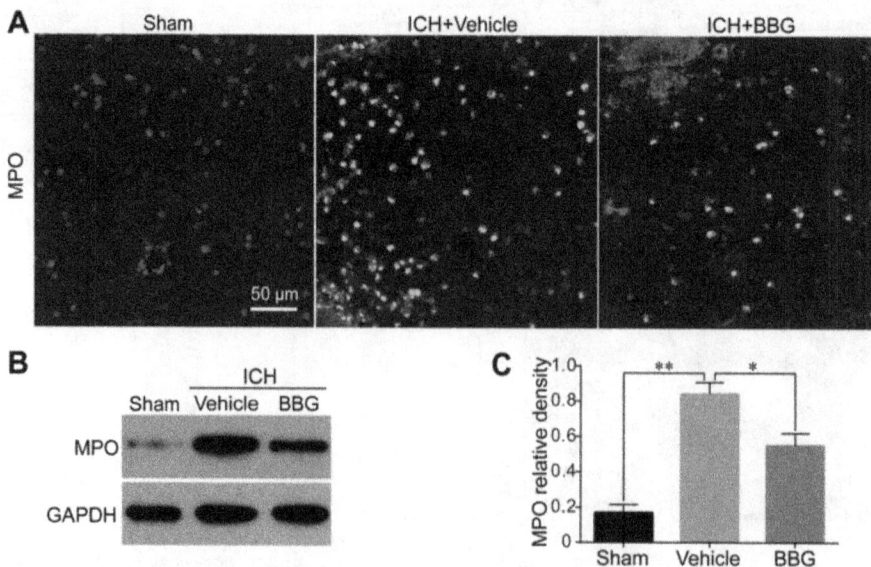

Fig. 8 Effects of BBG on neutrophils infiltration after ICH. Representative photographs of immunofluorescence staining (**a**) for MPO (neutrophil marker)-positive cells in perihematomal area in the Sham, Vehicle, and BBG (50 mg/kg) groups at 24 h following operation, $n = 6$ rats per group. Representative western blot (**b**) and effects of BBG on MPO levels (**c**) at 24 h after ICH, $n = 4$ rats per group. Scale bar = 50 μm. Data represent means ± SD. *$P < 0.05$, **$P < 0.01$. BBG brilliant blue G, ICH intracerebral hemorrhage

processing of IL-1β/IL-18. P2X7R siRNA treatment significantly reduced NLRP3 mRNA expression ($P < 0.01$) (Fig. 4a). The protein levels of NLRP3 inflammasome component and IL-1β/IL-18 production were evidently elevated in the Vehicle and Scramble siRNA groups at 24 h after ICH ($P < 0.01$). P2X7R siRNA treatment significantly suppressed caspase-1 activation and the subsequent secretion of mature IL-1β/IL-18 ($P < 0.05$) (Fig. 4b–f).

BBG deceased post-ICH neurological deficits, brain water content, and neuronal apoptosis

Next, we investigated the effects of the selective P2X7R inhibitor, BBG. Both doses (50 and 100 mg/kg) significantly attenuated brain water content at 24 h (50 mg/kg, 81.76 ± 0.32 % vs. Vehicle, 82.54 ± 0.66 %, $P < 0.05$; 100 mg/kg, 81.67 ± 0.43 % vs. Vehicle, 82.54 ± 0.66 %, $P < 0.05$) and 72 h (50 mg/kg, 81.59 ± 1.15 % vs. Vehicle, 82.94 ± 1.00 %, $P < 0.05$; 100 mg/kg, 81.74 ± 1.12 % vs. Vehicle, 82.94 ± 1.00 %, $P < 0.05$) after ICH (Fig. 5d, h). The hemorrhagic lesion volume at 24 h post-ICH for the Vehicle and BBG groups were 91.17 ± 23.54 and 82.77 ± 21.31, respectively ($P > 0.05$) (Fig. 5a, b), indicating that BBG did not affect bleeding. However, the hemorrhagic lesion volume for the BBG group (37.79 + 15.56) was significantly decreased compared with the Vehicle (73.03 + 19.34) group at 72 h

post-ICH ($P < 0.01$) (Fig. 5e, f), indicating that BBG could promote tissue reconstruction. Meanwhile, the tissue damage around the lesion site was evidently mitigated by BBG treatment at both 24 and 72 h (Fig. 5c, d, g, h). Consistently, neurological deficits (Fig. 6c) at both 24 h (50 mg/kg, 8.83 ± 1.64 vs. Vehicle, 10.00 ± 1.95, $P < 0.05$; 100 mg/kg, 8.66 ± 1.55 vs. Vehicle, 10.00 ± 1.95, $P < 0.05$) and 72 h (50 mg/kg, 6.40 ± 1.64 vs. Vehicle, 8.10 ± 1.96, $P < 0.05$; 100 mg/kg, 7.00 ± 1.78 vs. Vehicle, 8.10 ± 1.96, $P < 0.05$) after ICH were improved by BBG treatment. However, there was no difference between animals that received 50 and 100 mg/kg doses of BBG treatment with regard to mNSS scores or brain water contents. Thus, the 50 mg/kg dose was applied in further studies.

The number of apoptotic neurons was significantly increased at 24 h after ICH compared with the Sham group ($P < 0.01$), and BBG treatment significantly reduced the number of apoptotic neurons ($P < 0.01$) relative to the Vehicle group (Fig. 6a, b).

BBG decreased P2X7R expression, NLRP3/ASC/caspase-1 activation, and subsequent IL-1β/IL-18 production following ICH

BBG treatment significantly reduced NLRP3 mRNA levels (Fig. 7a). Western blot analysis revealed that BBG

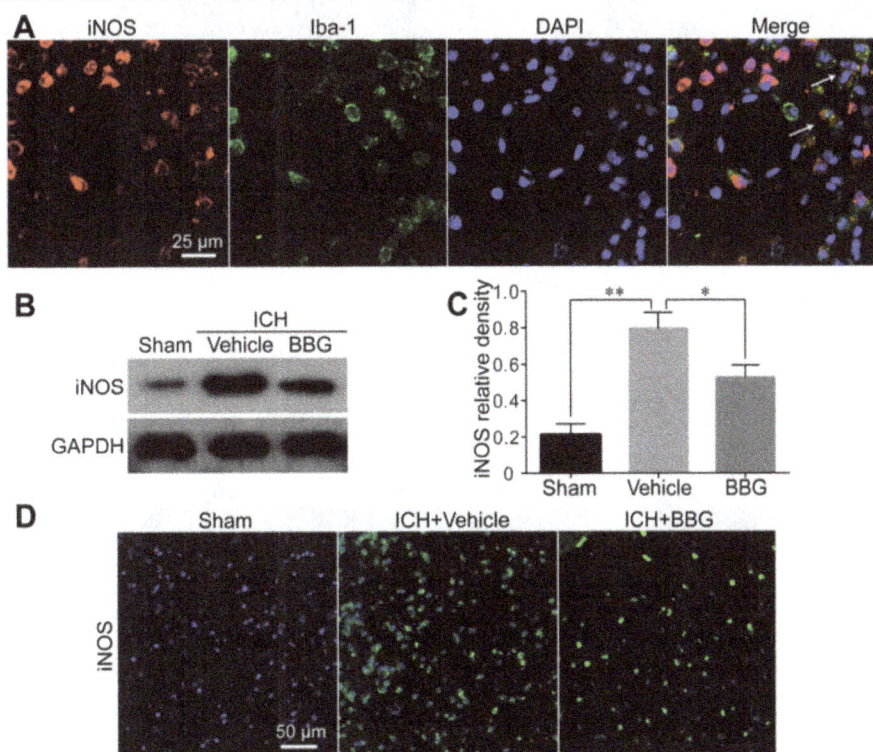

Fig. 9 Effects of BBG on ICH-induced iNOS expression in the striatum. Most iNOS signals overlapped with Iba-1 positive microglia (**a**). Western blot (**b, c**) and immunofluorescence labeling (**d**) showing that BBG treatment significantly decreased striatal iNOS expression 24 h after ICH compared with the Vehicle group. $n = 4$ (**b, c**) or $n = 6$ (**a, d**) rats per group. Scale bar = 25 μm (**a**) or 50 μm (**d**). Data represent means ± SD. $^{*}P < 0.05$, $^{**}P < 0.01$. *BBG* brilliant blue G, *GAPDH* glyceraldehyde 3-phosphate dehydrogenase, *ICH* intracerebral hemorrhage, *iNOS* inducible nitric oxide synthase

(50 mg/kg) treatment attenuated the expressions of P2X7R ($P < 0.05$ vs. Vehicle), NLRP3 ($P < 0.05$ vs. Vehicle), ASC ($P < 0.01$ vs. Vehicle), and cleaved caspase-1 ($P < 0.05$ vs. Vehicle). Furthermore, the levels of mature IL-1β ($P < 0.05$ vs. Vehicle) and IL-18 ($P < 0.05$ vs. Vehicle) were distinctly reduced after BBG treatment (Fig. 7b–h).

BBG reduced neutrophils infiltration after ICH.

We detected MPO levels in brain tissue by IF (Fig. 8a) and western blot (Fig. 8b, c) at 24 h following ICH to determine the effect of P2X7R/NLRP3 inflammasome axis activation on neutrophil infiltration. Striatal MPO levels were evidently increased following ICH

compared with the Sham group ($P < 0.01$ vs. Sham). BBG (50 mg/kg) significantly suppressed MPO expression compared to the Vehicle group ($P < 0.05$ vs. Vehicle).

BBG suppressed ICH-induced iNOS expression

iNOS is upregulated in both blood infusion and collagenase-induced ICH rat models [31, 35]. The role of P2X7R in iNOS signaling was next investigated using IF and western blot analysis. iNOS expression was weak in Sham-operated rats but was dramatically elevated 24 h after ICH induction ($P < 0.01$ vs. Sham). To further trace the source of iNOS, double IF was performed and found that iNOS was mainly expressed in Iba-1-positive microglia (Fig. 9a). Western

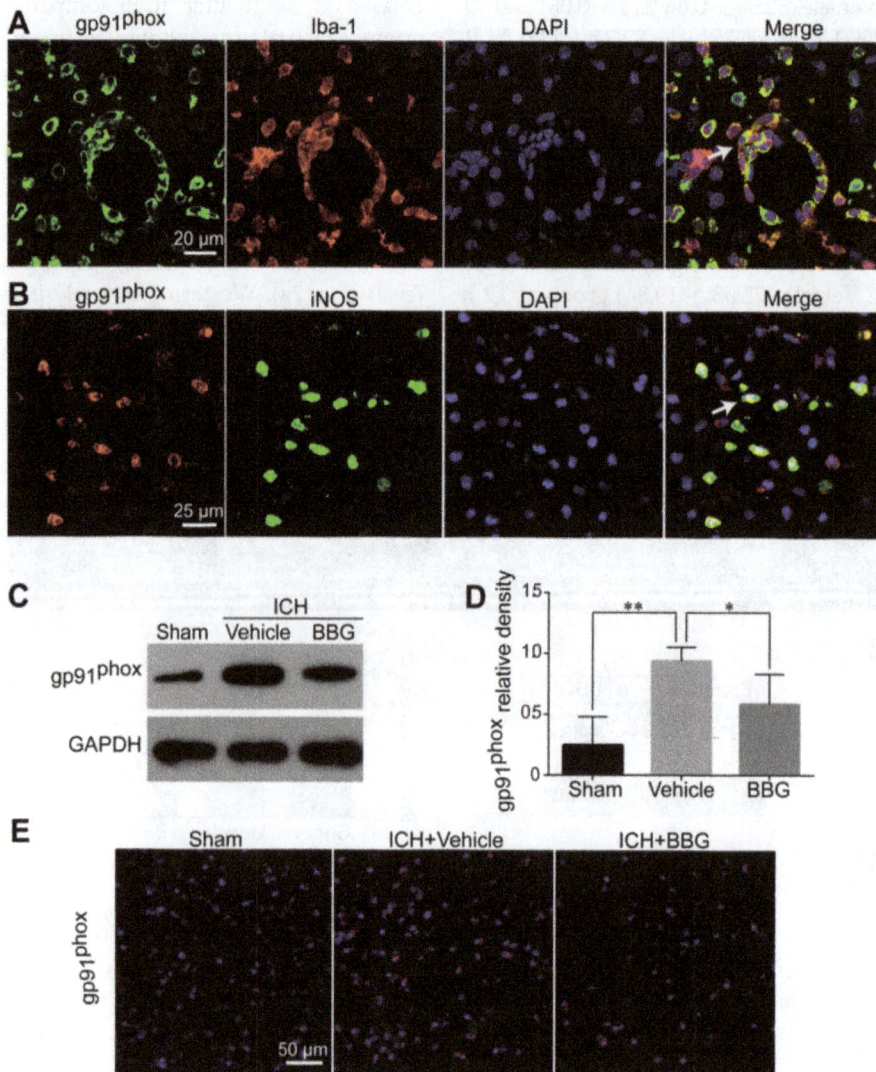

Fig. 10 Effects of BBG on ICH-induced gp91^{phox} expression in the striatum. Gp91^{phox} significantly colocalized with Iba-1 (**a**). Most gp91^{phox} signals overlapped with iNOS (**b**). Western blot (**c, d**) and immunofluorescence labeling (**e**) showing that BBG treatment significantly reduced the striatal gp91^{phox} expression 24 h after ICH compared with the Vehicle group. $n = 4$ (**d**) or $n = 6$ (**e**) rats per group. Scale bar = 20 μm (**a**) or 25 μm (**b**) or 50 μm (**e**). Data represent means ± SD. $^{*}P < 0.05$; $^{**}P < 0.01$. *BBG* brilliant blue G, *GAPDH* glyceraldehyde 3-phosphate dehydrogenase, *ICH* intracerebral hemorrhage, *iNOS* inducible nitric oxide synthase

blots and IF showed that the enhanced iNOS levels were markedly attenuated in BBG-treated rats ($P < 0.05$ vs. Vehicle) (Fig. 9b–d).

BBG reduced ICH-induced NOX2 expression

NOX2, a primary source of O_2^-, is actively involved in ICH-induced brain injury [15]. We studied the expression of gp91[phox], a membrane subunit of NOX2, by IF and western blotting. Double IF showed that gp91[phox] was also mainly expressed in Iba-1-positive areas (Fig. 10a) and most overlapped with iNOS expression (Fig. 10b), implying a close connection between them. Consistent with iNOS, gp91[phox] was significantly increased after ICH in ipsilateral hemisphere brain tissues as compared with the Sham group ($P < 0.01$ vs. Sham) at 24 h after ICH. BBG treatment significantly downregulated gp91[phox] overexpression ($P < 0.05$ vs. Vehicle) (Fig. 10c–e).

BBG attenuated peroxynitrite formation following ICH

The enhancement of iNOS and NOX2 after ICH induction prompted us to examine the involvement of P2X7R in $ONOO^-$ formation. Double IF demonstrated a high degree of colocalization with Iba-1 (Fig. 11a). Moreover, 3-NT and gp91[phox] expressions were almost completely overlapped (Fig. 11b), implying that peroxynitrite production is NOX2 dependent. However, BBG treatment significantly downregulated 3-NT overexpression ($P < 0.05$ vs. Vehicle) (Fig. 11c–e).

The $ONOO^-$ decomposition catalyst FeTPPS inhibited NLRP3/ASC/Caspase-1 activation and subsequent production of mature IL-1β/IL-18 following ICH

Our findings suggested a pivotal role for microglia-expressed P2X7R in mediating $ONOO^-$ formation in an iNOS and NOX2-dependent way, which further prompted

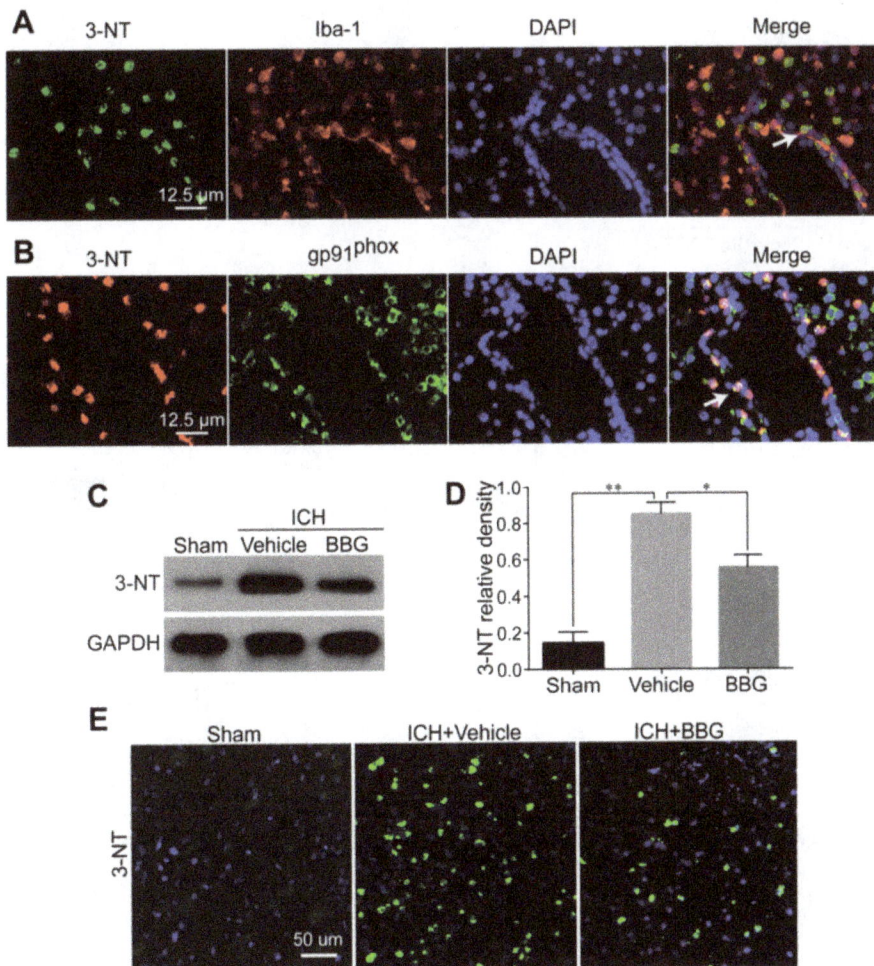

Fig. 11 Effects of BBG on ICH-induced 3-NT expression in the striatum. 3-NT significantly colocalized with Iba-1 (**a**). Most 3-NT signals overlapped with gp91[phox] (**b**). Western blot (**c, d**) and immunofluorescence staining (**e**) showing that BBG treatment significantly suppressed striatal 3-NT expression 24 h after ICH compared with the Vehicle group. $n = 4$ (**a, b, e**) or $n = 6$ (**c, d**) rats per group. Bar = 12.5 μm (**a, b**) or 50 μm (**e**). Data represent means ± SD. $^*P < 0.05$, $^{**}P < 0.01$. *BBG* brilliant blue G, *GAPDH* glyceraldehyde 3-phosphate dehydrogenase, *ICH* intracerebral hemorrhage, *3-NT* 3-nitrotyrosine

us to explore whether ONOO⁻ served as the key bridge between P2X7R and NLRP3 inflammasome activation. To answer this question, the ONOO⁻ decomposition catalyst FeTPPS was applied in vivo. Firstly, FeTPPS significantly reduced 3-NT levels ($P < 0.01$ vs. Vehicle) on western blot (Fig. 12a, b). Thereafter, the expression levels of P2X7R and NLRP3 inflammasome components were measured by western blot at 24 h following ICH. The results indicated that FeTPPS significantly downregulated the enhanced levels of NLRP3 ($P < 0.05$ vs. Vehicle), ASC ($P < 0.05$ vs. Vehicle), and cleaved caspase-1 ($P < 0.05$ vs. Vehicle) after ICH. Moreover, the upregulation of IL-1β/IL-18 was also attenuated by FeTPPS ($P < 0.05$ vs. Vehicle) (Fig. 12c–h).

However, FeTPPS had no influence on P2X7R expressions (Additional file 3). FeTPPS treatment significantly reduced NLRP3 mRNA expression. Together, these results reveal that P2X7R-dependent synthesis of ONOO⁻ may be a key activator of the NLRP3 inflammasome.

Discussion

Innate immune and inflammatory responses are increasingly recognized as important factors in the pathophysiology of secondary brain injury following ICH. The NLRP3 inflammasome, the most characterized pattern recognition receptor (PRR) in innate immune response initiation, is

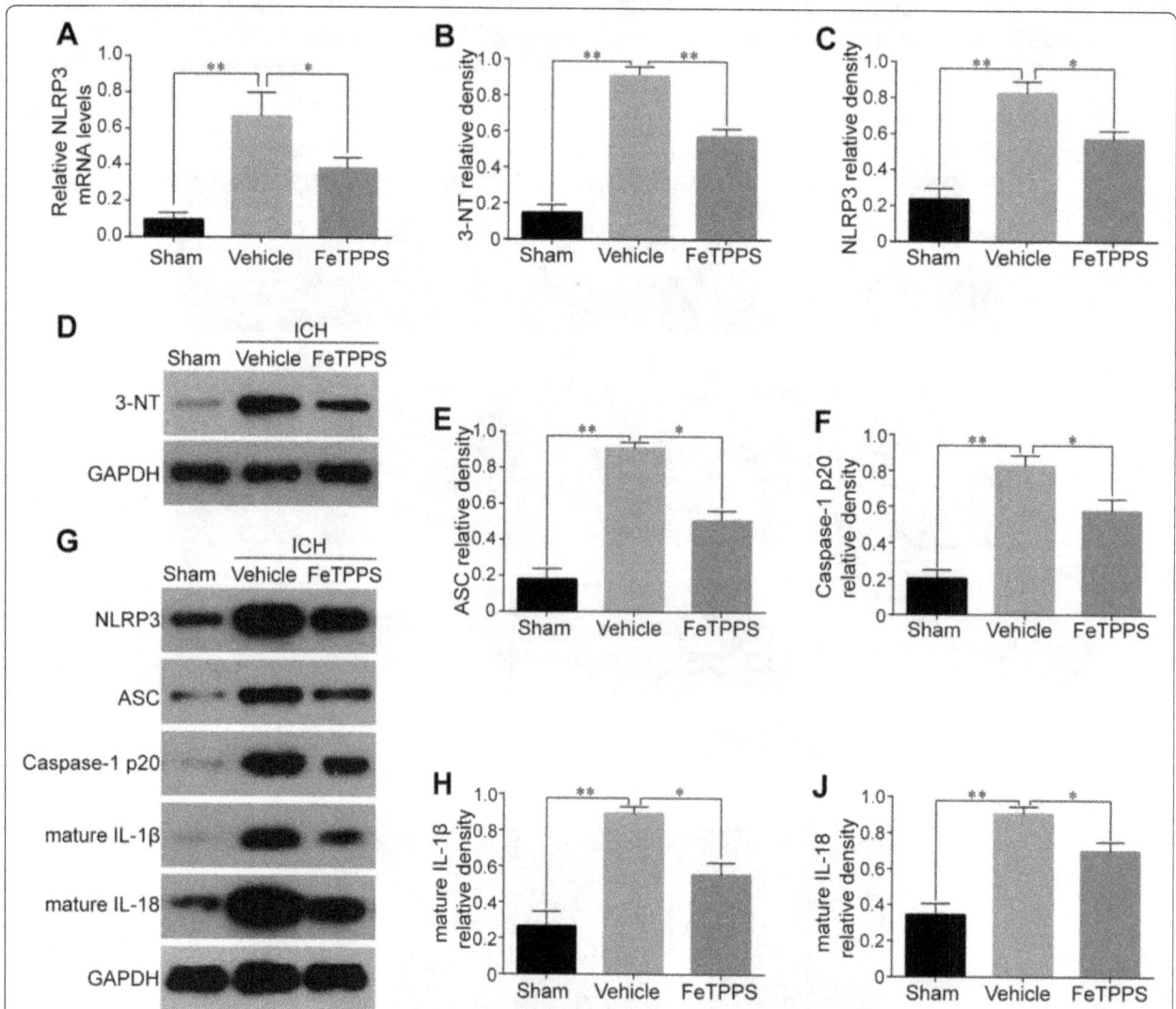

Fig. 12 Effects of FeTPPS on NLRP3 inflammasome activation and IL-1β/IL-18 maturation. RT-PCR of NLRP3 after FeTPPS treatment 24 h following ICH, $n = 6$ rats per group (**a**). Western blot (**d**, **b**) showed that FeTPPS significantly reduced striatal 3-NT expression 24 h after ICH compared with the Vehicle group. Western blot assay (**g**) and quantification of NLRP3 (**c**), ASC (**e**), caspase-1 p20 subunit (**f**), mature IL-1β (**h**), and mature IL-18 (**j**) after FeTPPS treatment 24 h following ICH, $n = 5$ rats per group. Data represent means ± SD. $^*P < 0.05$, $^{**}P < 0.01$. *ASC* adaptor protein apoptosis-associated speck-like protein containing a CARD, *GAPDH* glyceraldehyde 3-phosphate dehydrogenase, *ICH* intracerebral hemorrhage, *IL* interleukin, *NLRP3* pyrin domain-containing 3, *3-NT* 3-nitrotyrosine

strongly involved in ICH-induced inflammation and produces pro-inflammatory factors such as IL-1β [2].

Several distinct mechanisms have been proposed to account for NLRP3 activation, including potassium (K^+) efflux, intracellular calcium alteration, ubiquitination, and reactive oxygen species (ROS) generation [36]. It was recently reported that extracellular ATP-induced P2X7R activation could directly mediate K^+ efflux through the hemichannel pannexin 1 to activate the NLRP3 inflammasome [5, 28, 36]. However, pannexin 1-deficient mice do not show diminished caspase-1 activation [37], implying that pannexin-1 is dispensable for the assembly of caspase-1 activating inflammasome complexes. This raises the hypothesis that other signaling pathways may be involved in P2X7R-mediated NLRP3 inflammasome activation or that something besides pannexin 1 is necessary for P2X7R-dependent K^+ efflux. NOX2-derived ROS after ATP release-mediated P2X7R activation is well established in a growing body of in vitro and in vivo disease models [23–25]. Importantly, there are a number of reports supporting that high ROS levels, particularly NOX2-derived ROS, are critical for NLRP3 inflammasome activation [36]. RNS also play an important role as evidenced by the fact that both an $ONOO^-$ scavenger and NOX2 inhibitor suppressed nigericin-induced caspase-1 activation and IL-1β secretion in human monocytes [28]. Additionally, K^+ efflux can be positively regulated by ROS [14] and RNS (e.g., $ONOO^-$) [38]. In this regard, we propose that NOX2-mediated $ONOO^-$ formation may link P2X7R and NLRP3 inflammasome activation.

P2X7R activation in the ICH brain is a novel finding of this study. ATP is released in large quantities following any kind of cell injury [39], and cell death occurs 3 to 6 h after collagenase- induced ICH [40]. Elevated extracellular ATP is necessary for P2X7R activation [13]. In the present study, increased P2X7R was observed as early as 6 h after ICH in the perihematomal tissue along with expression of the microglia marker Iba-1, suggesting that P2X7R may act as a signal in the process of microglia activation as previously reported [41].

Microglia are believed to be one of the first non-neuronal cells to respond to brain injury [42], much earlier than neutrophil invasion [43]. Activated microglia then release pro-inflammatory cytokines, such as IL-1β [44] and IL-18 [45], which recruit leukocytes especially neutrophils. The infiltrated neutrophils amplify neuroinflammation by releasing and expressing neurotoxic factors or even by stimulating microglia to secrete neurotoxic factors, creating a vicious cycle [46]. In the present study, upregulated P2X7R was closely associated with increased NLRP3/ASC/caspase-1 inflammasome expression; siRNA interference or pharmacological blockage of P2X7R impaired inflammasome activation and IL-1β/IL-18 secretion, which had a pronounced neuroprotective effect. Moreover, infiltrated

neutrophils were also diminished in the BBG group compared with the Vehicle group. These results indicate that P2X7R may be responsible for ICH-induced inflammation, possibly by NLRP3 inflammasome-dependent IL-1β/IL-18 release and subsequent neutrophil infiltration signals. In accordance with our results, Ma and colleagues [2] found that NLRP3 mainly colocalized with microglia but not with other cell types, providing further support for a tight relationship between P2X7R and NLRP3.

In response to microglia activation, large amounts O_2^- and NO are released through activated NADPH oxidase and iNOS [17], both of which play pivotal roles in ICH-induced brain damage [15, 16]. In our study, enhanced $gp91^{phox}$ in microglia largely colocalized with iNOS, prompting us to consider $ONOO^-$. Double IF revealed that increased 3-NT was also expressed in microglia and mostly overlapped with $gp91^{phox}$. Consistently with this, Mander and Brown [47] reported that activation of NOX or iNOS alone was relatively harmless, but their simultaneous activation was lethal because it spurred $ONOO^-$ production. Inhibition of either iNOS [48] or NOX2 [49] significantly reduced $ONOO^-$ production in CNS disease models. Collectively, we can infer that NOX2-derived O_2^- and iNOS-derived NO may contribute to $ONOO^-$ formation upon microglia activation after ICH.

We also found that ICH-induced upregulations of NOX2, iNOS, and $ONOO^-$ were diminished in BBG treated ICH rats, indicating that they may be downstream of P2X7R as previously reported [26, 29]. We next explored the role of $ONOO^-$ in NLRP3 inflammasome activation. As a highly active and relatively specific $ONOO^-$ decomposition catalyst, FeTPPS exerts neuroprotective effects in many CNS disease models [20, 50] because it catalyzes peroxynitrite to become a harmless nitrate [51]. Our results show that overexpression of NLRP3 inflammasome components and mature IL-1β/IL-18 was reduced by FeTPPS. These findings suggest that $ONOO^-$ may be involved in inflammasome activation following ICH. Consistent with our results, an early report found that FeTPPS inhibited nigericin-induced caspase-1 activation and IL-1β secretion in human monocytes [28].

Although we did not attempt to explore the exact mechanisms of $ONOO^-$ in modulating NLRP3 inflammasome activation, $ONOO^-$ may act as a key mediator for inflammasome activation through several mechanisms. Firstly, direct oxidation of mitochondria and the release of mitochondrial DNA (mtDNA) activate the NLRP3 inflammasome; a recent study showed that oxidized mtDNA released into the cytosol from injured mitochondria could bind to and activate the NLRP3 inflammasome [52]. $ONOO^-$ is a potent ROS with strong abilities to oxidize and nitrate proteins, lipids, and DNA. Mitochondria are a primary target for peroxynitrite [18]. Secondly, nitration can inactivate thioredoxin (Trx), leading to the dissociation of thioredoxin interaction protein (TXNIP) from Trx. Zhou et al. [53] reported that TXNIP could dissociate from Trx in an ROS-sensitive way, allowing it to bind and activate NLRP3. Thirdly, $ONOO^-$ may mediate K^+ efflux and then activate NLRP3. K^+ efflux is a well-characterized activator for NLRP3 inflammasome, and $ONOO^-$ is a positive modulator for K^+ efflux [38]. Therefore, $ONOO^-$ may be responsible for NLRP3 inflammasome activation.

Of translational significance, we investigated the effect of BBG in an ICH rat model. Previous studies have demonstrated a neuroprotective effect of BBG in many acute CNS diseases such as ischemic stroke [54], subarachnoid hemorrhage [6], traumatic brain injury [55], and spinal cord injury [56]. BBG is a derivative of the widely used and Food and Drug Administration-approved food additive FD&C Blue number 1 [57]. With its low toxicity and high selectivity, BBG is considered to be an attractive drug for CNS diseases [56]. We found that BBG treatment inhibited the inflammatory response via the P2X7R/NLRP3 axis following ICH, and this was associated with significantly improved neurological function and less brain edema.

Several potential limitations deserve mention. Firstly, although we employed the most commonly used ICH model and injected sterile-filtered collagenase, the extra-inflammatory responses induced by the collagenase itself seemed unavoidable. Secondly, our observation period was 72 h but it appears that ASC and caspase-1 activation may undergo a second peak at 72 h; we speculate that other signaling pathways may be involved in ASC and caspase-1 activation in a later phase. Finally, although it was significant, the effect of P2X7R siRNA and BBG on changes in brain water content and neurobehavioral scores was relatively small. Thus, further experiments are necessary to address these problems.

Conclusion

In summary, our results indicate that P2X7R contributes to NLRP3 inflammasome activation and subsequent IL-1β/IL-18 release to drive brain inflammation and neuronal damage in an ICH rat model. NOX2/iNOS-dependent $ONOO^-$ formation, a potential downstream signaling component of P2X7R, may be a key trigger of NLRP3 inflammasome activation. Thus, inhibition of P2X7R or $ONOO^-$ could be a potential therapeutic target for secondary brain injury accompanying ICH.

Additional files

Additional file 1: Experiment design and animal group classification. ICH = intracerebral hemorrhage; WB = western blotting; BWC = brain water content; IF = immunofluorescence; BBG = brilliant blue G. (TIFF 891 kb)

Additional file 2: No evident immunostaining for P2X7R was found in astrocytes and neurons. Double immunostaining showed that P2X7R was not expressed in GFAP positive astrocytes (A). Double immunostaining showed that P2X7R was not expressed in NeuN positive neurons (B). (TIFF 4781 kb)

Additional file 3: FeTPPS treatment had no influence on P2X7R expressions. Western blot (A,B) showed that FeTPPS did not affect the protein expressions of P2X7R. $^*P < 0.05$, $^{**}P < 0.01$ (TIFF 494 kb)

Abbreviations
3-NT: 3-nitrotyrosine; ASC: apoptosis-associated speck-like protein containing a CARD; ATP: adenosine triphosphate; BBG: brilliant blue G; CNS: central nervous system; ICH: intracerebral hemorrhage; IL: interleukin; iNOS: inducible nitric oxide synthase; LPS: lipopolysaccharide; mNSS: modified Neurological Severity Score; MPO: myeloperoxidase; mtDNA: mitochondrial DNA; NLRP3: NLR family, pyrin domain-containing 3; NO: nitric oxide; NOX2: NADPH oxidase 2; O_2^-: superoxide anion; $ONOO^-$: peroxynitrite; P2X7R: purinergic 2X7 receptor; RNS: reactive nitrogen species; ROS: reactive oxygen species; SD: Sprague–Dawley; Sham: sham-operated animals; siRNA: small interfering RNA; TUNEL: terminal deoxynucleotidyl transferase-mediated dUTP nick 3'-end labeling.

Competing interests
The authors declare that they have no competing interests.

Authors' contributions
Conceived and designed the experiments: YZC and LF. Performed the experiments: LF. Analyzed the data: YZC and LF. Wrote the paper: LF. Paper revision: YZC. RD, ZHF, SY, XQD, and JZ provided experimental technical support and assisted in completing the study at different stages. All authors read and approved the final manuscript.

Acknowledgements
This study was supported by the National Natural Science Foundation of China (Nos. 81271314 and 30500526), Natural Science Foundation of Guangdong (No. 5300468), Special Project on the Integration of Industry, Education and Research of Guangdong Province and Ministry of Education (No. 2012B091100154), Natural Science Foundation of Guangdong (No.2014A030313346), and The Guangdong Provincial Clinical Medical Centre For Neurosurgery (No. 2013B020400005).

Author details
[1]The National Key Clinical Specialty, The Engineering Technology Research Center of Education Ministry of China, Guangdong Provincial Key Laboratory on Brain Function Repair and Regeneration, Department of Neurosurgery, Zhujiang Hospital, Southern Medical University, Guangzhou 510282, China. [2]Department of Neurosurgery, Jingmen No. 1 People's Hospital, Jingmen 448000Hubei, China. [3]Department of Neurosurgery, The Fifth Affiliated Hospital of Southern Medical University, Guangzhou 510900, China. [4]Department of Neurosurgery, Gaoqing Campus of Central Hospital of Zibo, Gaoqing People's Hospital, Gaoqing, Zibo 256300 Shandong, China. [5]Department of Neurosurgery, 999 Brain Hospital, Jinan University, Guangzhou 510510 Guangdong, China.

References
1. Keep RF, Hua Y, Xi G. Intracerebral haemorrhage: mechanisms of injury and therapeutic targets. Lancet Neurol. 2012;11:720–31.
2. Ma Q, Chen S, Hu Q, Feng H, Zhang JH, Tang J. NLRP3 inflammasome contributes to inflammation after intracerebral hemorrhage. Ann Neurol. 2014;75:209–19.
3. Wang YC, Zhou Y, Fang H, Lin S, Wang PF, Xiong RP, et al. Toll-like receptor 2/4 heterodimer mediates inflammatory injury in intracerebral hemorrhage. Ann Neurol. 2014;75:876–89.
4. Rathinam VA, Vanaja SK, Fitzgerald KA. Regulation of inflammasome signaling. Nat Immunol. 2012;13:333–42.
5. Latz E, Xiao TS, Stutz A. Activation and regulation of the inflammasomes. Nat Rev Immunol. 2013;13:397–411.

6. Chen S, Ma Q, Krafft PR, Hu Q, Rolland 2nd W, Sherchan P, et al. P2X7R/cryopyrin inflammasome axis inhibition reduces neuroinflammation after SAH. Neurobiol Dis. 2013;58:296–307.

7. Yang F, Wang Z, Wei X, Han H, Meng X, Zhang Y, et al. NLRP3 deficiency ameliorates neurovascular damage in experimental ischemic stroke. J Cereb Blood Flow Metab. 2014;34:660–7.

8. Liu HD, Li W, Chen ZR, Hu YC, Zhang DD, Shen W, et al. Expression of the NLRP3 inflammasome in cerebral cortex after traumatic brain injury in a rat model. Neurochem Res. 2013;38:2072–83.

9. Bigford GE, Bracchi-Ricard VC, Keane RW, Nash MS, Bethea JR. Neuroendocrine and cardiac metabolic dysfunction and NLRP3 inflammasome activation in adipose tissue and pancreas following chronic spinal cord injury in the mouse. ASN Neuro. 2013;5:243–55.

10. Meng XF, Tan L, Tan MS, Jiang T, Tan CC, Li MM, et al. Inhibition of the NLRP3 inflammasome provides neuroprotection in rats following amygdala kindling-induced status epilepticus. J Neuroinflammation. 2014;11:212.

11. Parajuli B, Sonobe Y, Horiuchi H, Takeuchi H, Mizuno T, Suzumura A. Oligomeric amyloid beta induces IL-1beta processing via production of ROS: implication in Alzheimer's disease. Cell Death Dis. 2013;4:e975.

12. Di Virgilio F. Liaisons dangereuses: P2X(7) and the inflammasome. Trends Pharmacol Sci. 2007;28:465–72.

13. Sperlagh B, Illes P. P2X7 receptor: an emerging target in central nervous system diseases. Trends Pharmacol Sci. 2014;35:537–47.

14. Bartlett R, Stokes L, Sluyter R. The P2X7 receptor channel: recent developments and the use of P2X7 antagonists in models of disease. Pharmacol Rev. 2014;66:638–75.

15. Tang J, Liu J, Zhou C, Ostanin D, Grisham MB, Neil Granger D, et al. Role of NADPH oxidase in the brain injury of intracerebral hemorrhage. J Neurochem. 2005;94:1342–50.

16. Kim DW, Im SH, Kim JY, Kim DE, Oh GT, Jeong SW. Decreased brain edema after collagenase-induced intracerebral hemorrhage in mice lacking the inducible nitric oxide synthase gene. Laboratory investigation. J Neurosurg. 2009;111:995–1000.

17. Heneka MT, Kummer MP, Latz E. Innate immune activation in neurodegenerative disease. Nat Rev Immunol. 2014;14:463–77.

18. Szabo C, Ischiropoulos H, Radi R. Peroxynitrite: biochemistry, pathophysiology and development of therapeutics. Nat Rev Drug Discov. 2007;6:662–80.

19. Deng-Bryant Y, Singh IN, Carrico KM, Hall ED. Neuroprotective effects of tempol, a catalytic scavenger of peroxynitrite-derived free radicals, in a mouse traumatic brain injury model. J Cereb Blood Flow Metab. 2008;28:1114–26.

20. Genovese T, Mazzon E, Esposito E, Muia C, Di Paola R, Bramanti P, et al. Beneficial effects of FeTSPP, a peroxynitrite decomposition catalyst, in a mouse model of spinal cord injury. Free Radic Biol Med. 2007;43:763–80.

21. Ding R, Chen Y, Yang S, Deng X, Fu Z, Feng L, et al. Blood-brain barrier disruption induced by hemoglobin in vivo: involvement of up-regulation of nitric oxide synthase and peroxynitrite formation. Brain Res. 2014;1571:25–38.

22. Little JW, Cuzzocrea S, Bryant L, Esposito E, Doyle T, Rausaria S, et al. Spinal mitochondrial-derived peroxynitrite enhances neuroimmune activation during morphine hyperalgesia and antinociceptive tolerance. Pain. 2013;154:978–86.

23. Doyle T, Chen Z, Muscoli C, Bryant L, Esposito E, Cuzzocrea S, et al. Targeting the overproduction of peroxynitrite for the prevention and reversal of paclitaxel-induced neuropathic pain. J Neurosci. 2012;32:6149–60.

24. Pacher P, Beckman JS, Liaudet L. Nitric oxide and peroxynitrite in health and disease. Physiol Rev. 2007;87:315–424.

25. Apolloni S, Amadio S, Parisi C, Matteucci A, Potenza RL, Armida M, et al. Spinal cord pathology is ameliorated by P2X7 antagonism in a SOD1-mutant mouse model of amyotrophic lateral sclerosis. Dis Model Mech. 2014;7:1101–9.

26. Chatterjee S, Rana R, Corbett J, Kadiiska MB, Goldstein J, Mason RP. P2X7 receptor-NADPH oxidase axis mediates protein radical formation and Kupffer cell activation in carbon tetrachloride-mediated steatohepatitis in obese mice. Free Radic Biol Med. 2012;52:1666–79.

27. Parvathenani LK, Tertyshnikova S, Greco CR, Roberts SB, Robertson B, Posmantur R. P2X7 mediates superoxide production in primary microglia and is up-regulated in a transgenic mouse model of Alzheimer's disease. J Biol Chem. 2003;278:13309–17.

28. Hewinson J, Moore SF, Glover C, Watts AG, MacKenzie AB. A key role for redox signaling in rapid P2X7 receptor-induced IL-1 beta processing in human monocytes. J Immunol. 2008;180:8410–20.

29. Choi HB, Ryu JK, Kim SU, McLarnon JG. Modulation of the purinergic P2X7 receptor attenuates lipopolysaccharide-mediated microglial activation and neuronal damage in inflamed brain. J Neurosci. 2007;27:4957–68.

30. Ding R, Feng L, He L, Chen Y, Wen P, Fu Z, et al. Peroxynitrite decomposition catalyst prevents matrix metalloproteinase-9 activation and neurovascular injury after hemoglobin injection into the caudate nucleus of rats. Neuroscience. 2015;297:182–93.

31. Jung KH, Chu K, Jeong SW, Han SY, Lee ST, Kim JY, et al. HMG-CoA reductase inhibitor, atorvastatin, promotes sensorimotor recovery, suppressing acute inflammatory reaction after experimental intracerebral hemorrhage. Stroke. 2004;35:1744–9.

32. Rynkowski MA, Kim GH, Komotar RJ, Otten ML, Ducruet AF, Zacharia BE, et al. A mouse model of intracerebral hemorrhage using autologous blood infusion. Nat Protoc. 2008;3:122–8.

33. Chu K, Jeong SW, Jung KH, Han SY, Lee ST, Kim M, et al. Celecoxib induces functional recovery after intracerebral hemorrhage with reduction of brain edema and perihematomal cell death. J Cereb Blood Flow Metab. 2004;24:926–33.

34. Chen J, Sanberg PR, Li Y, Wang L, Lu M, Willing AE, et al. Intravenous administration of human umbilical cord blood reduces behavioral deficits after stroke in rats. Stroke. 2001;32:2682–8.

35. Zhao X, Zhang Y, Strong R, Zhang J, Grotta JC, Aronowski J. Distinct patterns of intracerebral hemorrhage-induced alterations in NF-kappaB subunit, iNOS, and COX-2 expression. J Neurochem. 2007;101:652–63.

36. Abais JM, Xia M, Zhang Y, Boini KM, Li PL. Redox regulation of NLRP3 inflammasomes: ROS as trigger or effector? Antioxid Redox Signal. 2015;22:1111–29.

37. Qu Y, Misaghi S, Newton K, Gilmour LL, Louie S, Cupp JE, et al. Pannexin-1 is required for ATP release during apoptosis but not for inflammasome activation. J Immunol. 2011;186:6553–61.

38. Bossy-Wetzel E, Talantova MV, Lee WD, Scholzke MN, Harrop A, Mathews E, et al. Crosstalk between nitric oxide and zinc pathways to neuronal cell death involving mitochondrial dysfunction and p38-activated K+ channels. Neuron. 2004;41:351–65.

39. Eltzschig HK, Sitkovsky MV, Robson SC. Purinergic signaling during inflammation. N Engl J Med. 2012;367:2322–33.

40. Zhu X, Tao L, Tejima-Mandeville E, Qiu J, Park J, Garber K, et al. Plasmalemma permeability and necrotic cell death phenotypes after intracerebral hemorrhage in mice. Stroke. 2012;43:524–31.

41. Benarroch EE. Microglia: multiple roles in surveillance, circuit shaping, and response to injury. Neurology. 2013;81:1079–88.

42. Wang J, Dore S. Inflammation after intracerebral hemorrhage. J Cereb Blood Flow Metab. 2007;27:894–908.

43. Wang J. Preclinical and clinical research on inflammation after intracerebral hemorrhage. Prog Neurobiol. 2010;92:463–77.

44. Lu A, Tang Y, Ran R, Ardizzone TL, Wagner KR, Sharp FR. Brain genomics of intracerebral hemorrhage. J Cereb Blood Flow Metab. 2006;26:230–52.

45. Felderhoff-Mueser U, Schmidt OI, Oberholzer A, Buhrer C, Stahel PF. IL-18: a key player in neuroinflammation and neurodegeneration? Trends Neurosci. 2005;28:487–93.

46. Ziai WC. Hematology and inflammatory signaling of intracerebral hemorrhage. Stroke. 2013;44:S74–8.

47. Mander P, Brown GC. Activation of microglial NADPH oxidase is synergistic with glial iNOS expression in inducing neuronal death: a dual-key mechanism of inflammatory neurodegeneration. J Neuroinflammation. 2005;2:20.

48. Ryu JK, McLarnon JG. Minocycline or iNOS inhibition block 3-nitrotyrosine increases and blood-brain barrier leakiness in amyloid beta-peptide-injected rat hippocampus. Exp Neurol. 2006;198:552–7.

49. Dohi K, Ohtaki H, Nakamachi T, Yofu S, Satoh K, Miyamoto K, et al. Gp91phox (NOX2) in classically activated microglia exacerbates traumatic brain injury. J Neuroinflammation. 2010;7:41.

50. Thiyagarajan M, Kaul CL, Sharma SS. Neuroprotective efficacy and therapeutic time window of peroxynitrite decomposition catalysts in focal cerebral ischemia in rats. Br J Pharmacol. 2004;142:899–911.

51. Salvemini D, Wang ZQ, Stern MK, Currie MG, Misko TP. Peroxynitrite decomposition catalysts: therapeutics for peroxynitrite-mediated pathology. Proc Natl Acad Sci U S A. 1998;95:2659–63.

52. Shimada K, Crother TR, Karlin J, Dagvadorj J, Chiba N, Chen S, et al. Oxidized mitochondrial DNA activates the NLRP3 inflammasome during apoptosis. Immunity. 2012;36:401–14.

53. Zhou R, Tardivel A, Thorens B, Choi I, Tschopp J. Thioredoxin-interacting protein links oxidative stress to inflammasome activation. Nat Immunol. 2010;11:136–40.

54. Arbeloa J, Perez-Samartin A, Gottlieb M, Matute C. P2X7 receptor blockade prevents ATP excitotoxicity in neurons and reduces brain damage after ischemia. Neurobiol Dis. 2012;45:954–61.

55. Kimbler DE, Shields J, Yanasak N, Vender JR, Dhandapani KM. Activation of P2X7 promotes cerebral edema and neurological injury after traumatic brain injury in mice. PLoS ONE. 2012;7:e41229.

56. Peng W, Cotrina ML, Han X, Yu H, Bekar L, Blum L, et al. Systemic administration of an antagonist of the ATP-sensitive receptor P2X7 improves recovery after spinal cord injury. Proc Natl Acad Sci U S A. 2009;106:12489–93.

57. Wang J, Jackson DG, Dahl G. The food dye FD&C Blue No. 1 is a selective inhibitor of the ATP release channel Panx1. J Gen Physiol. 2013;141:649–56.

Endogenous hydrogen sulphide attenuates NLRP3 inflammasome-mediated neuroinflammation by suppressing the P2X7 receptor after intracerebral haemorrhage in rats

Hengli Zhao, Pengyu Pan, Yang Yang, Hongfei Ge, Weixiang Chen, Jie Qu, Jiantao Shi, Gaoyu Cui, Xin Liu, Hua Feng* and Yujie Chen*

Abstract

Background: Emerging studies have demonstrated the important physiological and pathophysiological roles of hydrogen sulphide (H_2S) as a gasotransmitter for NOD-like receptor family pyrin domain-containing 3 (NLRP3) inflammasome-associated neuroinflammation in the central nervous system. However, the effects of H_2S on neuroinflammation after intracerebral haemorrhage (ICH), especially on the NLRP3 inflammasome, remain unknown.

Methods: We employed a Sprague–Dawley rat of collagenase-induced ICH in the present study. The time course of H_2S content and the spatial expression of cystathionine-β-synthase (CBS) after ICH, the effects of endogenous and exogenous H_2S after ICH, the effects of endogenous and exogenous H_2S on NLRP3 inflammasome activation under P2X7 receptor (P2X7R) overexpression after ICH, and the involvement of the P2X7R in the mechanism by which microglia-derived H_2S prevented NLRP3 inflammasome activation were investigated.

Results: We found ICH induced significant downregulation of endogenous H_2S production in the brain, which may be the result of decreasing in CBS, the predominant cerebral H_2S-generating enzyme. Administration of S-adenosyl-L-methionine (SAM), a CBS-specific agonist, or sodium hydrosulfide (NaHS), a classical exogenous H_2S donor, not only restored brain and plasma H_2S content but also attenuated brain oedema, microglial accumulation and neurological deficits at 1 day post-ICH by inhibiting the P2X7R/NLRP3 inflammasome cascade. Endogenous H_2S production, which was derived mainly by microglia and above treatments, was verified by adenovirus-overexpressed P2X7R and in vitro primary microglia studies.

Conclusions: These results indicated endogenous H_2S synthesis was impaired after ICH, which plays a pivotal role in the P2X7R/NLRP3 inflammasome-associated neuroinflammatory response in the pathogenesis of secondary brain injury. Maintaining appropriate H_2S concentrations in the central nervous system may represent a potential therapeutic strategy for managing post-ICH secondary brain injury and associated neurological deficits.

Keywords: Hydrogen sulfide, Intracerebral haemorrhage, NLRP3 inflammasome, P2X7 receptor, Microglia

* Correspondence: fenghua8888@vip.163.com; yujiechen6886@foxmail.com
Department of Neurosurgery, Southwest Hospital, Third Military Medical
University, 29 Gaotanyan Street, Shapingba District, Chongqing 400038,
China

Background

Intracerebral haemorrhage (ICH) is a devastating stroke subtype with high mortality and morbidity rates. Numerous forms of evidence from preclinical and clinical studies suggest that inflammatory mechanisms are involved in the pathophysiologic progression of ICH-induced secondary brain injury [1, 2]. Our previous study demonstrated that NOD-like receptor (NLR) family pyrin domain-containing 3 (NLRP3) inflammasome activation contributes greatly to neuroinflammation development after ICH [3]. Despite the performance of several recent studies, in which the NLRP3 inflammasome was manipulated in experimental ICH animals [4–6], the fundamental mechanisms underlying NLRP3 inflammasome-mediated neuroinflammation are still unclear.

Hydrogen sulphide (H_2S) is a colourless gas with a special rotten egg odour. H_2S has been considered a toxic and potentially lethal gas for centuries, but emerging studies have demonstrated its important physiological and pathophysiological roles as a gasotransmitter in the central nervous system and in other tissues [7]. Relatively high H_2S concentrations (50–160 mol/L) have been observed in the brain tissues of many species, including humans [8]. H_2S plays a significant neuroprotective role in central nervous system diseases, including Alzheimer's disease, Parkinson's disease, traumatic brain injury, subarachnoid haemorrhage and ischaemic stroke, as a result of its anti-inflammatory and anti-oxidative effects [7, 9, 10]. However, the effects of H_2S on neuroinflammation after ICH, especially its effects on the NLRP3 inflammasome, remain unknown.

The purinergic P2X7 receptor (P2X7R) is an ATP-gated, non-selective cation channel that belongs to the ionotropic P2X receptor family. The P2X7R is mainly expressed on immune cells, can be activated by high concentrations of extracellular ATP released by any type of cell injury and can regulate innate immune and inflammatory responses [11]. It was reported that the P2X7R directly interacted with NLRP3 inflammasome scaffold protein and was responsible for NLRP3 recruitment and activation [12]. In the case of ICH, P2X7R levels and NLRP3 inflammasome component levels were both significantly elevated and reached their peak at 1 day after ICH onset [13].

Based on these findings and the results of our previous study, we postulate that endogenous H_2S attenuates NLRP3 inflammasome-mediated inflammatory injury and may be involved in the P2X7R signalling pathway. To explore this hypothesis, we sought to investigate the anti-inflammatory effects of microglia-derived endogenous H_2S in the setting of ICH, both in vivo and in vitro, as well as the involvement of P2X7R signalling in this process.

Methods

Experimental animals

A total of 299 Sprague–Dawley (SD) male rats weighing 280–320 g and 40 1-day-old post-natal Sprague–Dawley male rats were provided by the Experimental Animal Centre of the Third Military Medical University (Chongqing, China). All experimental procedures and animal care procedures were approved by the Ethics Committee of Southwest Hospital, performed in accordance with the guidelines by the National Institutes of Health Guide for the Care and Use of Laboratory Animals, and reported following the ARRIVE guidelines (Animal Research: Reporting in Vivo Experiments, https://www.nc3rs.org.uk/arrive-guidelines). The rats were housed in a temperature- and humidity-controlled environment, were provided food and water ad libitum, were maintained under a 12-h light/dark cycle and were acclimatized for more than 1 week before undergoing surgery.

Experimental protocol

In the present study, the following four separate experiments were conducted:

Experiment 1

To investigate the time course of H_2S content and the spatial expression of cystathionine-β-synthase (CBS) after ICH, we divided 50 rats into eight groups (sham and 3, 6, 12 h, 1 2, 3 and 7 days after ICH, $n = 6$). Brain striatum H_2S content and plasma and protein CBS expression were assessed by methylene blue assay and western blotting, respectively. Tissue samples for immunofluorescence were collected from two additional rats 1 day after ICH induction.

Experiment 2

To evaluate the effects of endogenous and exogenous H_2S after ICH, we randomized 149 rats into the following four groups: sham, vehicle (ICH + saline, intraperitoneal injection), S-adenosyl-L-methionine (SAM), and sodium hydrosulfide (NaHS). The sham group did not undergo the measurements of H_2S content and haemorrhagic volume and the detection of leukocyte infiltration and microglia accumulation ($n = 4$). Methylene blue testing ($n = 6$), haemoglobin assay ($n = 5$), western blotting ($n = 6$), quantitative polymerase chain reaction (qPCR, $n = 6$), Fluoro-Jade C staining ($n = 5$), immunofluorescence ($n = 4$) and terminal deoxynucleotidyl transferase dUTP nick end-labelling (TUNEL) staining ($n = 4$) were carried out 1 day after ICH induction, and Modified Neurological Severity Scores (mNSSs, $n = 6$) and brain water content ($n = 6$) were assessed at both 1 and 3 days after ICH.

Experiment 3

To evaluate the effects of endogenous and exogenous H_2S on NLRP3 inflammasome activation under P2X7R overexpression after ICH, 100 rats were randomized into the following five groups: vehicle (ICH + saline, intracerebroventricular injection), adenovirus GFP (Ad-GFP) (as a control to adenovirus P2X7R (Ad-P2X7R)), Ad-P2X7R, Ad-P2X7R + SAM, and Ad-P2X7R + NaHS. For the 3-day study, mNSSs (n = 5 for the 1-day or 3-day time point) and brain water content (n = 5 for the 1-day or 3-day time point) were assessed. qPCR (n = 5) and western blotting (n = 5) were performed at 1 day after ICH.

Experiment 4

To validate the involvement of the P2X7R in the mechanism by which microglia-derived H_2S prevented NLRP3 inflammasome activation, we harvested rat primary microglial cells from 40 1-day-old post-natal rats, cultured the cells and randomized them into the following four groups: control, LPS + ATP, LPS + ATP + SAM and LPS + ATP + NaHS. qPCR (n = 3) and western blotting (n = 3) were performed, and the effects of different SAM and NaHS concentrations on cell viability (n = 3) were measured by Cell Counting Kit-8 (CCK-8) under lipopolysaccharide (LPS) and ATP stimulation.

Drug and adenovirus administration

S-adenosyl-L-methionine, a CBS-specific agonist (SAM, Sigma-Aldrich, St. Louis, MO, USA), and sodium hydrosulfide, a classical exogenous H_2S donor (NaHS, Aladdin, Shanghai, China), were diluted to concentrations of 100 mg/kg [14, 15] and 5.6 mg/kg [7], respectively, in vehicle (saline) solution. The rats were treated intraperitoneally with SAM, NaHS or vehicle at 0.5 h after ICH. For the 72-h study, SAM, NaHS and vehicle were administered three times at 0.5, 24, and 48 h after ICH.

For in vivo adenovirus administration, the following two types of recombinant adenoviruses were used for gene transfer: (1) a replication-deficient human adenovirus containing the rat P2X7R (adenovirus P2X7R, Ad-P2X7R), which was used to upregulate P2X7R expression, and (2) an adenovirus containing human GFP (Ad-GFP), which served as a control for Ad-P2X7R. Ad-P2X7R (6×10^{10} pfu/mL) and Ad-GFP (2×10^{10} pfu/mL) were produced by Genechem in Shanghai, China. Both adenoviruses were stored at $- 80$ °C until use and were diluted to 1.3×10^{10} pfu/mL in an enhanced transfection solution (Genechem, Shanghai, China) before intracerebroventricular injection. A total volume of 10 μL was used for each adenovirus administration to the animals.

Intracerebroventricular injection and ICH model establishment

The adenoviruses were injected into the left lateral ventricle 6 days before ICH, according to the previous procedure [16]. The rats were anaesthetised with intraperitoneal injections of sodium pentobarbital (100 mg/kg, Sigma-Aldrich,

St. Louis, MO, USA) and then fixed onto a stereotaxic head apparatus. A 26-gauge needle in a 10-μL Hamilton syringe (Microliter 701; Hamilton Company, Reno, NV, USA) was inserted into the left lateral ventricle through a cranial burr hole at the following coordinates relative to the bregma: 1.5 mm posterior, 3.0 mm lateral and 5.5 mm below the horizontal plane of the bregma. Then, the abovementioned formulated solution was slowly injected by a microinfusion pump (Harvard Apparatus, Holliston, MA, USA) at a rate of 0.5 μL/min. The needle was kept in place for 10 min after injection before being slowly withdrawn, and then, the head of the rat was tilted nose-down at a 30° angle for 30 min after suture placement. The animals in the sham and vehicle groups were injected with equal volumes of saline into their left lateral ventricle, and then, their incisions were closed with sutures.

The experimental ICH model was established as described in our previous study [17]. Briefly, the rats were anaesthetised and positioned prone in a stereotactic head frame (Kopf Instruments, Tujunga, CA, USA). A scalp incision was made along the midline, and a burr hole (1 mm) was drilled on the right side of the skull at 3 mm lateral to the bregma and 5 mm ventral to the cortical surface. One microliter (0.2 μL/min) of saline containing 0.2 units of bacterial collagenase (type VII; Sigma-Aldrich, St. Louis, MO, USA) was injected stereotaxically into the striatum (6 mm ventral from the skull surface) using a Nanomite Syringe Pump (Harvard Apparatus, Holliston, MA, USA). After injection, the syringe was left in place for 5 min. The needle was slowly removed over an additional 5 min to prevent backflow. The hole was sealed with bone wax, and the wound was sutured closed. In the sham group, the rats were subjected to only the needle insertion procedure described above. The rats were allowed to recover in separate cages, with free access to food and water.

Primary microglial cultures and drug treatment

Primary cultured rat microglial cells were prepared as described in our previous study [18], with minor modifications. Briefly, the meninges, choroidal plexus, brainstem and cerebellum were carefully separated from the cerebral hemispheres of 1-day-old post-natal Sprague–Dawley rats. Then, the cortices of the cerebral hemispheres were dissected and digested with 0.25% trypsin. The fragments were washed twice with D-Hank's solution, and the resuspended cells were then collected and seeded in uncoated culture flasks containing the indicated medium (DMEM/F12 supplemented with 10% foetal bovine serum, 1×10^5 U/L penicillin, 1×10^5 U/L streptomycin sulphate, pH 7.2) at a concentration of 1×10^6 cells/mL. The cells were cultured at 37 °C in humidified 5% CO_2/95% air, and the medium was changed every 4–5 days. Upon reaching confluence (14 days), the microglial cells were separated from the underlying astrocytic monolayer via gentle shaking of the flasks overnight, a separation made possible by the differential adhesive properties of the two cell lines. The floating microglia were subsequently collected and plated on sterile culture dishes at a density of 1×10^5 cells/cm^2. After 24 h of culture, the microglial cells were ready for use. The cells were verified via immunohistochemical staining with microglia-specific Iba1 antibodies.

To induce inflammasome activation, we plated 1×10^5 cells in a 6-well plate overnight. The medium was changed to serum-free medium the following morning, and then, the cells were treated with 1 µg/mL lipopolysaccharide (LPS, Sigma, St. Louis, MO, USA) with SAM or NaHS for 12 h. We administered dimethylsulfoxide (DMSO, Sigma, St. Louis, MO, USA)-only treatment as a control. Then, the microglial cells were exposed to 5 mM adenosine triphosphate (ATP) for 1 h. The cell extracts and precipitated supernatants were analysed by immunoblotting.

Neurobehavioural evaluation

Neurobehavioural function was assessed with the Modified Neurological Severity Scores (mNSSs) at 1 and 3 days after ICH by an investigator who was blinded to the experimental groups. The mNSS (normal score, 0; maximal deficit score, 18) is determined by summing the scores of motor, sensory, reflex and balance assessments [19], with higher scores signifying more severe neurological deficits.

Brain water content

Brain water content was evaluated for the brain edema as previously reported [16]. Briefly, the brain specimens were quickly divided into the ipsilateral cortex (Ipsi-CX), ipsilateral basal ganglia (Ipsi-BG), contralateral cortex (Cont-CX) and contralateral basal ganglia (Cont-BG). Brain water content was calculated as (wet weight – dry weight)/wet weight × 100%.

Methylene blue assay

Methylene blue assay was performed for the H$_2$S concentration. The rats were deeply anaesthetised, and their brains were removed post-operatively. The ipsilateral striatum was dissected out on an ice-cold operating table and immediately frozen at −80 °C until assayed. The tissues from the striatum of the injured hemisphere were collected for determination of their H$_2$S concentrations by the spectro-luminosity method. The brain tissues were homogenized in ice-cold 50 mmol/L potassium phosphate buffer, pH 8.0 (12% wt/vol), with a Polytron homogenizer. The tissue homogenates were centrifuged (47,000g, 10 min, 4 °C), and the cell supernatants were collected to evaluate H$_2$S levels. Blood samples were collected from the abdominal aorta and were immediately centrifuged to obtain plasma to test H$_2$S levels. The cell supernatants or plasma samples (75 µL) were mixed with 0.25 mL of Zn acetate (1%) and 0.45 mL of water for 10 min at room temperature. Trichloroacetic acid (TCA; 10%, 0.25 mL) was then added to the mixture, which was centrifuged under the indicated conditions (14,000g, 10 min, 4 °C). The clear supernatant was collected and mixed with N,N-dimethyl-p-phenylenediamine sulphate (20 mmol/L; 133 µL) in 7.2 mol/L hydrogen chloride (HCl) and ferric trichloride (FeCl$_3$; 30 mmol/L, 133 µL) in 1.2 mol/L HCl. After the resulting solution had incubated for 20 min at room temperature, we measured its absorbance at 670 nm with a spectrophotometer. A calibration curve of absorbance versus sulphide concentrations was constructed using defined concentrations of NaHS solution. When NaHS is dissolved in water, HS− is released and forms H$_2$S with H+. The H$_2$S concentration was taken as 30% of the NaHS concentration in each calculation.

Haemoglobin assay

The rats were perfused transcranially with phosphate-buffered saline under anaesthesia, and their ipsilateral hemispheres were collected for the following haemoglobin assay to indicate the hematoma volume, as previously reported [20]. Briefly, the rat ipsilateral hemispheres were homogenized in 3 mL of distilled water for 60 s. Then, the homogenized specimens were centrifuged at 13,000g for 30 min, after which 400 µL of Drabkin's reagent (Sigma-Aldrich, St Louis, MO, USA) was added to 100 µL of supernatant and stored at room temperature for 15 min. The haemoglobin absorbance was measured at 540 nm by a spectrophotometer and quantified using a standard curve. The results are presented as microliters of blood to represent the haemoglobin content in the ipsilateral hemispheres.

Fluoro-Jade C staining

Perihaematomal neuronal degeneration was examined by Fluoro-Jade C staining (Millipore, Temecula, CA, USA), as described previously [17]. The brain tissue sections were rinsed in basic alcohol for 5 min before being rinsed for 2 min in 70% alcohol. Distilled water was used to remove the alcohol, after which the sections were incubated in 0.06% potassium permanganate (KMnO$_4$) for 10 min, stained with 0.0001% Fluoro-Jade C in 0.1% acetic for 10 min and rinsed in distilled water for 5 min. After being triple-rinsed with distilled water, the sections were air-dried for 10 min, cleared in xylene and then covered with slips. Four perihaematomal images in each section were captured by a Zeiss microscope (Zeiss AxioCam, Germany), and Fluoro-Jade C-positive neurons were counted by ImageJ (National Institutes of Health, Bethesda, MD, USA).

CCK-8 assay

Primary microglial cells (1×10^5 cells/mL) were seeded into 96-well plates (100 µL/well) and grouped according to the different concentrations of SAM (0, 10, 100, 20, 400 µmol/L) and NaHS (0, 10, 100, 20, 400, 600 µmol/L) with which they were treated under LPS and ATP stimulation. Cell viability was evaluated by CCK-8 assay (Dojindo Laboratories, Kumamoto, Japan). At the end of each time point, the medium in the 96-well culture plates was changed to DMEM/F12 to avoid background interference, and then, CCK-8 (10 µL) was added to each well. Absorbance was measured at 450 nm using a spectrophotometer, and 620 nm was used as a reference wavelength.

qPCR

Total RNA was extracted from perihaematomal brain tissue specimens or primary microglial cells using TRIzol reagent (Invitrogen, Camarillo, CA, USA). Isolated RNA was reverse-transcribed into complementary DNA (cDNA) using a cDNA synthesis kit (Vazyme, Jiangsu, China) in accordance with the manufacturer's protocols. qPCR was performed using synthetic primers and SYBR Green (Thermo, Rockford, IL, USA) with an IQ5 Detection System. After incubating at 50 °C for 2 min and 95 °C for 10 min, the samples were subjected to 40 cycles of 95 °C for 15 s and 60 °C for 1 min. GAPDH was used as an endogenous control gene. The sequences of the primers specific for the P2X7R, NLRP3 and GADPH were as follows:

P2X7R, 5′-CTACTCTTCGGTGGGGGCTT-3′ (forward primer),
P2X7R, 5′-CTCTGGATCCGGGTGACTTT-3′ (reverse primer);
NLRP3, 5′-CTGCATGCCGTATCTGGTTG-3′ (forward primer),
NLRP3, 5′-GCTGAGCAAGCTAAAGGCTTC-3′ (reverse primer);
GAPDH, 5′-AGACAGCCGCATCTTCTTGT-3′ (forward primer),
GAPDH, 5′- TGATGGCAACAATGTCCACT-3′ (reverse primer).

Western blot analysis

Samples, including perihaematomal brain tissues, cell lysates and medium, were collected and subjected to western blot analysis, as described in our previous studies [16, 17]. The following primary antibodies were used: rabbit polyclonal anti-CBS antibody (1:200, Santa Cruz Biotechnology, Santa Cruz, CA, USA), rabbit polyclonal anti-P2X7R antibody (1:1000, Alomone Labs, Jerusalem, Israel), rabbit polyclonal anti-NLRP3 antibody (1:200, Santa Cruz Biotechnology, Santa Cruz, CA, USA), rabbit polyclonal anti-ASC antibody (1:500, Abcam, Cambridge, MA, USA), mouse monoclonal anti-caspase-1 p20 antibody (1:200, Santa Cruz Biotechnology, CA, USA), rabbit polyclonal anti-IL-1β antibody (1:1000, Millipore, Billerica, MA, USA), rabbit polyclonal anti-myeloperoxidase antibody (anti-MPO, 1:500, Abcam, Cambridge, MA, USA) and goat polyclonal anti-Iba1 antibody (1:600, Abcam, Cambridge, MA, USA). GAPDH (1:1000, Cell Signalling Technology, Danvers, MA, USA) was used as a loading control. The proteins were detected on nitrocellulose membranes with enhanced chemiluminescence reagents (GE Healthcare, Beijing, China), and the blot bands were quantified by densitometry with Image J software (National Institutes of Health, Bethesda, MD, USA). The results are expressed as a relative density ratio, which was normalized to the mean value of the vehicle or control group.

Immunofluorescence staining

Frozen sections (20-µm thickness) were obtained from each group at 1 day after ICH, for immunofluorescence staining as described previously [17], and washed with a 0.01 M phosphate buffer solution after 30 min of heating at 37 °C. The sections were incubated for 30 min in 5% bovine serum albumin and then incubated at 4 °C overnight with the following primary antibodies: rabbit polyclonal anti-CBS antibody (1:100, Santa Cruz Biotechnology, Santa Cruz, CA, USA), rabbit polyclonal anti-P2X7R antibody (1:500, Alomone Labs, Jerusalem, Israel), goat polyclonal anti-Iba1 antibody (1:300, Abcam, Cambridge, MA, USA), and rabbit polyclonal anti-MPO antibody (1:50, Abcam, Cambridge, MA, USA).

The microglial cultures were fixed for 30 min in 4% paraformaldehyde. The cells were blocked with 1% bovine serum for 60 min and then incubated overnight at 4 °C with the following primary antibodies: goat polyclonal anti-Iba1 antibody (1:300, Abcam, Cambridge, MA, USA) and rabbit polyclonal anti-P2X7R antibody (1:500, Alomone Labs, Jerusalem, Israel). For the double-staining experiments, the cells were incubated with the above primary antibodies overnight at 4 °C before undergoing a separate incubation with Alexa 488 and Alexa 568 secondary fluorescent antibodies (1:400, Invitrogen, Carlsbad, CA, USA) for 60 min at 37 °C. The nuclei were stained with 4′,6-diamidino-2-phenylindole (DAPI, Thermo Fisher Scientific, Waltham, MA, USA) for 10 min. The sections and cells were observed by microscopy (Zeiss, AxioCam, Germany) or confocal microscopy (LSM780, Zeiss, Jena, Germany).

TUNEL staining

TUNEL staining was performed to evaluate the cell apoptosis in perihaematomal brain tissues. At 1 day after ICH, TUNEL staining was performed with an in situ apoptosis detection kit (Roche Molecular Biochemicals, Mannheim, Germany), according to the manufacturer's instruction. Briefly, selected sections were pretreated with 20 mg/mL proteinase-K in 10 mM Tris-HCl at 37 °C for 15 min and then incubated in 0.3% hydrogen peroxide dissolved in anhydrous methanol for 10 min after being rinsed in phosphate-buffered saline. The sections were then incubated in 0.1% sodium citrate and 0.1% Triton X-100 solution for 2 min at 4 °C. After several washes with phosphate-buffered saline, the sections were incubated with 50 μL of TUNEL reaction mixture with terminal deoxynucleotidyl transferase (TdT) for 60 min at 37 °C under humidified conditions, and the neuronal nuclei were stained with DAPI. Then, the sections were visualized by a confocal microscope. Negative controls were prepared by omitting the TdT enzyme. To evaluate the extent of cell injury, we examined and photographed six microscopic fields in parallel for TUNEL-positive cell counting.

Statistical analysis

All data are expressed as the mean ± SEM. SPSS 11.5 (SPSS Inc., Chicago, IL, USA) was used for statistical analysis. The Mann–Whitney U test was used to compare behaviour and activity scores among the groups. Other data were analysed by one-way ANOVA followed by the Scheffé F test for post hoc analysis. $p < 0.05$ was considered statistically significant.

Results

Endogenous H₂S production after ICH

To assess the changes in H₂S production after ICH, we measured H₂S concentrations in the brain striatum and blood plasma at 3, 6 and 12 h and 1, 2, 3 and 7 days after ICH (Fig. 1a). We found that H₂S concentrations in the brain striatum and blood plasma were significantly decreased in ICH-treated rats compared with sham-operated rats at all post-ICH time points ($p < 0.05$ vs. sham) and reached a nadir at 1 and 2 days after ICH, respectively ($p < 0.01$ vs. sham). The western blotting results indicated that CBS, a key enzyme involved in endogenous H₂S synthesis, exhibited the same trend in its protein levels as H₂S concentrations in the ipsilateral/right hemisphere after ICH (Fig. 1b). Further investigation with double-immunofluorescence staining revealed that CBS was colocalized with perihaematoma microglia in the ipsilateral striatum, as demonstrated by the presence of Iba1 (Fig. 1c). These data demonstrated that microglia produce endogenous H₂S after ICH and that ICH significantly inhibits CBS activity.

Artificial regulation of H₂S after ICH

Since H₂S production decreased significantly after ICH, we employed an agonist of CBS, SAM or the classical exogenous H₂S donor, NaHS, to assess the fundamental functions of H₂S. Our data indicated that both SAM administration and NaHS administration significantly increased H₂S content in the brain striatum ($p < 0.05$ vs. vehicle, Fig. 1d) and blood plasma ($p < 0.05$ vs. vehicle, Fig. 1e) at 1 day after ICH. These data also demonstrated that SAM and NaHS administration significantly increased endogenous and exogenous H2S content, respectively, at 1 day after ICH.

There was no significant difference in haemorrhage volume among the vehicle group, SAM group and NaHS group ($p > 0.05$ vs. vehicle, Fig. 1f), demonstrating that our ICH rat models were reproducible and consistent and that the artificial interventions used in this study had no influence on haematoma formation or absorption.

H₂S attenuated neurological deficits after ICH

Fluoro-Jade C staining demonstrated significantly reduced perihaematomal neuronal cell injury as a result of SAM or NaHS administration at 1 day after ICH ($p < 0.05$ vs. vehicle, Fig. 2a, b, d). In addition, compared with the sham group, the vehicle group exhibited an increased number of TUNEL-positive cells in the perihaematomal area ($p < 0.01$, Fig. 2a, c, e). Remarkably, both SAM treatment and NaHS treatment induced a significant reduction in the number of TUNEL-positive cells in the perihaematomal area ($p < 0.05$ vs. vehicle, Fig. 2a, c, e). SAM and NaHS administration significantly revered the neurological deficits assessed at 1 and 3 days after ICH ($p < 0.01$ vs. sham, Fig. 2f) at both time points ($p < 0.05$ vs. vehicle, Fig. 2f).

At 1 day after ICH, brain water content was significantly increased in the ipsilateral basal ganglia ($p < 0.01$) and ipsilateral cortex ($p < 0.05$) of the ICH-treated groups compared with the sham group (Fig. 2g). SAM or NaHS treatment significantly reduced brain water content in the ipsilateral basal ganglia ($p < 0.05$ vs. vehicle, Fig. 2g), but not in the contralateral basal ganglia and ipsilateral cortex ($p > 0.05$ vs. vehicle, Fig. 2g). Moreover, there were no significant differences in brain water content in the contralateral basal ganglia and ipsilateral cortex in the ICH-treated groups compared to the vehicle group ($p > 0.05$, Fig. 2g). At 3 days after ICH, brain water content was increased only in the ipsilateral basal ganglia after ICH ($p < 0.01$ vs. sham, Fig. 2h) and was significantly reduced by both SAM administration and NaHS administration ($p < 0.05$ vs. vehicle, Fig. 2h).

H₂S inhibited ICH-induced microglia accumulation, NLRP3 inflammasome activation and subsequent IL-1β release

Since the key enzyme for the endogenous synthesis of H2S, CBS, colocalized with microglia, as illustrated above, we investigated the effects of SAM and NaHS administration on neutrophil infiltration and microglia

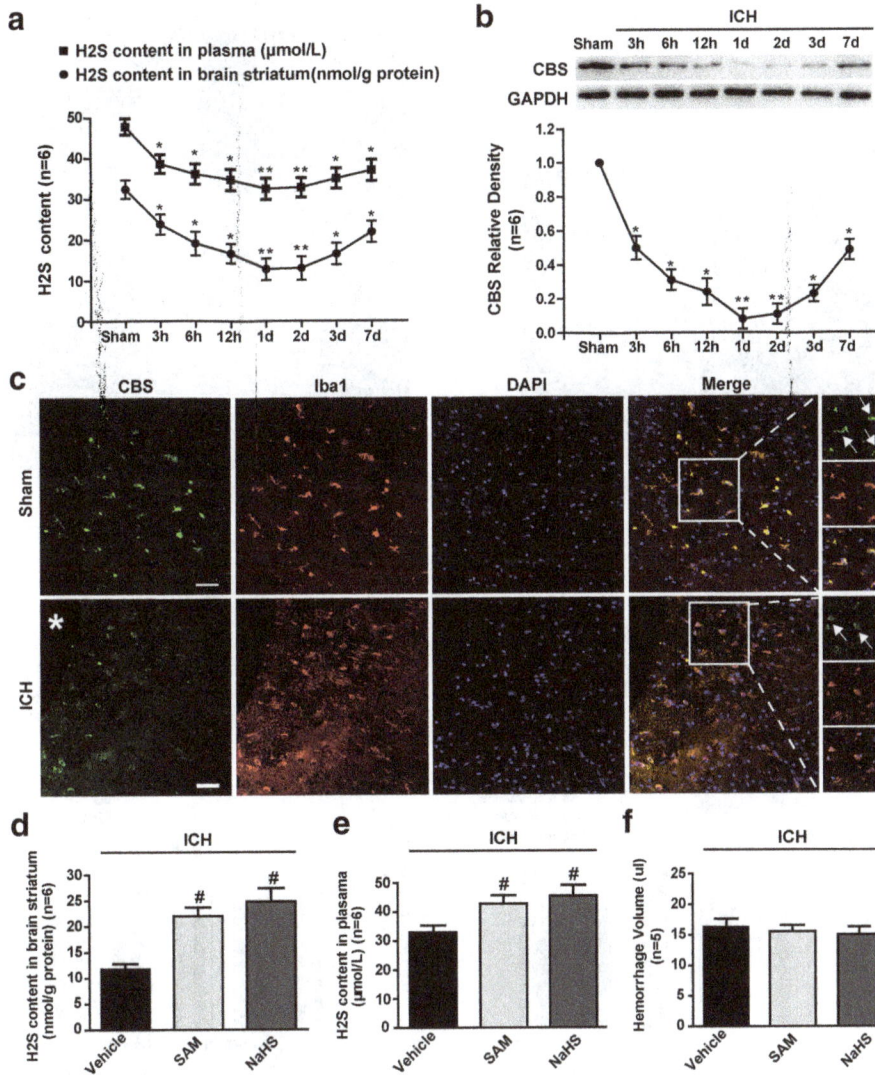

Fig. 1 Time course of H_2S content and CBS expression after ICH in rats. **a** Time course of H_2S content in the brain striatum and blood plasma at different time points after ICH. H_2S concentrations in the brain striatum and blood plasma were significantly decreased in ICH-treated rats compared with those in sham-operated rats at all post-ICH time points ($p < 0.05$ vs. sham) and reached a nadir at 1 and 2 days after ICH, respectively ($p < 0.01$ vs. sham). **b** Representative bands and quantitative analysis of the time course of CBS in perihaematomal brain tissues after ICH. CBS, a key enzyme involved in endogenous H_2S synthesis, exhibited the same trend in its protein levels as H_2S concentrations in the ipsilateral/right hemisphere after ICH. The relative densities of each protein have been normalized against those of the sham group. **c** Representative photographs of immunofluorescence staining for CBS (green) expression in microglia (Iba-1, red) in sham and the perihaematomal area, as the arrow indicates, at 1 day after ICH. CBS was colocalized with perihaematoma microglia in the ipsilateral striatum, as demonstrated by the presence of Iba1. **d, e** H_2S content in the brain striatum and plasma at 1 day after ICH in the vehicle, SAM and NaHS groups. Both SAM administration and NaHS administration significantly increased H_2S content in brain striatum ($p < 0.05$ vs. vehicle) and blood plasma ($p < 0.05$ vs. vehicle) at 1 day after ICH. These data also demonstrated that SAM and NaHS administration significantly increased endogenous and exogenous H2S content, respectively, at 1 day after ICH. **f** Quantitative analyses of haemorrhage volume in the vehicle, SAM and NaHS groups at 1 day after ICH. There was no significant difference in haemorrhage volume among the vehicle group, SAM group and NaHS group ($p > 0.05$ vs. vehicle). For haemorrhage volume, $n = 5$ rats per group; for others, $n = 6$ rats per group and time point. Scale bar = 12.5 μm. Data are presented as the mean ± SEM. $*p < 0.05$ vs. sham, $**p < 0.01$ vs. sham, $\#p < 0.05$ vs. vehicle. CBS cystathionine-β-synthase, DAPI 4′,6-diamidino-2-phenylindole, GAPDH glyceraldehyde 3-phosphate dehydrogenase, ICH intracerebral haemorrhage, SAM S-adenosyl-L-methionine

accumulation. We detected myeloperoxidase (MPO) and Iba1 levels in brain tissue by immunostaining, as well as western blotting, 1 day following ICH. Immunostaining (Fig. 3a) indicated that SAM and NaHS treatment significantly reduced the number of MPO-positive and

Iba1-positive cells in the perihaematomal area in the ICH-treated groups compared to the vehicle group ($p < 0.05$, Fig. 3b, c). Consistently, the western blotting results showed that MPO and Iba1 protein levels in the ipsilateral hemisphere were markedly reduced after SAM

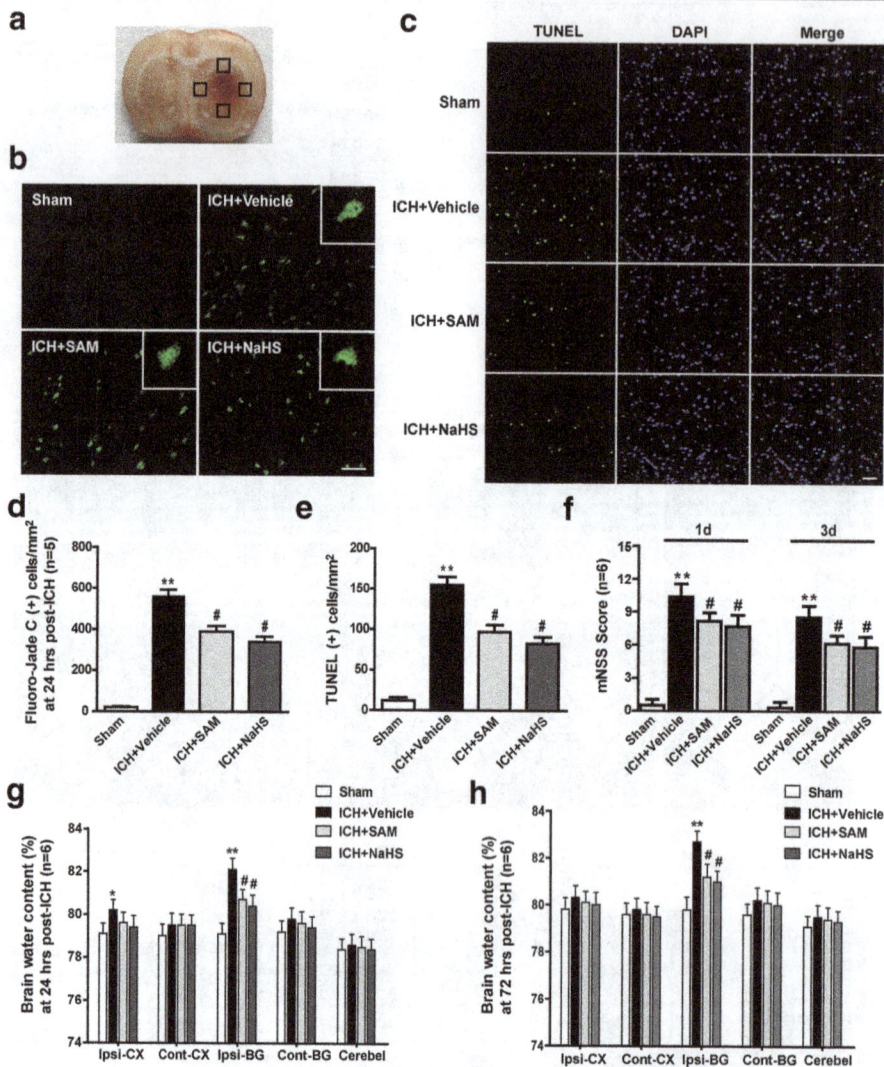

Fig. 2 The effects of SAM and NaHS administration on neurological deficits and brain edema at 1 and 3 days after ICH. **a** The schematic diagram shows the four areas (black squares) for Fluoro-Jade C- and TUNEL-positive cell counting in the perihaematomal region. **b** Representative Fluoro-Jade C staining images and quantitative analyses of Fluoro-Jade C-positive neurons surrounding the haematoma in the sham, vehicle, SAM and NaHS groups at 1 day after ICH. **c** Representative images of TUNEL-stained (green) and DAPI-stained (blue) brain sections in the perihaematomal area in the sham, vehicle, SAM and NaHS groups at 1 day following operation. **d**, **e** Quantitative analyses of Fluoro-Jade C-positive neurons and TUNEL-positive cells surrounding the haematoma in the sham, vehicle, SAM and NaHS groups at 1 day after ICH. Fluoro-Jade C staining demonstrated significantly reduced perihaematomal neuronal cell injury as a result of SAM or NaHS administration at 1 day after ICH ($p < 0.05$ vs. vehicle). Compared with the sham group, the vehicle group exhibited an increased number of TUNEL-positive cells in the perihaematomal area ($p < 0.01$). Remarkably, both SAM treatment and NaHS treatment induced a significant reduction in the number TUNEL-positive cells in the perihaematomal area ($p < 0.05$ vs. vehicle). **f** Modified Neurological Severity Scores in the sham, vehicle, SAM and NaHS groups at 1 and 3 days after ICH. SAM and NaHS administration significantly revered the neurological deficits assessed at 1 and 3 days after ICH ($p < 0.01$ vs. sham) at both time points ($p < 0.05$ vs. vehicle). **g**, **h** Brain water content assessment in the sham, vehicle, SAM and NaHS groups at 1 and 3 days after operation. At 1 day after ICH, brain water content was significantly increased in the ipsilateral basal ganglia ($p < 0.01$) and ipsilateral cortex ($p < 0.05$) of the ICH-treated groups compared with that in the sham group. SAM or NaHS treatment significantly reduced brain water content in the ipsilateral basal ganglia ($p < 0.05$ vs. vehicle), but not in the contralateral basal ganglia and ipsilateral cortex ($p > 0.05$ vs. vehicle). Moreover, there were no significant differences in brain water content in the contralateral basal ganglia and ipsilateral cortex in the ICH-treated groups compared to the vehicle group ($p > 0.05$). At 3 days after ICH, brain water content was increased only in the ipsilateral basal ganglia after ICH ($p < 0.01$ vs. sham) and was significantly reduced by both SAM administration and NaHS administration ($p < 0.05$ vs. vehicle). $N = 6$ for mNSS and brain water content assessment; $n = 5$ for Fluoro-Jade C staining; $n = 4$ for TUNEL staining. Scale bar = 50 μm. Data are presented as the mean ± SEM. *$p < 0.05$ vs. sham; **$p < 0.01$ vs. sham; #$p < 0.05$ vs. vehicle. SAM S-adenosyl-L-methionine, mNSS Modified Neurological Severity Score, ICH intracerebral haemorrhage, TUNEL terminal deoxynucleotidyl transferase dUTP nick end-labelling, DAPI 4′,6-diamidino-2-phenylindole, Ipsi-CX ipsilateral cortex, Cont-CX contralateral cortex, Ipsi-BG ipsilateral basal ganglia, Cont-BG contralateral basal ganglia, Cerebel cerebellum

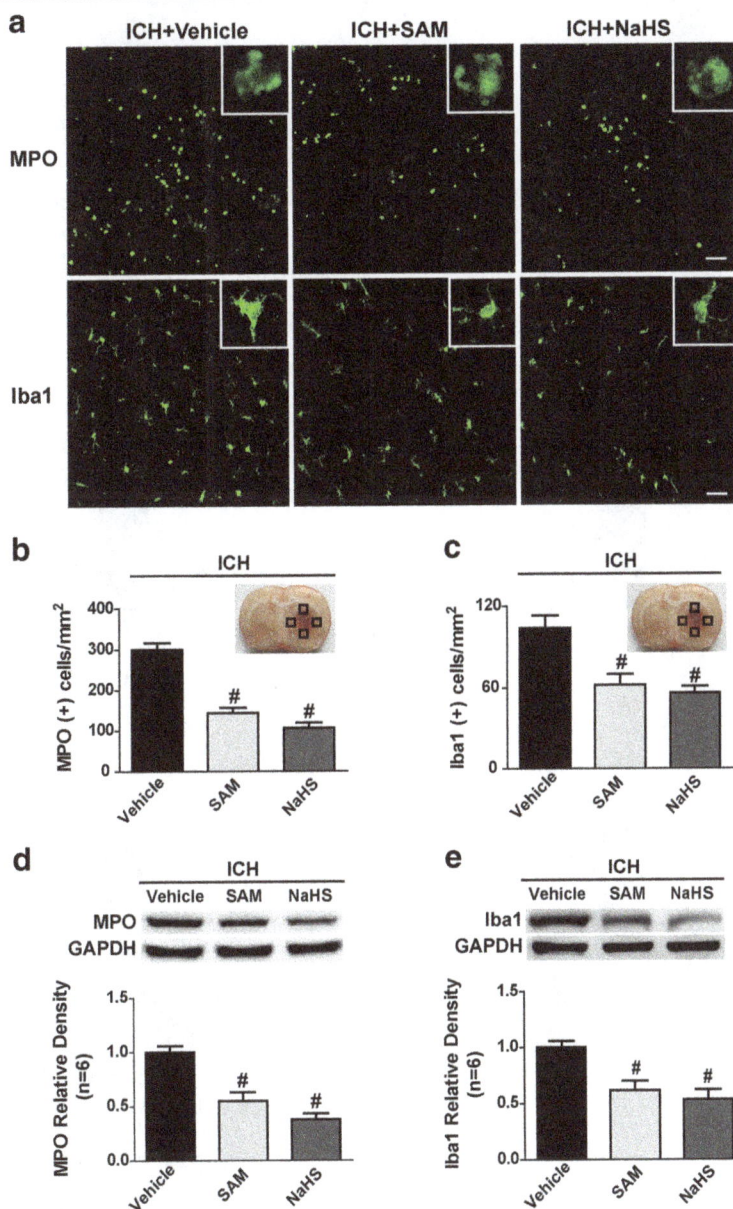

Fig. 3 The effects of SAM and NaHS administration on neutrophil infiltration and microglia accumulation at 1 day after ICH. **a** Representative photographs of immunofluorescence staining of MPO immuno-labelled neutrophils (green) and Iba1 immuno-labelled microglia (green) in the perihaematomal area in the vehicle, SAM and NaHS groups at 1 day after ICH. **b**, **c** Quantitative analysis of MPO and Iba1-positive cells in the perihaematomal region in the vehicle, SAM and NaHS groups at 1 day after ICH. SAM and NaHS treatment significantly reduced the number of MPO-positive and Iba1-positive cells in the perihaematomal area in the ICH-treated groups compared to the vehicle group. **d**, **e** Representative bands and quantitative analysis of MPO and Iba1 protein levels in the perihaematomal tissues in the vehicle, SAM and NaHS groups at 1 day after ICH. MPO and Iba1 protein levels in the ipsilateral hemisphere were markedly reduced after SAM and NaHS treatment in the ICH-treated groups compared to the vehicle group. The relative densities of each protein have been normalized against those of the vehicle group. For western blotting, $n = 6$ rats per group; for others, $n = 4$ rats per group. Scale bar = 25 μm. Data are presented as the mean ± SEM. #$p < 0.05$ vs. vehicle. MPO myeloperoxidase, SAM S-adenosyl-L-methionine, ICH intracerebral haemorrhage

and NaHS treatment in the ICH-treated groups compared to the vehicle group ($p < 0.05$, Fig. 3d, e).

To investigate the effects of SAM and NaHS on NLRP3 inflammasome activation, we first detected NLRP3 messenger RNA (mRNA) levels by qPCR. NLRP3 mRNA levels were apparently increased in the vehicle group at 1 day after ICH ($p < 0.01$ vs. sham, Fig. 4a). SAM and NaHS treatment significantly reduced NLRP3 mRNA expression in their respective treatment groups compared to the vehicle group ($p < 0.05$, Fig. 4a). Then, we detected the protein levels of the NLRP3 inflammasome components and mature IL-1β by western blotting. The protein

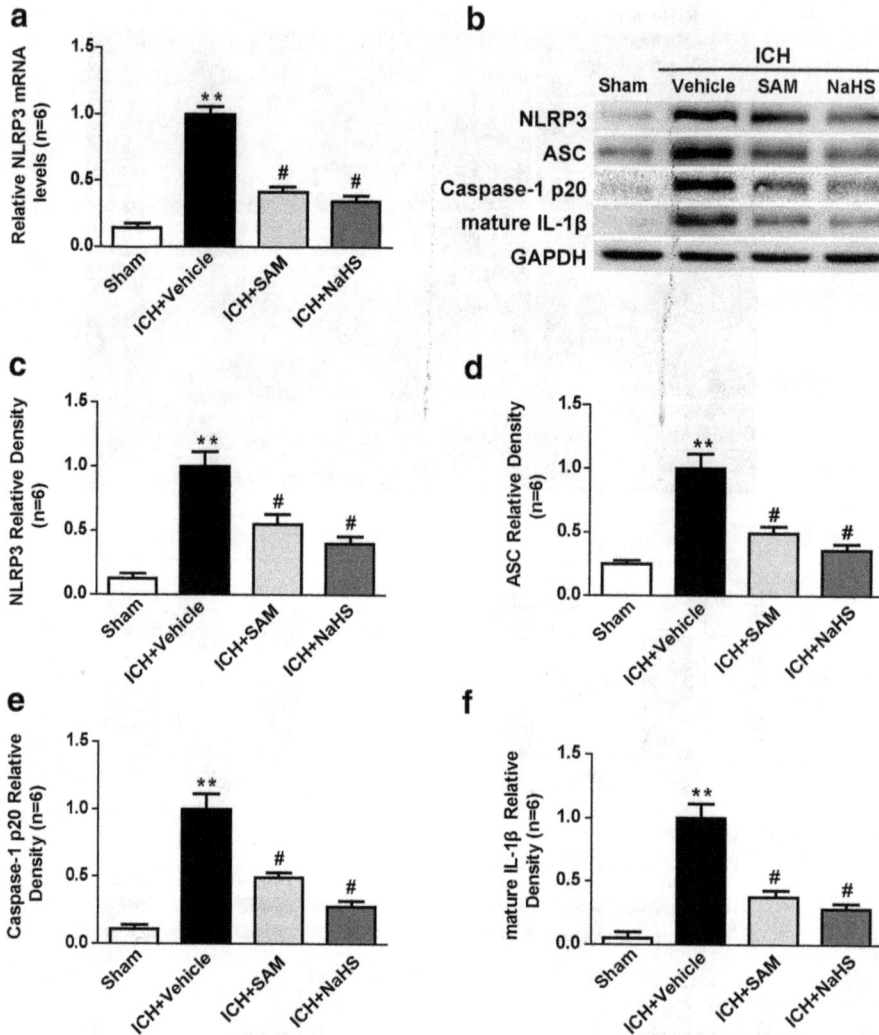

Fig. 4 The effects of SAM and NaHS administration on NLRP3 inflammasome activation and IL-1β maturation. **a** Quantitative analysis of NLRP3 mRNA levels by qPCR in the sham, vehicle, SAM and NaHS groups at 1 day after ICH. NLRP3 mRNA levels were apparently increased in the vehicle group at 1 day after ICH ($p < 0.01$ vs. sham). SAM and NaHS treatment significantly reduced NLRP3 mRNA expression in their respective treatment groups compared to the vehicle group ($p < 0.05$). The relative densities of each mRNA have been normalized against those of the vehicle group. **b–f** Representative bands and quantitative analysis of NLRP3, ASC, caspase-1 p20 subunit and mature IL-1β levels in the perihaematomal tissues of the sham, vehicle, SAM and NaHS groups at 1 day after ICH. The protein levels of the NLRP3 inflammasome components, including the protein levels of NLRP3, ASC and caspase-1, and the levels of IL-1β production were evidently elevated in the vehicle group at 1 day after ICH ($p < 0.01$ vs. sham). SAM and NaHS treatment significantly suppressed NLRP3 inflammasome component expression and the subsequent secretion of mature IL-1β ($p < 0.05$ vs. vehicle). The relative densities of each protein have been normalized against those of the vehicle group. $N = 6$ rats per group. Data are presented as the mean ± SEM. **$p < 0.01$ vs. sham; #$p < 0.05$ vs. vehicle. SAM S-adenosyl-L-methionine, GAPDH glyceraldehyde 3-phosphate dehydrogenase, ICH intracerebral haemorrhage, IL interleukin, NLRP3 pyrin domain-containing 3, ASC adaptor protein apoptosis-associated speck-like protein containing a CARD

levels of the NLRP3 inflammasome components, including the protein levels of NLRP3, ASC and caspase-1, and the levels of IL-1β production were evidently elevated in the vehicle group at 1 day after ICH ($p < 0.01$ vs. sham, Fig. 4b–f). SAM and NaHS treatment significantly suppressed NLRP3 inflammasome component expression and the subsequent secretion of mature IL-1β ($p < 0.05$ vs. vehicle, Fig. 4b–f).

H₂S suppressed P2X7R expression on microglia after ICH

The qPCR results revealed that ICH-induced P2X7R mRNA expression was evidently elevated in the periphery of the haemorrhage at 1 day after injury ($p < 0.01$ vs. sham, Fig. 5a). Both SAM treatment and NaHS treatment significantly reduced P2X7R mRNA expression in their respective treatment groups compared to the vehicle group ($p < 0.05$, Fig. 5a). Likewise, P2X7R protein expression

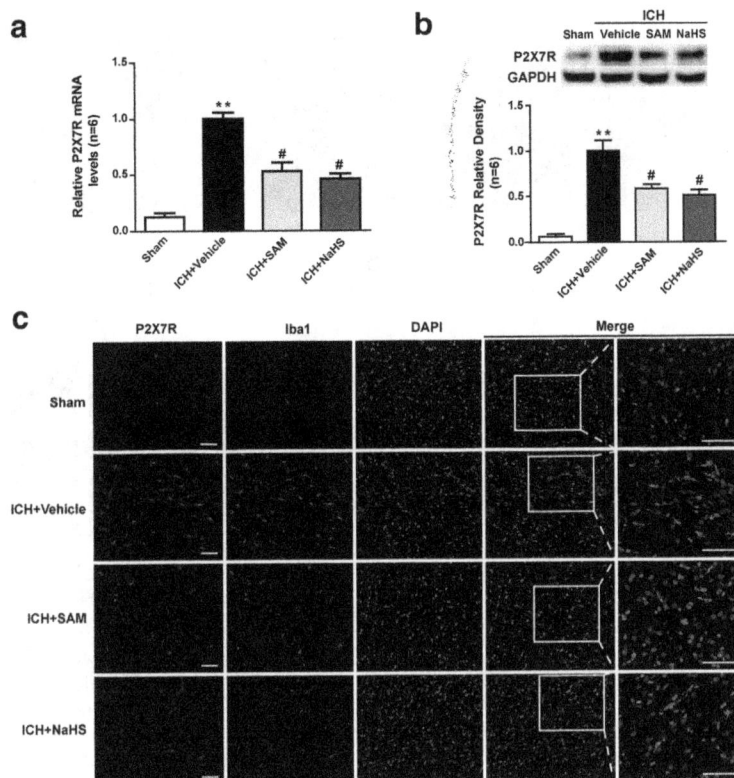

Fig. 5 The effects of SAM and NaHS administration on P2X7R expression at 1 day after ICH. **a** Quantitative analysis of P2X7R mRNA levels by qPCR in the sham, vehicle, SAM and NaHS groups at 1 day after ICH. The qPCR results revealed that ICH-induced P2X7R mRNA expression was evidently elevated in the periphery of the haemorrhage at 1 day after injury ($p < 0.01$ vs. sham). Both SAM treatment and NaHS treatment significantly reduced P2X7R mRNA expression in their respective treatment groups compared to the vehicle group ($p < 0.05$). The relative densities of each mRNA have been normalized against those of the vehicle group. **b** Representative bands and quantitative analysis of P2X7R expression in the perihaematomal tissues in the sham, vehicle, SAM and NaHS groups at 1 day after ICH. P2X7R protein expression was upregulated at 1 day after ICH induction ($p < 0.01$ vs. sham) and SAM and NaHS administration reversed this trend, as demonstrated by western blot analysis ($p < 0.05$ vs. vehicle). The relative densities of each protein have been normalized against those of the vehicle group. **c** Representative photographs of Iba1-positive cells co-labelled with P2X7R in the perihaematomal tissues of the sham, vehicle, SAM and NaHS groups at 1 day after ICH. Few P2X7R-positive microglia (Iba1-positive cells) were detected in the sham group. However, many more activated P2X7R-positive microglia were observed in the ICH-treated groups post-ICH. SAM and NaHS administration inhibited the increases in the numbers of P2X7R-positive microglia that occurred after ICH induction. $N = 6$ rats per group, scale bar = 40 μm. Data are the mean ± SEM. **$p < 0.01$ vs. sham, #$p < 0.05$ vs. vehicle. SAM S-adenosyl-L-methionine, GAPDH glyceraldehyde 3-phosphate dehydrogenase, ICH intracerebral haemorrhage, DAPI 4′,6-diamidino-2-phenylindole

was upregulated at 1 day after ICH induction ($p < 0.01$ vs. sham, Fig. 5b), and SAM and NaHS administration reversed this trend, as demonstrated by western blot analysis ($p < 0.05$ vs. vehicle, Fig. 5b).

Immunofluorescent characterization of the brain sections at 1 day after ICH and subsequent confocal analyses were performed to evaluate P2X7R and microglia cell colocalization. Few P2X7R-positive microglia (Iba1-positive cells) were detected in the sham group. However, many more activated P2X7R-positive microglia were observed in the ICH-treated groups post-ICH. SAM and NaHS administration inhibited the increases in the numbers of P2X7R-positive microglia that occurred after ICH induction (Fig. 5c).

To verify the involvement of the P2X7R in the suppression of NLRP3 inflammasome activation by H2S in microglia, we cultured primary microglial cells under in vitro conditions characterized by artificial inflammation and P2X7R activation facilitated by combining LPS and ATP in the culture mediums. First, to verify the primary cultured rat microglial cells, we seeded a subset of cells onto glass slides for characterization by immunofluorescence, which showed that the primary microglial cells were Iba1-positive cells (Fig. 6a, b). LPS and ATP stimulation substantially inhibited cell viability, as demonstrated by the CCK-8 assay ($p < 0.01$ vs. control, Fig. 6c). These cytotoxic effects were attenuated in a concentration-dependent manner by SAM at concentrations ranging from 50 to 400 μM, and the maximum response was achieved at a concentration of 200 μM ($p < 0.01$ vs. control, Fig. 6c). Similar effects were observed with NaHS administration. NaHS exerted its maximal effect at a concentration of 400 μM ($p < 0.01$ vs. control, Fig. 6d). These data suggested

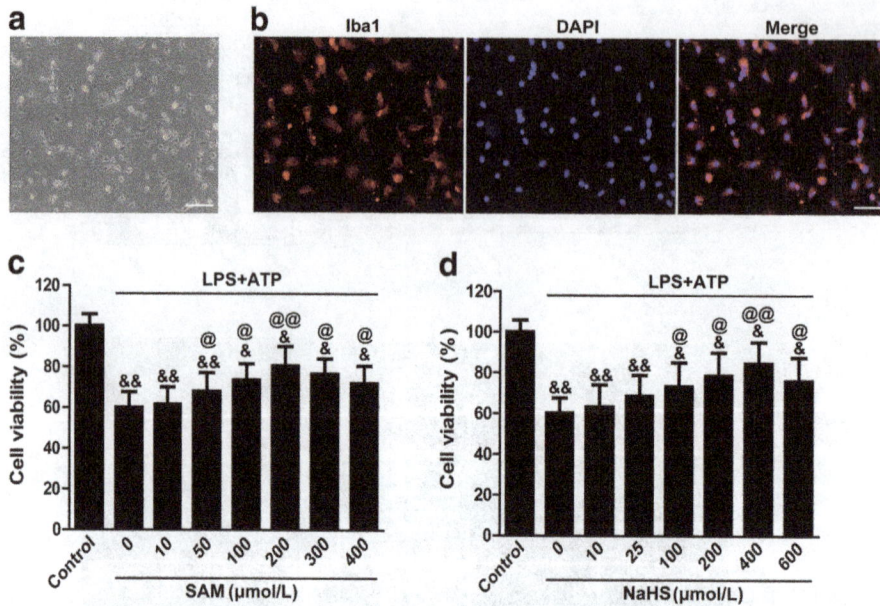

Fig. 6 Primary cultured rat microglial cells and the effects of SAM and NaHS on cell viability following LPS and ATP stimulation. **a** Microscope-captured image of microglial cells and **b** representative photographs of immunofluorescence staining for Iba-1-positive primary cultured rat microglia. **c, d** The effects of different concentrations of SAM and NaHS on the viability of rat primary cultured microglial cells. LPS and ATP stimulation substantially inhibited cell viability, as demonstrated by CCK-8 assay ($p < 0.01$ vs. control). These cytotoxic effects were attenuated in a concentration-dependent manner by SAM at concentrations ranging from 50 to 400 μM, and the maximum response was achieved at a concentration of 200 μM ($p < 0.01$ vs. control). Similar effects were observed with NaHS administration. NaHS exerted its maximal effect at a concentration of 400 μM ($p < 0.01$ vs. control). $N = 3$ per group, scale bars = 75 μm. Data are presented as the mean ± SEM. &&$p < 0.01$ vs. control; &$p < 0.05$ vs. control; @@$p < 0.01$ vs. LPS + ATP (with 0 μmol SAM); @$p < 0.05$ vs. LPS + ATP (with 0 μmol SAM). SAM S-adenosyl-L-methionine, DAPI 4′,6-diamidino-2-phenylindole

that H_2S protected the microglial cells against LPS and ATP stimulation-induced cell injury, results consistent with those of our in vivo study, especially the results of our TUNEL staining assay. SAM (at a concentration of 200 μM) or NaHS (at a concentration of 400 μM) was added to produce endogenous and exogenous H2S for the following in vitro study.

Subsequently, qPCR and western blotting were carried out to detect P2X7R mRNA and protein expression. The results of those experiments revealed that both P2X7R mRNA and P2X7R protein levels were evidently elevated after LPS and ATP stimulation ($p < 0.01$ vs. control, Fig. 7a, b) and that both SAM treatment and NaHS treatment significantly suppressed these upregulations ($p < 0.05$, Fig. 7a, b). Immunostaining also indicated that the numbers of P2X7R-positive cells were increased and that the cells were visually identical to activated microglia after LPS and ATP stimulation (Fig. 7c). Both SAM treatment and NaHS treatment significantly alleviated these changes (Fig. 7c).

H₂S reversed the detrimental effects of P2X7R overexpression

To study the effects of H2S on microglial NLRP3 inflammasome activation in vitro, we applied qPCR to detect NLRP3 mRNA levels in the microglial cell lysates, and then, we carried out western blotting to detect NLRP3

and ASC protein levels in the microglial cell lysates, as well as caspase-1 p20 and mature IL-1β levels in the medium, under LPS and ATP stimulation. LPS and ATP stimulation significantly enhanced NLRP3 mRNA levels ($p < 0.01$ vs. control, Fig. 8a). Both SAM and NaHS treatment inhibited this enhancement ($p < 0.05$ vs. LPS + ATP, Fig. 8a). Compared with the control group, LPS and ATP stimulation increased the protein levels of the NLRP3 inflammasome components in the LPS + ATP group, leading to increased levels of IL-1β and caspase-1 release in the medium ($p < 0.01$, Fig. 6b–f), but SAM and NaHS treatment significantly suppressed these upregulations ($p < 0.05$, Fig. 8b–f).

To clarify the role of the P2X7R in the activation of the NLRP3 inflammasome and the subsequent processing of IL-1β, we generated recombinant adenoviruses to overexpress the P2X7R in vivo. The qPCR results revealed that the mRNA levels of the P2X7R and NLRP3 were upregulated in the Ad-P2X7R group ($p < 0.05$ vs. vehicle, Fig. 9a, b), but not in the Ad-GFP group ($p > 0.05$ vs. vehicle, Fig. 9a, b), at 1 day after ICH. Administration of both SAM and NaHS inhibited the increase in P2X7R expression ($p < 0.05$ vs. Ad-P2X7R, Fig. 9a, b). Western blotting performed at 1 day after ICH indicated that similar increases in the protein levels of the P2X7R and NLRP3 were induced by

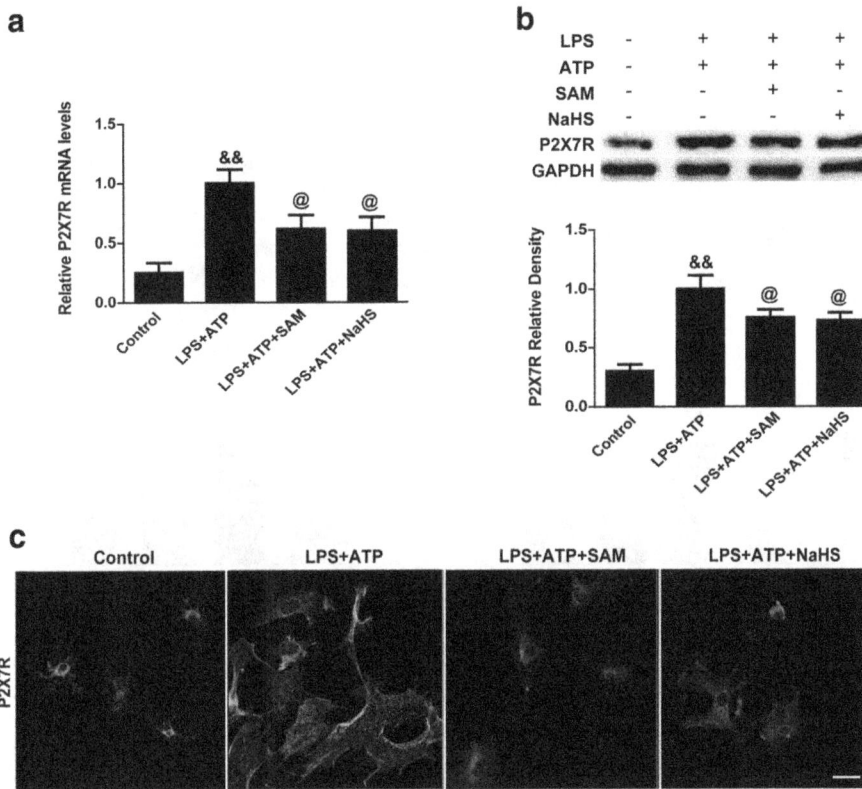

Fig. 7 The effects of SAM and NaHS administration on P2X7R expression in primary microglial cells. **a** Quantitative analysis of P2X7R mRNA levels by qPCR in the control, LPS + ATP, LPS + ATP + SAM and LPS + ATP + NaHS groups. P2X7R mRNAs were evidently elevated after LPS and ATP stimulation ($p < 0.01$ vs. control) and that both SAM treatment and NaHS treatment significantly suppressed these upregulations ($p < 0.05$ (**a, b**)). The relative densities of each mRNA have been normalized against those of the LPS + ATP group. **b** Representative bands and quantitative analysis of P2X7R in the control, LPS + ATP, LPS + ATP + SAM and LPS + ATP + NaHS groups. P2X7R protein levels were evidently elevated after LPS and ATP stimulation ($p < 0.01$ vs. control) and that both SAM treatment and NaHS treatment significantly suppressed these upregulations ($p < 0.05$). The relative densities of each protein have been normalized against those of the LPS + ATP group. **c** Representative photographs of P2X7R-positive cells in the control, LPS + ATP, LPS + ATP + SAM and LPS + ATP + NaHS groups. The numbers of P2X7R-positive cells were increased and that the cells were visually identical to activated microglia after LPS and ATP stimulation. Both SAM treatment and NaHS treatment significantly alleviated these changes. $N = 3$ per group, scale bar = 50 μm. Data are the mean ± SEM. $**p < 0.01$ vs. sham, $#p < 0.05$ vs. vehicle, $&&p < 0.01$ vs. control, $@p < 0.05$ vs. LPS + ATP. SAM S-adenosyl-L-methionine, DAPI 4′,6-diamidino-2-phenylindole

P2X7R overexpression and were suppressed by SAM and NaHS administration (Fig. 9c, d). Moreover, the protein levels of mature IL-1β and MPO were significantly elevated by overexpressing P2X7R at 1 day after ICH in the indicated group compared to the vehicle group ($p < 0.05$, Fig. 9e, f), but SAM or NaHS administration inhibited these increases ($p < 0.05$ vs. Ad-P2X7R, Fig. 9e, f).

Additionally, regarding the 3-day study of neurological outcomes and brain oedema in the setting of P2X7R overexpression after ICH, we found that neurological deficits (Fig. 10a, b) and brain oedema (Fig. 10c, d) were worse in the Ad-P2X7R group ($p < 0.05$), but not in the Ad-GFP group ($p > 0.05$ vs. vehicle, Fig. 10a–d), than in the vehicle group. Neurological deficits and brain oedema were significantly alleviated in the Ad-P2X7R + SAM and Ad-P2X7R + NaHS groups ($p < 0.05$ vs. Ad-P2X7R, Fig. 10a–d). These results indicated that the P2X7R played a pivotal

role in H$_2$S-mediated anti-NLRP3 inflammasome activation and neuroprotection after ICH.

Discussion

In this study, we demonstrated that ICH induced significant downregulation of endogenous H$_2$S production in the rat brain. This downregulation may be the result of a decrease in CBS protein levels. Administration of SAM, the CBS-specific agonist, or NaHS, a classical exogenous H$_2$S donor, not only restored brain and plasma H$_2$S content but also attenuated brain oedema, neutrophil infiltration, microglial accumulation, neurological deficits and neuronal apoptosis at 1 day post-ICH by inhibiting the P2X7R/NLRP3 inflammasome signalling cascade. Endogenous H$_2$S production, which was mainly driven by microglial cells and the above treatments, was verified by adenovirus-mediated P2X7 receptor overexpression and an in vitro study involving a primary microglial cell

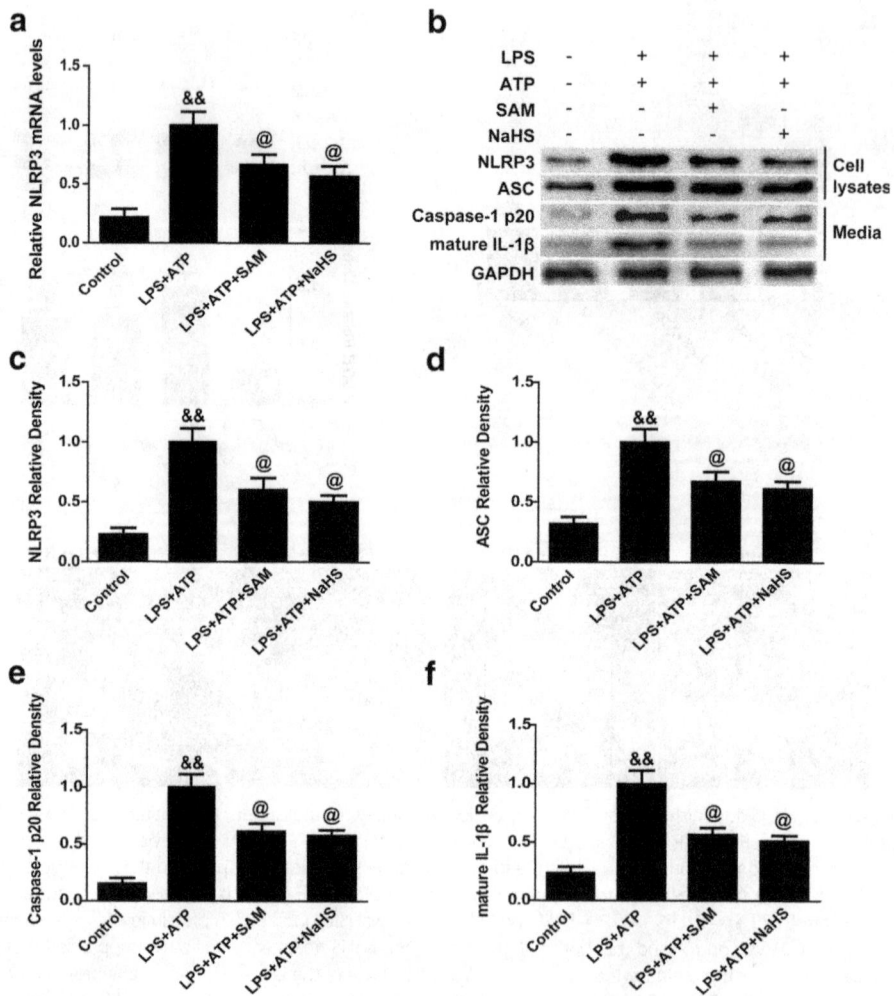

Fig. 8 The effects of SAM and NaHS administration on NLRP3 inflammasome activation in primary microglial cells. **a** Quantitative analysis of NLRP3 mRNA levels by qPCR in the control, LPS + ATP, LPS + ATP + SAM and LPS + ATP + NaHS groups. The relative densities of each mRNA have been normalized against those of the LPS + ATP group. LPS and ATP stimulation significantly enhanced NLRP3 mRNA levels ($p < 0.01$ vs. control). Both SAM and NaHS treatment inhibited this enhancement ($p < 0.05$ vs. LPS + ATP). **b–f** Representative bands and quantitative analysis of NLRP3 and ASC expression in the microglial cell lysates and caspase-1 p20 subunit and mature IL-1β levels in the medium and in the control, LPS + ATP, LPS + ATP + SAM and LPS + ATP + NaHS groups. Compared with the control group, LPS and ATP stimulation increased the protein levels of the NLRP3 inflammasome components in the LPS + ATP group, leading to increased levels of IL-1β and caspase-1 release in the medium ($p < 0.01$), but SAM and NaHS treatment significantly suppressed these upregulations ($p < 0.05$). The relative densities of each protein have been normalized against those of the LPS + ATP group. $N = 3$ per group, Data are presented as the mean ± SEM. &&$p < 0.01$ vs. control; @$p < 0.05$ vs. LPS + ATP. SAM S-adenosyl-L-methionine, GAPDH glyceraldehyde 3-phosphate dehydrogenase, IL interleukin, NLRP3 pyrin domain-containing 3, ASC adaptor protein apoptosis-associated speck-like protein containing a CARD

system. To our knowledge, we are the first to report that endogenous H_2S served as an anti-neuroinflammatory gasotransmitter in microglia to attenuate secondary brain injury mediated by the P2X7R/NLRP3 inflammasome signalling pathway after experimental ICH.

It is well known that the neuroinflammatory response plays an important role in the pathogenesis of ICH and that this response involves cell–cell connections between activated glial cells and neurons in the vascular neural network [21, 22]. Microglia are specialized macrophages residing in the central nervous system. Ample amounts

of evidence indicate that they play a crucial role in neuroinflammation. Activated microglia produce and release some pro-inflammatory factors, such as nitric oxide, tumour necrosis factor-α and IL-1β, which aggravate cell death and brain tissue injury further [23, 24]. Previous studies have shown that H_2S attenuated the inflammatory response in microglia exposed to lipopolysaccharides [25, 26] and demonstrated the ability to attenuate blood-brain barrier permeability and brain oedema after cardiac arrest and resuscitation [27]. However, the origin of endogenous H_2S has not been fully elucidated.

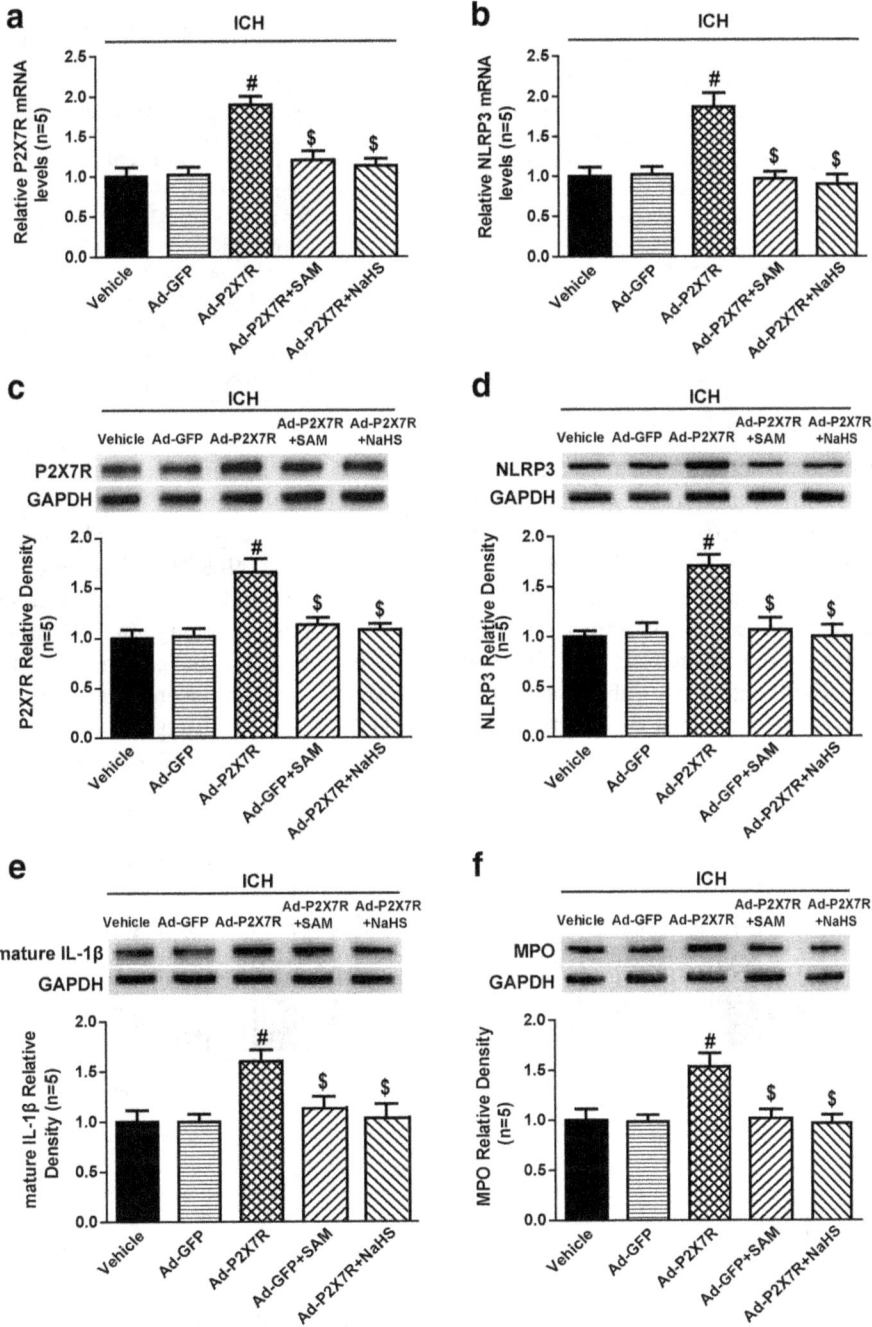

Fig. 9 (See legend on next page.)

Fig. 9 The effects of SAM and NaHS administration on NLRP3 inflammasome activation and MPO expression in P2X7R-overexpressing rats at 1 day after ICH. **a**, **b** Quantitative analysis of P2X7R and NLRP3 mRNA levels by qPCR in the vehicle, Ad-GFP, Ad-P2X7R, Ad-P2X7R + SAM and Ad-P2X7R + NaHS groups at 1 day after ICH. The mRNA levels of the P2X7R and NLRP3 were upregulated in Ad-P2X7R group ($p < 0.05$ vs. vehicle), but not in Ad-GFP group ($p > 0.05$ vs. vehicle), at 1 day after ICH. Administration of both SAM and NaHS inhibited the increase in P2X7R expression ($p < 0.05$ vs. Ad-P2X7R). The relative densities of each mRNA have been normalized against those of the vehicle group. **c–e** Representative bands and quantitative analysis of P2X7R, NLRP3 and mature IL-1β levels in the vehicle, Ad-GFP, Ad-P2X7R, Ad-P2X7R + SAM and Ad-P2X7R + NaHS groups at 1 day after ICH. The relative densities of each protein have been normalized against those of the vehicle group. **f** Representative bands and quantitative analysis of MPO levels in the vehicle, Ad-GFP, Ad-P2X7R, Ad-P2X7R + SAM and Ad-P2X7R + NaHS groups at 1 day after ICH. The relative densities of each protein have been normalized against those of the vehicle group. Western blotting performed at 1 day after ICH indicated that similar increases in the protein levels of the P2X7R and NLRP3 were induced by P2X7R overexpression and were suppressed by SAM and NaHS administration. Moreover, the protein levels of mature IL-1β and MPO were significantly elevated by overexpressing P2X7R at 1 day after ICH in the indicated group compared to the vehicle group ($p < 0.05$), but SAM or NaHS administration inhibited these increases ($p < 0.05$ vs. Ad-P2X7R). $N = 5$ rats per group. Data are presented as the mean ± SEM. #$p < 0.05$ vs. vehicle; $$p < 0.05$ vs. Ad-P2X7R. SAM S-adenosyl-L-methionine, NLRP3 pyrin domain-containing 3, GAPDH glyceraldehyde 3-phosphate dehydrogenase, ICH intracerebral haemorrhage, IL interleukin, Ad adenovirus, GFP green fluorescent protein, MPO myeloperoxidase

Increasing amounts of attention have been focused on the intestinal microbiome, which produces H₂S with the ability to cross the blood–brain barrier [28, 29]. In the present study, we found that the predominant H₂S-generating enzyme, CBS, colocalized with microglia after ICH, which suggested that microglia are sources of endogenous H₂S in the central neural system. Moreover, the aforementioned reductions in H₂S content and inhibition of CBS may indicate that the anti-inflammatory effects of H₂S were impaired after ICH.

The inflammasome is a multiprotein complex that serves as a platform for caspase-1 activation and IL-1β maturation. Our previous study demonstrated that activation of the NLRP3 inflammasome, which contains NLRP3, ASC and caspase-1, makes great contributions to neuroinflammation after ICH [3]. Recently, the NLRP3 inflammasome was reported to be expressed exclusively on microglia and exerts detrimental effects after ICH [4, 6]. Li et al. reported that NaHS administration prevented and partially reversed ozone-induced features

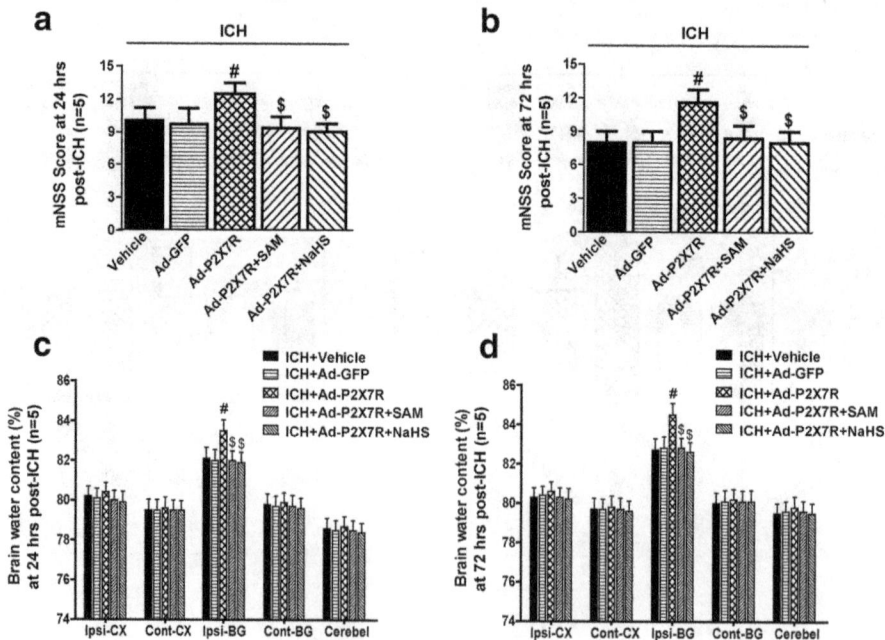

Fig. 10 The effects of SAM and NaHS administration on neurological outcomes and brain edema in P2X7R-overexpressing rats at 1 and 3 days after ICH. **a**, **b** Modified Neurological Severity Score in the vehicle, Ad-GFP, Ad-P2X7R, Ad-P2X7R + SAM and Ad-P2X7R + NaHS groups at 1 and 3 days after ICH. **c**, **d** Brain water content assessment in the vehicle, Ad-GFP, Ad-P2X7R, Ad-P2X7R + SAM and Ad-P2X7R + NaHS groups at 1 and 3 days after ICH. Regarding the 3-day study of neurological outcomes and brain oedema in the setting of P2X7R overexpression after ICH, the neurological deficits and brain oedema were worse in the Ad-P2X7R group ($p < 0.05$), but not in the Ad-GFP group ($p > 0.05$ vs. vehicle), than in the vehicle group. Neurological deficits and brain oedema were significantly alleviated in the Ad-P2X7R + SAM and Ad-P2X7R + NaHS groups ($p < 0.05$ vs. Ad-P2X7R). $N = 5$ rats per group. Data are presented as the mean ± SEM. #$p < 0.05$ vs. vehicle; $$p < 0.05$ vs. Ad-P2X7R. SAM S-adenosyl-L-methionine, ICH intracerebral haemorrhage, Ad adenovirus, GFP green fluorescent protein

of lung inflammation and emphysema by regulating NLRP3 inflammasome activation [30]. Toldo et al. demonstrated that exogenous H_2S attenuates myocardial ischaemic and inflammatory injury in mice [31]. However, whether H_2S influences NLRP3 inflammasome activation following ICH remains unclear. In the present study, we employed SAM and NaHS to upregulate endogenous and exogenous H_2S to examine the effects H_2S on NLRP3 inflammasome activation both in vivo and in vitro. We demonstrated that both treatments inhibited ICH-induced neutrophil infiltration, microglia accumulation and cell injury, as well as NLRP3 inflammasome activation.

The NLRP3 inflammasome can be activated by many stimuli, including potassium efflux, intracellular calcium level alterations, ubiquitination and reactive oxygen species generation [32]. After ICH, extracellular ATP binds to the P2X7R and triggers potassium efflux, which is a sufficient signal for NLRP3 activation [12, 33]. Recent studies have linked the P2X7R to NLRP3 inflammasome activation in response to diverse inflammatory danger signals [12]. Coincidentally, Gustin et al. demonstrated that the NLRP3 inflammasome is expressed and functional in mouse brain microglia, the same cell in which endogenous H_2S is produced, but not in astrocytes [34]. Our previous study demonstrated that P2X7R suppression could preserve the blood–brain barrier after ICH [17], and another study found that P2X7R suppression could inhibit ICH-induced NLRP3 inflammasome activation [6]. Therefore, we investigated the involvement of the P2X7R in the effects of H_2S on NLRP3 inflammasome activation after ICH. The results of this investigation supported our hypothesis.

Moreover, we employed primary microglial cells to identify the specific cell involved in this mechanism. LPS is a classical means of mimicking artificial inflammation in vitro but failed to generate ATP and activate the P2X7R. Thus, we added ATP for the present in vitro studies, which were based on the complications of ICH pathophysiology. We found that LPS + ATP exposure could successfully activate the P2X7R on primary microglia following NLRP3 inflammasome activation, findings consistent with those of the in vitro model of NLRP3 inflammasome activation, which was described previously [35]. Both SAM treatment and NaHS treatment attenuated the increased expression of P2X7R induced by LPS + ATP exposure and alleviated the changes in P2X7R-positive cells exhibiting morphology characteristic of activated microglia, as reported previously [36]. All these data greatly supported the observations of our in vivo study.

Several potential weaknesses of our study should be mentioned. First, apart from facilitating H_2S formation, SAM exerts a spectrum of biological effects, a number of which have been attributed to its methyl donor properties [37]. For example, a previous study reported that striatal adenosine A2A receptor expression is controlled by SAM-mediated methylation [14]. Therefore, we could not exclude the possibility that other mechanisms contribute to the regulation of P2X7R expression and NLRP3 inflammasome activation by SAM after ICH. Second, H_2S is known to play an important role in antioxidation; thus, it is reasonable to speculate that H_2S could inactivate the NLRP3 inflammasome by directly clearing reactive oxygen species after ICH, in addition to suppressing P2X7R expression, as was noted in the present study. Finally, although the increased expression of the P2X7R is believed to be the result of accumulation of extracellular ATP from damaged or dying cells after ICH, ATP overflow has not been measured in vivo and in vitro. Further exploration of how H_2S affects ATP overflow and the subsequent elevations in P2X7R expression is still needed.

Conclusions

Endogenous H_2S synthesis, which plays a pivotal role in the P2X7R/NLRP3 inflammasome-associated neuroinflammatory response in the pathogenesis of secondary brain injury, was impaired after ICH. Maintaining appropriate H_2S concentrations in the central nervous system may represent a potential therapeutic strategy for managing secondary brain injury and its associated neurological deficits after ICH.

Abbreviations

Ad-GFP: Adenovirus GFP; Ad-P2X7R: Adenovirus P2X7R; ARRIVE: Animal Research: Reporting in Vivo Experiments; ATP: Adenosine triphosphate; CBS: Cystathionine-β-synthase; CCK-8: Cell Counting Kit-8; Cont-BG: Contralateral basal ganglia; Cont-CX: Contralateral cortex; DAPI: 4′,6-Diamidino-2-phenylindole; DMSO: Dimethylsulfoxide; H_2S: Hydrogen sulphide; HCl: Hydrogen chloride; ICH: Intracerebral haemorrhage; Ipsi-BG: Ipsilateral basal ganglia; Ipsi-CX: Ipsilateral cortex; $KMnO_4$: Potassium permanganate; LPS: Lipopolysaccharide; mNSSs: Modified Neurological Severity Scores; NaHS: Sodium hydrosulfide; P2X7R: P2X7 receptor; qPCR: Quantitative polymerase chain reaction; SAM: S-adenosyl-L-methionine; SD: Sprague–Dawley; TCA: Trichloroacetic acid; TdT: Terminal deoxynucleotidyl transferase; TUNEL: Terminal deoxynucleotidyl transferase dUTP nick end-labelling

Acknowledgements

Not applicable.

Funding

This work was supported by the National Basic Research Program of China (973 Program, grant number 2014CB541600), the National Natural Science Foundation of China (grant numbers 81501002 and 81220108009) and the Basic Science and Advanced Technology Research Project of Chongqing (grant number cstc2016jcyjA1730). The funders were not involved in the study design; in the collection, analysis and interpretation of the data; in the writing of the report; and in the decision to submit the article for publication.

Authors' contributions

YC, HF and XL conceived and designed the experiments; HZ, PP, YY, HG, WC, JQ and JS performed the experiments; HZ, YC and GC analysed the data; and YC and HZ wrote and revised the manuscript. All authors read and approved the final manuscript.

Competing interests

The authors declare that they have no competing interests.

References

1.   Wang J. Preclinical and clinical research on inflammation after intracerebral hemorrhage. Prog Neurobiol. 2010;92:463–77.
2.   Chen S, Yang Q, Chen G, Zhang JH. An update on inflammation in the acute phase of intracerebral hemorrhage. Transl Stroke Res. 2015;6:4–8.
3.   Ma Q, Chen S, Hu Q, Feng H, Zhang JH, Tang J. NLRP3 inflammasome contributes to inflammation after intracerebral hemorrhage. Ann Neurol. 2014;75:209–19.
4.   Weng X, Tan Y, Chu X, Wu XF, Liu R, Tian Y, Li L, Guo F, Ouyang Q, Li L. N-methyl-D-aspartic acid receptor 1 (NMDAR1) aggravates secondary inflammatory damage induced by hemin-NLRP3 pathway after intracerebral hemorrhage. Chin J Traumatol. 2015;18:254–8.
5.   Yang Z, Zhong L, Xian R, Yuan B. MicroRNA-223 regulates inflammation and brain injury via feedback to NLRP3 inflammasome after intracerebral hemorrhage. Mol Immunol. 2015;65:267–76.
6.   Yuan B, Shen H, Lin L, Su T, Zhong S, Yang Z. Recombinant adenovirus encoding NLRP3 RNAi attenuate inflammation and brain injury after intracerebral hemorrhage. J Neuroimmunol. 2015;287:71–5.
7.   Cui Y, Duan X, Li H, Dang B, Yin J, Wang Y, Gao A, Yu Z, Chen G. Hydrogen sulfide ameliorates early brain injury following subarachnoid hemorrhage in rats. Mol Neurobiol. 2016;53:3646–57.
8.   Abe K, Kimura H. The possible role of hydrogen sulfide as an endogenous neuromodulator. J Neurosci. 1996;16:1066–71.
9.   Liu H, Wang Y, Xiao Y, Hua C, Cheng J, Jia J. Hydrogen sulfide attenuates tissue plasminogen activator-induced cerebral hemorrhage following experimental stroke. Transl Stroke Res. 2016;7:209–19.
10. Lee M, McGeer EG, McGeer PL. Sodium thiosulfate attenuates glial-mediated neuroinflammation in degenerative neurological diseases. J Neuroinflammation. 2016;13:32.
11. Tewari M, Seth P. Emerging role of P2X7 receptors in CNS health and disease. Ageing Res Rev. 2015;24:328–42.
12. Franceschini A, Capece M, Chiozzi P, Falzoni S, Sanz JM, Sarti AC, Bonora M, Pinton P, Di Virgilio F. The P2X7 receptor directly interacts with the NLRP3 inflammasome scaffold protein. FASEB J. 2015;29:2450–61.
13. Feng L, Chen Y, Ding R, Fu Z, Yang S, Deng X, Zeng J. P2X7R blockade prevents NLRP3 inflammasome activation and brain injury in a rat model of intracerebral hemorrhage: involvement of peroxynitrite. J Neuroinflammation. 2015;12:190.
14. Villar-Menendez I, Nunez F, Diaz-Sanchez S, Albasanz JL, Taura J, Fernandez-Duenas V, Ferrer I, Martin M, Ciruela F, Barrachina M. Striatal adenosine A2A receptor expression is controlled by S-adenosyl-L-methionine-mediated methylation. Purinergic Signal. 2014;10:523–8.
15. Dello Russo C, Tringali G, Ragazzoni E, Maggiano N, Menini E, Vairano M, Preziosi P, Navarra P. Evidence that hydrogen sulphide can modulate

hypothalamo-pituitary-adrenal axis function: in vitro and in vivo studies in the rat. J Neuroendocrinol. 2000;12:225–33.
16. Chen Y, Zhang Y, Tang J, Liu F, Hu Q, Luo C, Tang J, Feng H, Zhang JH. Norrin protected blood-brain barrier via frizzled-4/beta-catenin pathway after subarachnoid hemorrhage in rats. Stroke. 2015;46:529–36.
17. Zhao H, Zhang X, Dai Z, Feng Y, Li Q, Zhang JH, Liu X, Chen Y, Feng H. P2X7 receptor suppression preserves blood-brain barrier through inhibiting RhoA activation after experimental intracerebral hemorrhage in rats. Sci Rep. 2016;6:23286.
18. Tao Y, Li L, Jiang B, Feng Z, Yang L, Tang J, Chen Q, Zhang J, Tan Q, Feng H, et al. Cannabinoid receptor-2 stimulation suppresses neuroinflammation by regulating microglial M1/M2 polarization through the cAMP/PKA pathway in an experimental GMH rat model. Brain Behav Immun. 2016;58:118–29.
19. Wang L, Wang X, Su H, Han Z, Yu H, Wang D, Jiang R, Liu Z, Zhang J. Recombinant human erythropoietin improves the neurofunctional recovery of rats following traumatic brain injury via an increase in circulating endothelial progenitor cells. Transl Stroke Res. 2015;6:50–9.
20. Soejima Y, Ostrowski RP, Manaenko A, Fujii M, Tang J, Zhang JH. Hyperbaric oxygen preconditioning attenuates hyperglycemia enhanced hemorrhagic transformation after transient MCAO in rats. Med Gas Res. 2012;2:9.
21. Zhang JH, Badaut J, Tang J, Obenaus A, Hartman R, Pearce WJ. The vascular neural network—a new paradigm in stroke pathophysiology. Nat Rev Neurol. 2012;8:711–6.
22. Yin Y, Ge H, Zhang JH, Feng H. Targeting vascular neural network in intracerebral hemorrhage. Curr Pharm Des. 2017;23(15):2197–205.
23. Mracsko E, Veltkamp R. Neuroinflammation after intracerebral hemorrhage. Front Cell Neurosci. 2014;8:388.
24. Taylor RA, Sansing LH. Microglial responses after ischemic stroke and intracerebral hemorrhage. Clin Dev Immunol. 2013;2013:746068.
25. Kida K, Ichinose F. Hydrogen sulfide and neuroinflammation. Handb Exp Pharmacol. 2015;230:181–9.
26. Hu LF, Wong PT, Moore PK, Bian JS. Hydrogen sulfide attenuates lipopolysaccharide-induced inflammation by inhibition of p38 mitogen-activated protein kinase in microglia. J Neurochem. 2007;100:1121–8.
27. Geng Y, Li E, Mu Q, Zhang Y, Wei X, Li H, Cheng L, Zhang B. Hydrogen sulfide inhalation decreases early blood-brain barrier permeability and brain edema induced by cardiac arrest and resuscitation. J Cereb Blood Flow Metab. 2015;35:494–500.
28. Pouokam E, Althaus M. Epithelial electrolyte transport physiology and the gasotransmitter hydrogen sulfide. Oxidative Med Cell Longev. 2016;2016:4723416.
29. Motta JP, Flannigan KL, Agbor TA, Beatty JK, Blackler RW, Workentine ML, Da Silva GJ, Wang R, Buret AG, Wallace JL. Hydrogen sulfide protects from colitis and restores intestinal microbiota biofilm and mucus production. Inflamm Bowel Dis. 2015;21:1006–17.
30. Li F, Zhang P, Zhang M, Liang L, Sun X, Li M, Tang Y, Bao A, Gong J, Zhang J, et al. Hydrogen sulfide prevents and partially reverses ozone-induced features of lung inflammation and emphysema in mice. Am J Respir Cell Mol Biol. 2016;55:72–81.
31. Toldo S, Das A, Mezzaroma E, Chau VQ, Marchetti C, Durrant D, Samidurai A, Van Tassell BW, Yin C, Ockaili RA, et al. Induction of microRNA-21 with exogenous hydrogen sulfide attenuates myocardial ischemic and inflammatory injury in mice. Circ Cardiovasc Genet. 2014;7:311–20.
32. Yang F, Wang Z, Wei X, Han H, Meng X, Zhang Y, Shi W, Li F, Xin T, Pang Q, Yi F. NLRP3 deficiency ameliorates neurovascular damage in experimental ischemic stroke. J Cereb Blood Flow Metab. 2014;34:660–7.
33. Karmakar M, Katsnelson MA, Dubyak GR, Pearlman E. Neutrophil P2X7 receptors mediate NLRP3 inflammasome-dependent IL-1beta secretion in response to ATP. Nat Commun. 2016;7:10555.
34. Gustin A, Kirchmeyer M, Koncina E, Felten P, Losciuto S, Heurtaux T, Tardivel A, Heuschling P, Dostert C. NLRP3 inflammasome is expressed and functional in mouse brain microglia but not in astrocytes. PLoS One. 2015;10:e0130624.
35. Cai Y, Kong H, Pan YB, Jiang L, Pan XX, Hu L, Qian YN, Jiang CY, Liu WT. Procyanidins alleviates morphine tolerance by inhibiting activation of NLRP3 inflammasome in microglia. J Neuroinflammation. 2016;13:53.
36. Monif M, Reid CA, Powell KL, Smart ML, Williams DA. The P2X7 receptor drives microglial activation and proliferation: a trophic role for P2X7R pore. J Neurosci. 2009;29:3781–91.
37. Cantoni GL, Mudd SH, Andreoli V. Affective disorders and S-adenosylmethionine: a new hypothesis. Trends Neurosci. 1989;12:319–24.

Deletion of the hemopexin or heme oxygenase-2 gene aggravates brain injury following stroma-free hemoglobin-induced intracerebral hemorrhage

Bo Ma[1], Jason Patrick Day[1], Harrison Phillips[1], Bryan Slootsky[1], Emanuela Tolosano[2] and Sylvain Doré[1,3*]

Abstract

Background: Following intracerebral hemorrhage (ICH), red blood cells release massive amounts of toxic heme that causes local brain injury. Hemopexin (Hpx) has the highest binding affinity to heme and participates in its transport, while heme oxygenase 2 (HO2) is the rate-limiting enzyme for the degradation of heme. Microglia are the resident macrophages in the brain; however, the significance and role of HO2 and Hpx on microglial clearance of the toxic heme (iron-protoporphyrin IX) after ICH still remain understudied. Accordingly, we postulated that global deletion of constitutive HO2 or Hpx would lead to worsening of ICH outcomes.

Methods: Intracerebral injection of stroma-free hemoglobin (SFHb) was used in our study to induce ICH. Hpx knockout (Hpx$^{-/-}$) or HO2 knockout (HO2$^{-/-}$) mice were injected with 10 μL of SFHb in the striatum. After injection, behavioral/functional tests were performed, along with anatomical analyses. Iron deposition and neuronal degeneration were depicted by Perls' and Fluoro-Jade B staining, respectively. Immunohistochemistry with anti-ionized calcium-binding adapter protein 1 (Iba1) was used to estimate activated microglial cells around the injured site.

Results: This study shows that deleting Hpx or HO2 aggravated SFHb-induced brain injury. Compared to wild-type littermates, larger lesion volumes were observed in Hpx$^{-/-}$ and HO2$^{-/-}$ mice, which also bear more degenerating neurons in the peri-lesion area 24 h postinjection. Fewer Iba1-positive microglial cells were detected at the peri-lesion area in Hpx$^{-/-}$ and HO2$^{-/-}$ mice, interestingly, which is associated with markedly increased iron-positive microglial cells. Moreover, the Iba1-positive microglial cells increased from 24 to 72 h postinjection and were accompanied with improved neurologic deficits in Hpx$^{-/-}$ and HO2$^{-/-}$ mice. These results suggest that Iba1-positive microglial cells could engulf the extracellular SFHb and provide protective effects after ICH. We then treated cultured primary microglial cells with SFHb at low and high concentrations. The results show that microglial cells actively take up the extracellular SFHb. Of interest, we also found that iron overload in microglia significantly reduces the Iba1 expression level and resultantly inhibits microglial phagocytosis.

Conclusions: This study suggests that microglial cells contribute to hemoglobin-heme clearance after ICH; however, the resultant iron overloads in microglia appear to decrease Iba1 expression and to further inhibit microglial phagocytosis.

Keywords: Fluoro-Jade, Hemorrhagic stroke, Iron, Microglia, Perls, Phagocytosis

* Correspondence: sdore@ufl.edu
[1]Department of Anesthesiology, Center for Translational Research in Neurodegenerative Disease, University of Florida College of Medicine, P.O. Box 100159, Gainesville, FL 32610, USA
[3]Departments of Neuroscience, Neurology, Psychiatry, Psychology and Pharmaceutics, University of Florida College of Medicine, Gainesville, FL 32610, USA
Full list of author information is available at the end of the article

Background

Intracerebral hemorrhage (ICH) causes severe clinical disability and mortality [1]. During ICH, large amounts of erythrocytes are released into the extracellular spaces in the brain. When erythrocytes are lysed, extracellular hemoglobin is rapidly oxidized from ferrous (Fe^{2+}) to ferric (Fe^{3+}) hemoglobin (methemoglobin) [2, 3], which, in turn, readily releases heme [4, 5]. The free heme is extremely lipophilic and binds to lipids intercalating into cell membranes, which results in cellular oxidative damage [6, 7]. Understanding how the released heme is removed after ICH is important because excess free heme is highly toxic [8–11]. The hemoglobin and heme scavenger proteins haptoglobin (Hp) and hemopexin (Hpx) contribute to hematoma removal after ICH [12], and Hpx has the highest binding affinity to heme (Kd < 1 pM) [12, 13]. Hp and Hpx have been characterized as a sequential defense system with Hp as the primary protector and Hpx as a backup when Hp has been depleted during severe ICH. Interestingly, recent quantitative analysis defined an exponential relationship between Hp availability relative to hemoglobin and related protective activities, illustrating that large Hp quantities are required to prevent hemoglobin toxicity [14], perhaps because oxidatively modified hemoglobin loses its binding affinity to Hp and CD163 [15]. In contrast, the linear relationship between Hpx concentration and protection defined a highly efficient backup scavenger system during conditions of large excess of free hemoglobin [14]. These together suggest that Hpx could be more critical in hematoma removal after ICH than has been known before. One study also supports that another role of Hpx is to act as an antioxidant after blood-heme overload [16]. The heme-Hpx complex is endocytosed by cells expressing the CD91 receptor [17]. It is noteworthy that the CD91 receptor is highly expressed within the brain on vascular cells, microglia, and neurons [18]. The CD163 receptor is known for the uptake of the Hp-hemoglobin complex and is expressed on activated microglia [19]. In the brain, Hp is almost exclusively synthesized by oligodendrocytes [20], and Hpx is expressed on neurons and microglia [21–23]. Moreover, it has been suggested that Hp expression cannot be induced in the brain. For example, intraperitoneal injection of bacterial endotoxin has been shown to cause a robust increase in Hp expression in peripheral organs and blood serum, but not in the brain [15].

The heme oxygenase (HO) system is responsible for cellular heme degradation to biliverdin, iron, and carbon monoxide. Two main isoforms have been reported to date: homologous HO1 and HO2 are microsomal proteins that share more than 45 % residue identity and catalyze the same reaction. However, the HO1 isoform has been extensively studied mainly for its ability to respond to numerous cellular stresses such as oxidants, hemorrhage, or trauma [24–26]. On the contrary, HO2 has been less studied likely due to its apparent constitutive nature. Nevertheless, its particular abundance in the brain emphasizes the relevance of HO2 function [27, 28]. HO2 is constitutively expressed by most brain cells, notably neurons, and endothelial and glial cells [29–31] and accounts for the majority of HO activity in the brain [32]. Under oxidative stress conditions, HO2 can rapidly degrade heme [33, 34]. Further evidence for this concept came from experiments with HO2-deficient animals, demonstrating its involvement in brain cell damage produced by cerebral ischemia and ICH [35, 36]. HO2 is the abundant isoform in the adult rodent brain and has been detected in the forebrain, hippocampus, midbrain, basal ganglia, thalamic regions, cerebellum, and brain stem [37]. Additional effort is required to further clarify the physiological role of the Hpx-HO system in the brain. Also, it remains to be investigated which cell type plays the major role in hemoglobin clearance after ICH.

As the resident macrophages in the brain, microglial cells are purported effectors of the innate response after injuries. Growing evidence suggests a protective role for microglial activation in central nervous system pathologies, including ICH [38–41]. The possible mechanism underlying the beneficial effects of activated/migrating microglia may be phagocytosis. For example, it has been shown that microglial cells were activated and recruited to newly formed β-amyloid plaques within 1 to 2 days in animal models of Alzheimer's disease [42]. By stimulating the peroxisome proliferator-activated receptor, it has been demonstrated that activated microglia can promote the removal of hematomas after ICH [38]. Even in the resting state, microglial cells can be active and vigilant in the adult brain, and blood-brain barrier disruption provokes immediate activation of microglia [43].

In general, although Hpx and HO2 are important for the clearance of hemoglobin and heme, little is known about the role that the Hpx-HO system plays after ICH and notably in respect of the microglia phagocytosis properties. In this study, we investigated the role of Hpx and HO2 after ICH, using genetically modified mice that have separate deletions for Hpx and HO2, to establish whether Hpx is a critical factor for hematoma removal after ICH and whether HO2 is required for the removal. We also investigated the unique role of microglia in hematoma removal.

Methods
Animals

All procedures were approved by the Institutional Animal Care and Use Committee of the University of Florida. Adult male Hpx knockout ($Hpx^{-/-}$) mice (22–28 g) were descendants of those generated by Dr. Tolosano's lab [44], and HO2 knockout ($HO2^{-/-}$) mice were generated by Drs. Poss and Tonegawa [45]. The mouse genotype was assayed by polymerase chain reaction and was additionally confirmed by standard Western blot analysis. $Hpx^{-/-}$ and $HO2^{-/-}$ mice were backcrossed into the C57BL/6 background, and matched C57BL/6 mice were used as the wild-type (WT) controls. The knockout mice and the size of their litters were normal overall. No cognition or motor dysfunction was observed. When we examined the gross superficial cerebrovascular anatomy, no detectable changes were observed. Mice had access to food and water ad libitum and were housed under controlled conditions (23 ± 2 °C; 12-h light/dark periods).

Antibodies

The antibodies used for these studies included mouse monoclonal neuronal nuclei (NeuN; specific for neurons) antibody (Millipore, Billerica, MA), rabbit polyclonal ionized calcium-binding adapter protein 1 (Iba1) antibody (specific for microglial-like cells; Wako Bioproducts, Richmond, VA), and glial fibrillary acidic protein (GFAP) antibody (specific for astrocytic-like cells; DAKO, Carpinteria, CA). Secondary antibodies were conjugated with Alexa-488 (Jackson ImmunoResearch, Inc., West Grove, PA) or labeled with avidin-peroxidase-biotin complex (Vector Laboratories, Inc., Burlingame, CA).

ICH model

The procedure for preparing murine stroma-free hemoglobin (SFHb) has been described previously [46]. In brief, blood was taken by cardiac puncture in mice. After centrifugation (2500 r.p.m.) for 5 min at 4 °C, the supernatant was removed and the cell pellet was washed three times with sterile saline. Cells were then collected, suspended in sterile saline, and lysed by two freeze-thaw cycles. The sample was then centrifuged, the supernatant was removed, and the hemoglobin concentration was determined spectrophotometrically. SFHb was then diluted with sterile saline to 2 mM (expressed as the concentration of the hemoglobin tetramer), which approximates its concentration in whole blood. It was aliquoted and stored at −80 °C until used. For hemoglobin injection, age- and weight-matched male mice were anesthetized with halothane (3 % initial, 1–1.5 % maintenance) in O_2 and air (80 and 20 %, respectively). To model hemorrhage, we placed mice in a stereotaxic device (Stoelting, Wood Dale, IL) and introduced a 32-gauge stainless-steel needle through a burr hole into the right striatum at the following stereotactic coordinates: 0.5 mm anterior and 2.0 mm lateral of the bregma, 3.5 mm in depth. We then injected them unilaterally with 10 μL of 2 mM SFHb over a period of 30 min with a microinfusion apparatus. The injection

needle was slowly withdrawn 15 min later, and the wound was sutured. Mice in the sham group received sterile saline injection only. Rectal temperature was maintained at 37.0 ± 0.5 °C throughout the experimental and recovery periods. At 24 and 72 h after SFHb injection, behavioral tests were performed and brains were harvested for stroke injury analysis.

Locomotor activity

Locomotor activities were assessed before ICH and 24, 48, and 72 h after ICH by an automated system (MED Associates, Inc., St. Albans, VT). The mice were placed in four transparent acrylic cages at the same time every day and monitored for locomotor (horizontal activity), rearing (vertical activity), and stereotypy behaviors during a 30-min test period. The results are expressed as an activity ratio of the baseline for each mouse [47].

Neurological scoring

Neurological deficits were assessed at 24 and 72 h after SFHb injection. An experimenter blind to the mouse genotype scored all mice for neurological deficits with a 24-point neurological scoring system [48]. The tests included body symmetry, gait, climbing, circling behavior, front-limb symmetry, and compulsory circling and whisker response. Each test was graded from 0 to 4, establishing a maximum deficit score of 24. Immediately after the testing, the mice were sacrificed for injury analysis.

Histology and immunohistochemistry

At 24 and 72 h after ICH, mice were euthanized and perfused transcardially with phosphate-buffered saline (PBS; pH 7.4) and then ice-cold 4 % paraformaldehyde (PFA) in PBS. The brains were removed, postfixed, and cut into 30-μm coronal sections with a cryostat. The mounted sections were stained with cresyl violet to estimate the lesion volume. Six to eight coronal sections, including the entire injured hemorrhagic area, were summed, and the lesion volumes in cubic millimeters were calculated by multiplying the thickness with the measured areas [47]. All slides were scanned using ScanScope CS (Aperio Technologies, Inc., Vista, CA) and analyzed using ImageScope software (Aperio Technologies, Inc.). For immunohistochemistry, free-floating sections or primary microglial cells were rinsed in PBS after fixation and permeabilization and then incubated at room temperature in 5 % donkey or goat serum to block nonspecific binding. All primary antibodies were diluted in PBS and applied overnight at 4 °C. Antibody concentrations were as follows: rabbit anti-Iba1: 1:1000; rabbit anti-GFAP: 1:2000; mouse anti-NeuN: 1:500. Avidin-peroxidase-labeled biotin-complex secondary antibodies (1:1000) and Vectastain ABC and 3,3′-diaminobenzidine (DAB) SK-4100 kits (Vector Laboratories, Inc.) were then used according to the manufacturer's instructions. When followed with fluorescence staining, the sections were incubated with a secondary antibody conjugated with Alexa-488 (1:1000). After being rinsed, all sections were mounted in DAPI Hardest Reagent (Vector Laboratories, Inc.) under a glass coverslip. To use as negative controls, additional sections were incubated without the primary antibodies. Stained sections were examined with a Nikon TE2000-E Eclipse fluorescence microscope (Nikon Instruments, Inc., Melville, NY); the images were captured and analyzed by SPOT advanced image software (Diagnostic Instruments, Inc., Sterling Heights, MI). To quantify the numbers of positive cells, photos were taken of four regions of interest in each section containing the infarct sites.

Perls' iron and Fluoro-Jade B staining

Iron deposition was detected with Perls' staining for mainly nonheme ferric iron (Fe^{3+}) followed by DAB development. Briefly, brain sections or primary microglial cells were washed in PBS after fixation in 4 % PFA and then incubated with Perls' solution (10 % potassium ferrocyanide and 20 % HCl, equal parts in PBS) for 30 min. After washing in PBS, the sections or microglial cells were incubated with DAB and hydrogen peroxide for 5 min. Brain sections were finally counterstained with hematoxylin for 2 min. The DAB intensification and hematoxylin counterstaining were omitted when brain sections were co-stained with specific cellular markers.

To determine neuronal cell degeneration in brain tissue, Fluoro-Jade B staining was used according to published protocol [49]. In brief, the slides were first immersed in a solution containing 1 % sodium hydroxide in 80 % alcohol for 5 min. This was followed by 2 min in 70 % alcohol and 2 min in distilled water. The slides were then transferred to a solution of 0.06 % potassium permanganate for 10 min and then rinsed in distilled water for 2 min. The staining solution was prepared from a 0.01 % stock solution of Fluoro-Jade B (Histo-Chem, Inc., Jefferson, AR). After 20 min in the staining solution, the slides were washed in distilled water. The dry slides were then cleared by xylene before coverslipping.

Perls' iron and Fluoro-Jade B-positive cells were counted in three to four fields immediately adjacent to the hematoma in each section. At least three sections per animal over a magnification field of ×400 were averaged and expressed as cells per field. The images of stained sections were captured and analyzed by SPOT image software. Tissue sections were all processed and analyzed by an observer who was blind to the mouse genotype.

Primary microglial cell cultures

Primary microglial cultures were prepared as described previously [50]. In brief, the mixed cell culture was prepared from postnatal 2- to 4-day-old mice and then maintained at 37 °C and 5 % CO_2 for 10 to 15 days in Dulbecco's modified Eagle's medium (DMEM) containing 10 % heat-inactivated fetal bovine serum (FBS), 50 U/mL penicillin, and 50 µg/mL streptomycin. Microglial cells were collected as floating cells by gentle shaking and used for the following experiments.

In vitro phagocytosis assay

Primary microglial cells were plated in divided dishes (35 mm, four compartments; Greiner Bio-One, Monroe, NC) for 48 h at a density of 60,000 cells per well in DMEM with 10 % FBS. Latex beads (6 µm, internally dyed with the fluorophore flash green; Polysciences, Inc., Warrington, PA) were preopsonized in 50 % FBS and PBS. Cells were pretreated with SFHb (1 mM) or vehicle for 2 h. Microglial cell media were then replaced with DMEM alone, and preopsonized beads were added to the cells at a concentration of 10 beads per cell. Microglial cells and beads were incubated at 37 °C for 1 h and then subsequently washed with ice-cold PBS. After fixation with 4 % PFA, the images were taken using the EVOS digital inverted fluorescence microscope (Life Technologies, Grand Island, NY).

Statistics

Data are expressed as mean ± SEM. Prism 5 software (GraphPad) was used for statistical analysis. In all comparisons, a P value less than 0.05 was considered significant. The statistical comparisons among multiple groups were made by one-way ANOVA followed by Newman-Keuls multiple comparison tests or two-way ANOVA followed by Bonferroni multiple comparison tests, except for neurologic deficit scores, which were calculated by the nonparametric Kruskal-Wallis test followed by Dunn's multiple comparison tests. Differences between two groups were determined by unpaired two-tailed Student's t test.

Results
Mortality

Overall, injection of 10 µL of SFHb did not cause any mortality. Of note, we had one mouse die following anesthesia before performing the injection.

Deletion of Hpx and HO2 aggravates brain injury after SFHb injection

Our preliminary studies showed that backflow did not occur when mice were injected over a period of 30 min with 10 µL of SFHb. This concentration of 2 mM SFHb approximates that in whole blood [46]. To define the location and distribution of SFHb, a cohort of mice was injected with 6 or 10 µL of SFHb in the right striatum and sacrificed 5 h after injection. Brain sections revealed that the injected 10 μL of SFHb diffused to the whole striatum, which led to behavioral disability. This condition was reproducible and optimal to assess the removal capacity of the Hpx-HO2 system (Fig. 1a). Thus, we chose the 10-μL injections of SFHb for the following experiments. Cresyl violet staining was used to quantify the lesion volume after injection (Fig. 1b). The results illustrated that 10 μL of SFHb led to a lesion in the striatum at 24 h post-ICH. The Hpx$^{-/-}$ and HO2$^{-/-}$ mice had larger lesion volume compared to their WT controls (Hpx$^{-/-}$, 7.5 ± 1.4; HO2$^{-/-}$, 7.6 ± 0.5 vs. WT, 5.0 ± 0.3 mm^3; both $P < 0.05$; Fig. 1c). In addition, no obvious lesion was observed in the saline-injected group (data not shown).

Deletion of Hpx and HO2 aggravates behavioral deficits after SFHb injection

At the same time, behavioral tests were performed blindly on the mice until 72 h after SFHb injection. The data indicated that significant behavioral deficits were caused by injecting 10 μL of SFHb in mice. Moreover, deleting Hpx or HO2 exerted detrimental effects on the neurological deficit score and undermined the locomotor activities in contrast with their WT controls (Fig. 2b). Further, improved performance on behavioral tests over time suggested that the brain injury caused by injected SFHb was recovering from 24 to 72 h postinjection (Fig. 2a, b). In addition, the 10-μL SFHb injection reduced mouse body weight after surgery; however, this was not significant among genotypes and times (Fig. 2c).

Deletion of Hpx and HO2 causes more iron deposition and neuronal degeneration

It has been reported that the accumulated ferric iron after ICH produced oxidative stress and loss of neurons

[9]. To show whether the toxic iron deposition resulted in neuronal degeneration at 24 h postinjection, we performed Perls' iron and Fluoro-Jade B staining on a series of sections. Interestingly, we found that the two positively stained signals were colocalized on successive sections (Fig. 3a), supporting that iron overload contributes to neuronal degeneration after ICH. Quantitative results demonstrated that HO2$^{-/-}$ mice have a larger Perls' iron-positive area compared to WT controls after SFHb injection (Fig. 3b). Under light microscopy, we observed two types of Perls' iron staining: one was diffused and located in the lesion area, which is generally colocalized with the dense positive signals of Fluoro-Jade B, and the other was located inside glia-like cells (Fig. 3a). To better identify the cell type with iron accumulation, we performed the Perls' iron staining with various cellular markers: Iba1 for microglial cells, GFAP for astrocytes, and NeuN for neurons. The results showed that the Perls' iron-positive signals were mainly in microglial cells (Fig. 3c), suggesting that microglia would appear to be the main cells for heme clearance after ICH. However, the extracellular diffused irons are toxic and cause neuronal degeneration after ICH. It has been reported that macrophages recycle iron in the liver, spleen, and bone marrow [51]. A recent publication reported that proliferation of local resident microglia rather than recruitment of circulating myeloid cells would be the main source of microgliosis after stroke [52]. Our data are overall consistent with such observation, although we could not entirely exclude the role of infiltrating macrophages.

To further address the effects of Hpx or HO2 deletion on neuronal degeneration and iron overload, we then quantified the Fluoro-Jade B-positive neuronal cells and the Perls' iron-positive microglial cells around the lesion 24 h postinjection (Fig. 3d). Compared to the WT

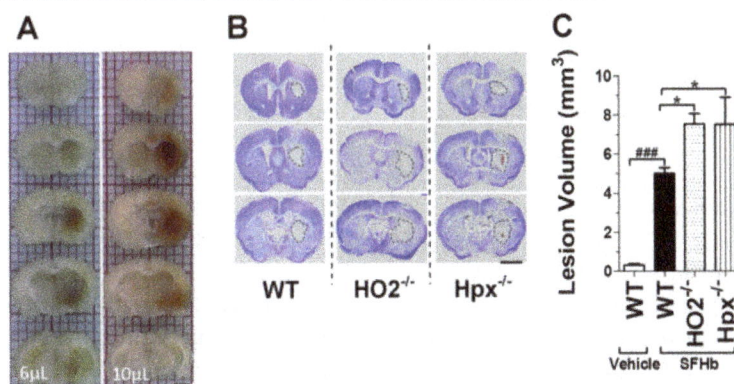

Fig. 1 Deleting Hpx and HO2 aggravates brain injury after SFHb injection. Photographs on the *left* are representative brain coronal sections without staining from WT mice illustrating the location of released hemoglobin 5 h after injection with 6 or 10 μL of SFHb (**a**). A separate cohort of age- and weight-matched WT, HO2$^{-/-}$, and Hpx$^{-/-}$ male mice were injected in the striatum with 10 μL of SFHb; brains were then sectioned and stained with cresyl violet 24 h after injection. The lesion perimeter is showed with a *dotted line* (**b**). The quantitative analysis shows that HO2$^{-/-}$ and Hpx$^{-/-}$ mice have markedly larger lesion volume than the WT mice (**c**). *Scale bar*, 2 mm. Values represent means ± SEM. *$P < 0.05$, ###$P < 0.001$ compared to WT mice, one-way ANOVA followed by Newman-Keuls multiple comparison tests ($n = 5$–6)

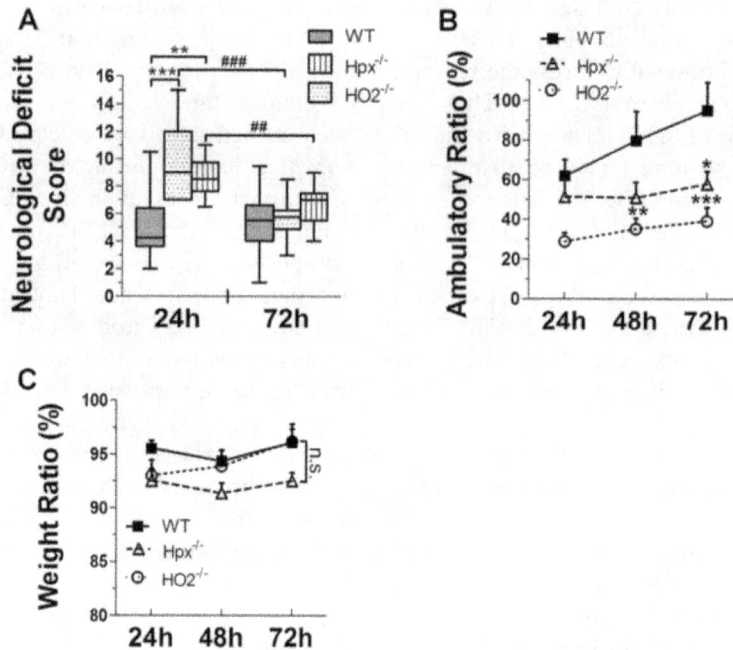

Fig. 2 Deleting Hpx and HO2 aggravates behavioral deficits after SFHb injection. Following SFHb injection, an investigator blind to the genotype assessed neurological function with neurological deficit score (**a**) and locomotor activity tests (**b**). All the mice showed recovery from the SFHb-induced injury 24 to 72 h after injection. The neurological deficit scores of HO2$^{-/-}$ and Hpx$^{-/-}$ mice are markedly higher than WT controls at 24 h, which suggests that neurological deficits were more severe in HO2$^{-/-}$ and Hpx$^{-/-}$ mice (**a**). In the locomotor test, the ambulatory distance of HO2$^{-/-}$ and Hpx$^{-/-}$ mice was significantly decreased compared with WT controls 72 h after injection (**b**). The body weight of all mice was decreased due to surgery; however, there was no significant difference among different genotypes after injection (**c**). Values represent means ± SEM, $n = 10$–12 per group. *$P < 0.05$, **$P < 0.01$, ***$P < 0.001$ compared to WT mice; ##$P < 0.01$, ###$P <0.001$ compared to 72 h, one-way or two-way ANOVA followed by Newman-Keuls or Bonferroni comparison tests except for neurological deficit scores, which were calculated by the nonparametric Kruskal-Wallis test followed by Dunn's multiple comparison test

controls, it was shown that Hpx$^{-/-}$ and HO2$^{-/-}$ mice had more degenerating neurons (Hpx$^{-/-}$, 455 ± 36; HO2$^{-/-}$, 486 ± 23 vs. WT, 318 ± 34 cells/mm^2; both $P < 0.01$; Fig. 3e) and Perls' iron-positive cells (Hpx$^{-/-}$, 1394 ± 109; HO2$^{-/-}$, 1532 ± 110 vs. WT, 788 ± 69 cells/mm^2; both $P < 0.001$; Fig. 3f). Therefore, we concluded that the resident microglial cells in the brain are actively involved in removing iron products after ICH. However, deleting Hpx and HO2 could attenuate this ability because of resultant iron overload in microglia, as indicated by Perls' staining.

Deletion of Hpx and HO2 reduces activated microglia after SFHb injection

It is known that microglia can be activated to exert migration and phagocytosis. We and others have postulated that activated microglial cells could play the critical role in hemoglobin clearance after ICH [38, 47]. However, activated microglia also release proinflammatory factors and reactive oxygen species, which can cause neuronal toxicity. Therefore, it is intriguing to check the net effect of microglial activation in this context of SFHb injection. Iba1 is widely accepted as a marker to show the resting and activated microglial cells in the brain, with an

increased expression level during activation. To assess the effects of Hpx or HO2 knockout on microglial activation, we immunostained brain sections with Iba1 antibody to observe microglial activation/morphology around the lesion 24 and 72 h after SFHb injection (Fig. 4a). The injected SFHb was able to induce microglial activation, and the quantitative data showed that Hpx$^{-/-}$ and HO2$^{-/-}$ mice had much less Iba1-positive cells around the lesion compared to WT controls at 24 h (Hpx$^{-/-}$, 476 ± 62, $P < 0.05$; HO2$^{-/-}$, 220 ± 48, $P < 0.001$ vs. WT, 704 ± 34 cells/mm^2) and 72 h postinjection (Hpx$^{-/-}$; 640 ± 41, $P > 0.05$; HO2$^{-/-}$; 416 ± 46, $P < 0.01$ vs. WT; 758 ± 95 cells/mm^2; Fig. 4b), suggesting that iron deposition within microglial cells could potentially reduce the Iba1 expression level after SFHb injection. Additionally, the numbers of activated microglial cells were increasing from 24 to 72 h postinjection, especially in Hpx$^{-/-}$ mice (from 476 ± 62 to 640 ± 41 cells/mm^2; $P < 0.05$) and HO2$^{-/-}$ mice (from 220 ± 48 to 416 ± 46 cells/mm^2; $P < 0.05$; Fig. 4b), which was accompanied with the improvement of behavioral tests during the same time period. Therefore, these results support that microglia could play a net protective role in this SFHb-injection ICH model.

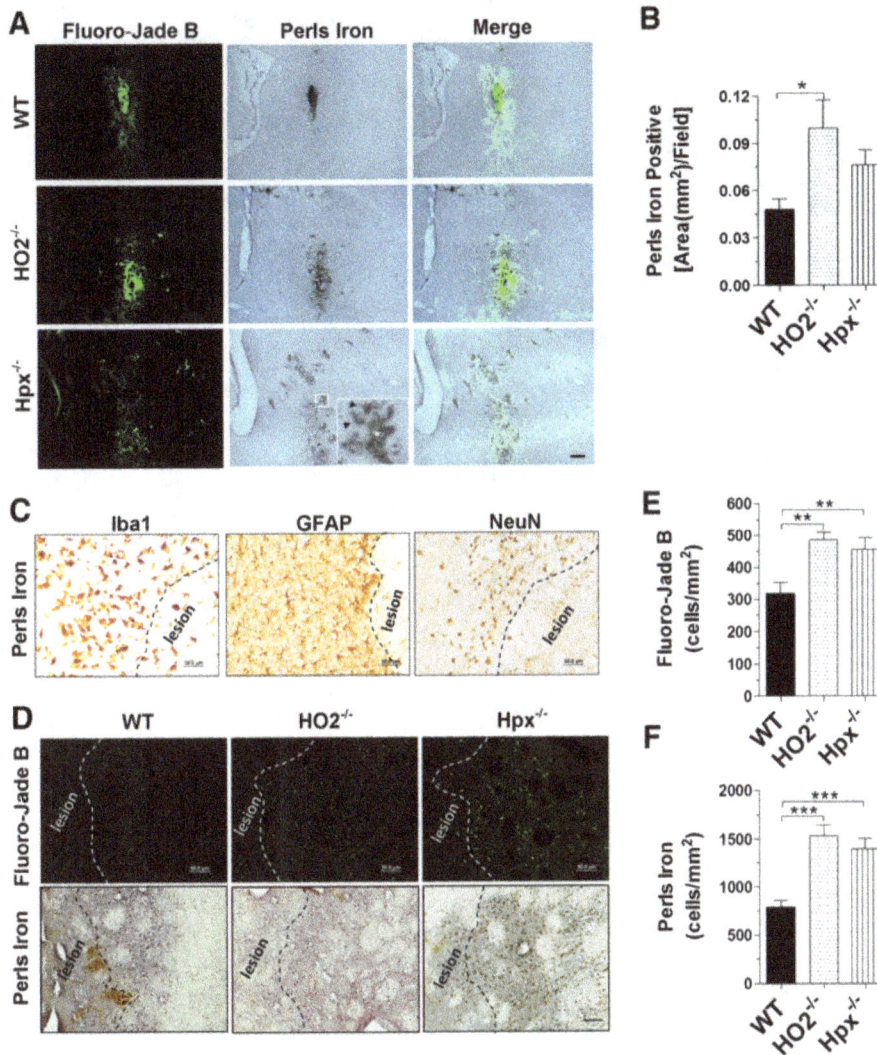

Fig. 3 Iron deposition causes neuronal degeneration. Age- and weight-matched WT, HO2$^{-/-}$, and Hpx$^{-/-}$ male mice were injected with 10 μL of SFHb, and brains were sectioned and stained with Fluoro-Jade B and Perls' iron staining 24 h after injection, respectively. Under microscopy, the positive signals of Fluoro-Jade B and Perls' iron staining were colocalized partially on continuous neighbor sections. The *inset image* shows that glia-like cells (*arrow head*) were activated around the lesion area (*star*). *Scale bar*, 200 μm (**a**). Quantitative data demonstrated that HO2$^{-/-}$ mice have a larger Perls' iron-positive area compared to WT controls after injection (**b**). Representative images were shown of the Perls' iron staining (*blue*) with various cellular markers (*brown*): Iba1 for microglial cells, GFAP for astrocytes, and NeuN for neurons, which illustrated that the Perls' iron-positive signals were mainly in microglial cells. *Scale bar*, 50 μm (**c**). The degenerating neurons and Perls' iron-positive cells are shown in coronal sections. *Scale bar*, 50 μm (**d**). The 10-μL SFHb injection produced significantly more degenerating neurons (**e**) and Perls' iron-positive microglial cells (**f**) in HO2$^{-/-}$ and Hpx$^{-/-}$ mice than those in WT controls. Values represent means ± SEM. *$P < 0.05$, **$P < 0.01$, and ***$P < 0.001$, compared to WT mice, one-way ANOVA followed by Newman-Keuls multiple comparison tests ($n = 5$–6)

Hemoglobin treatment induces iron deposition and reduces Iba1 expression

To further address whether microglial cells take up heme-hemoglobin and contribute to hemoglobin clearance, we treated cultured primarily microglial cells with two doses of SFHb for 2 h and then performed the Perls' iron and Iba1 double staining (Fig. 5a). First, we confirmed that hemoglobin can induce microglial activation. The areas of microglial cells treated with SFHb were markedly bigger than vehicle-treated cells (Fig. 5b).

Second, it was observed that SFHb treatment significantly increased the amount of iron accumulated in microglia and that higher SFHb treatment dosage resulted in more iron deposition within microglial cells (Fig. 5c). Further, we found that the accumulated iron in microglia reduced the Iba1 expression level, illustrating a significant negative correlation by linear-regression analysis (Fig. 5d). This observation supports our in vivo data that the injected SFHb may either directly or indirectly decrease the Iba1

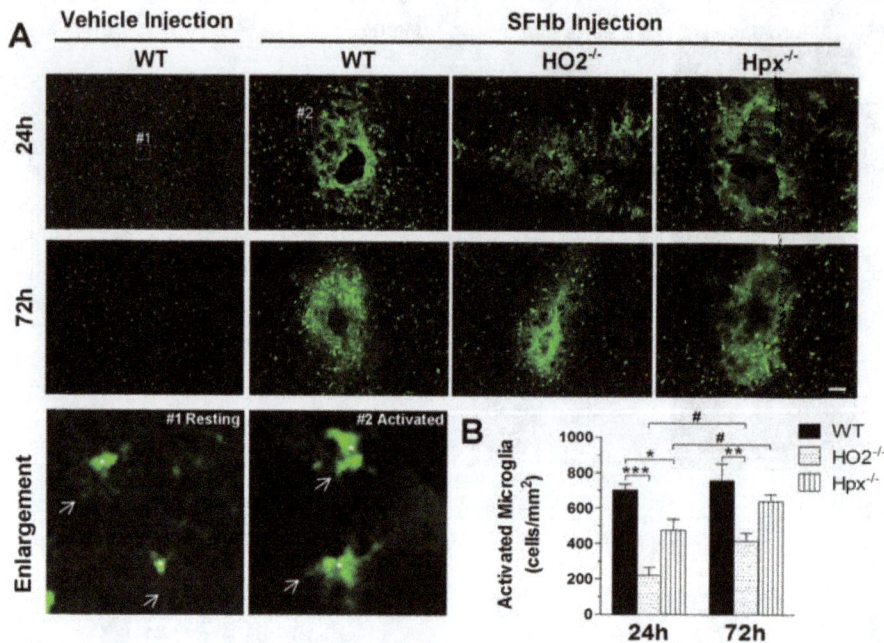

Fig. 4 Deleting Hpx and HO2 reduces activated microglia. The distribution and morphology of microglia (Iba1 positive) can be seen in coronal sections collected at 24 and 72 h from WT and Hpx$^{-/-}$ mice (**a**). Activated microglial cells were observed in and around the injury region after the SFHb injection (*#2*, with large cell bodies bearing short and thick processes) in contrast with resting microglia in the vehicle group (*#1*, with small cell bodies bearing ramified long and fine processes). *Stars* indicate cell bodies and *arrows* present cell processes. Quantitative analysis demonstrated that HO2$^{-/-}$ and Hpx$^{-/-}$ mice had less activated microglia at 24 and 72 h than WT mice. In addition, 72 h after injection, their activated microglia cells were significantly increased compared with those at 24 h (**b**). *Scale bar*, 50 μm; values represent means ± SEM.*$P < 0.05$, **$P < 0.01$, and ***$P < 0.001$, compared to WT mice; #$P < 0.05$ compared to 72 h, one-way or two-way ANOVA followed by Newman-Keuls or Bonferroni comparison tests ($n = 5$–6)

expression level and concurrently change Iba1-positive microglia to Perls' iron-positive microglia.

Hemoglobin treatment inhibits microglial phagocytosis

Iba1 is known to play an important role in microglia migration and phagocytosis [53, 54]. To determine the effect of iron overload on microglial phagocytosis, we treated primary microglial cells with SFHb (1 mM) or vehicle for 2 h and then incubated them with fluorescent latex beads for 1 h (Fig. 6a). The results showed that the hemoglobin pretreatment markedly reduced the percentage of phagocytic microglial cells (Fig. 6b) and the numbers of beads attached by microglia (Fig. 6c). This may suggest that following ICH, hemoglobin degradation within cells would affect microglial phagocytosis and delay resultant hematoma removal.

Discussion

By using the 10-μL SFHb-injection model, we found that Hpx or HO2 deletion leads to aggravated brain injury and Perls' iron deposition, which was consistent with the behavioral results showing the neurological and locomotor disability of the Hpx$^{-/-}$ and HO2$^{-/-}$ mice. Furthermore, by performing double staining of Perls' iron with various cellular markers, we showed that the Perls' iron-positive cells were mainly Iba1-positive microglial

cells. Using mouse primary microglial cultures, we also observed that the SFHb dose-dependently increased Perls' iron deposition within these cells and, interestingly, iron accumulation appeared to negatively correlate with Iba1 staining. Finally, using similar cultures, we observed that the rate of beads being phagocytosed within SFHb-treated microglia was drastically attenuated. These data suggest that (a) microglial cells contribute to hemoglobin-heme clearance after ICH; (b) however, the resultant heme/iron overloads in microglia appears to decrease Iba1 expression and further inhibit microglial phagocytosis. Therefore, microglial cells may have a sort of threshold for their hemoglobin-heme degradative capacity. Above this level, their activity, such as phagocytosis, is severely compromised.

The disparate effects of HO2 knockout have been shown in whole-blood and collagenase-injection models, which indicate the complexity in rodent ICH models and the necessity of a simplified ICH model [55, 56]. Here, in the 10-μL SFHb-injection model, the hemoglobin diffuses throughout the mouse striatum and produces a gradient distribution to induce the activation of microglia, which could be optimal to evaluate the hemoglobin-removal capacity of the Hpx-HO system. Also, hemoglobin injection excludes the intrinsic inflammatory influence of the erythrocyte debris and recombinant

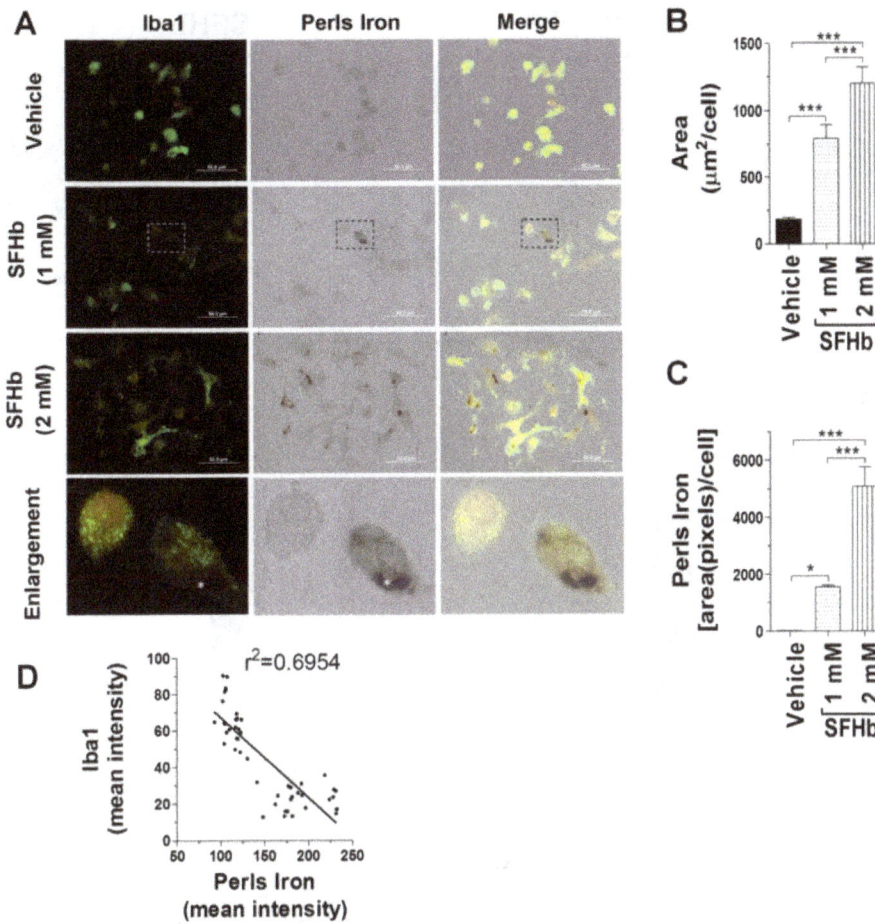

Fig. 5 Hemoglobin treatment induces iron deposition and reduces Iba1 expression. The primary microglia derived from WT mice were treated with SFHb for 2 h as indicated concentration. Distribution of Iba1 (*green*) and iron localization (*black*) was shown in microglia by double staining. The cells highlighted within the *dashed box* were demonstrated at a higher magnification in the enlargement. The asterisk (*) indicates that Iba1 signals were absent at the Perls' iron-positive area (**a**). The *bar graph* shows the significant changes in the size of microglia that are Perls' iron-positive. SFHb treatment greatly increases microglial size, which is dose-dependent (**b**). The SFHb-treated microglial cells have a larger area of positive Perls' iron staining, suggesting SFHb-induced iron deposition inside microglia (**c**). The *linear-regression graph* illustrates that Perls' iron-positive signals are negatively related to Iba1-positive signals, $n \geq 50$ cells (**d**). *Scale bar*, 50 μm. Values represent means ± SEM. Significant differences between the groups are expressed as follows: $*P < 0.05$; $***P < 0.001$, one-way ANOVA followed by Newman-Keuls multiple comparison tests. The experiment was repeated three times and in $n \geq 150$ cells

collagenase in whole-blood and collagenase-injection models. In our preliminary test, we had confirmed that minimal backflow happened over a very slow 30-min period of injection before withdrawing the needle. In addition, Hpx-deficient mice are viable and fertile [44]. Nevertheless, $Hpx^{-/-}$ mice were shown having iron deposits in oligodendrocytes [57, 58]. The Hp protein and mRNA levels are comparable in serum between naïve $Hpx^{-/-}$ and WT mice; however, after hemolytic stimulus, $Hpx^{-/-}$ mice showed persisted Hp levels in the circulation, suggesting compensatory expression of Hp induced by hemolysis [44]. It is well known that iron reacts with lipid hydroperoxides to produce free radicals. Free radicals attack DNA, lipids, and proteins, causing oxidative brain injury. In this study, the degradation of the injected SFHb caused two types of iron deposition in brain tissues: one appearing to be intensely diffused iron deposition in the lesion area and the other suggested to be iron overload in microglial cells. The results demonstrated that the distribution of Perls' iron staining was consistent with that of neuronal degeneration shown by Fluoro-Jade B staining, which suggested that iron overload mainly contributes to neuronal degeneration after SFHb injection. Under microscopy, we found that the Perls' iron-positive cells that were glia-like migrated around the lesion area. To further determine which cell type mainly contributes to this hemoglobin clearance and cellular iron accumulation around lesions, we performed double staining of various cellular markers with Perls' iron and showed that microglia mainly contribute to the clearance of hemoglobin

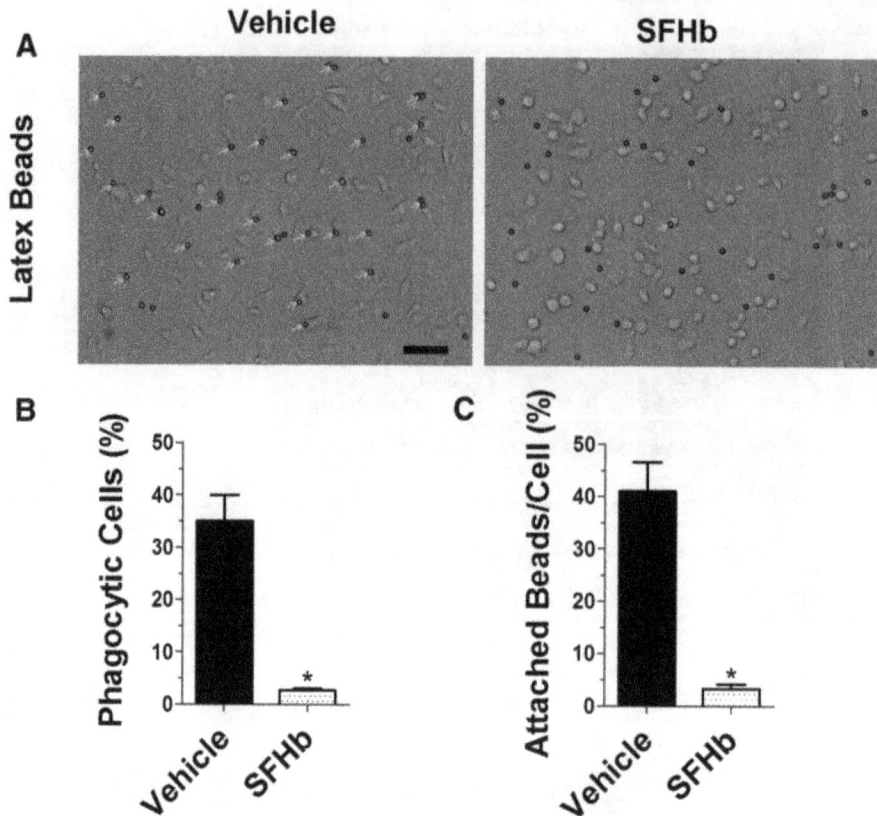

Fig. 6 Hemoglobin treatment inhibits microglial phagocytosis. Primary microglial cells were treated with SFHb (1 mM) or vehicle for 2 h and then incubated with fluorescent latex beads (diameter 6 μm) for 1 h. Representative images were taken and *white arrows* illustrate the attached beads to microglial cells (**a**). *Bar graphs* show that the hemoglobin pretreatment markedly reduces the percentage of phagocytic microglial cells (**b**) and the numbers of attached beads (**c**). *Scale bar*, 50 μm. Values represent means ± SEM. Differences between two groups were determined by unpaired two-tailed Student's *t* test. The experiment was repeated three times and in $n \geq 150$ cells

after ICH. This result was supported by the study from Keep's group [59], and it was also reported by Koeppen's group that most iron-positive cells around intracerebral hematoma were microglia [60].

It could be concluded that whether activated microglia exert protective or toxic effects might be context dependent, determined by both injury severity and duration [61, 62]. For example, the exogenous application of microglia was shown to protect against different types of ischemic injury in vivo [63–65] and in vitro [40]. On the other hand, brain microglial activation and its related inflammatory response had been shown to confer neurotoxicity in various models of neurodegeneration [66–69]. In this SFHb-injection model, compared to the toxicity of the large amount of hemoglobin, the harmful effects of the proinflammatory cytokines released from the activated microglial cells might remain minor within the experimental time frame and the beneficial potential of the neuroprotective factors might be limited. Therefore, we suggest that under our experimental protocol, it was the

effect of microglial phagocytosis that contributed to hemoglobin/heme clearance and behavioral improvement over time.

An interesting observation here was the suggestion that the iron overload appeared to reduce the Iba1 expression level, which could lead to reduced microglial phagocytosis. Also, it may be the reason why more Perls' iron-positive staining microglia were accompanied with less Iba1-positive microglia around the lesion area in $HO2^{-/-}$ and $Hpx^{-/-}$ mice. As mentioned, Iba1 proteins have been described as playing an essential role in microglia migration and phagocytosis [53, 70]. Thus, we speculate that the effect of HO2 deletion may be increasing the vulnerability of microglia to hemoglobin, potentially similar to the effect already reported for HO1 deficiency [71]. $Hpx^{-/-}$ mice could change the way heme was delivered to microglia and neurons from a controlled, receptor-based mechanism to uncontrolled intercalation into membranes and subsequent oxidative injury. Thus, it was not entirely surprising that it would result in a deleterious effect on microglia and neurons, while increasing iron staining.

Conclusions

Our findings suggest that microglial cells contribute to hemoglobin-heme clearance after ICH; however, the resultant iron overloads in microglia appear to decrease Iba1 expression and further inhibit microglial phagocytosis that warrants further investigation.

Abbreviations

DAB: 3,3'-diaminobenzidine; DMEM: Dulbecco's modified Eagle's medium; FBS: fetal bovine serum; GFAP: glial fibrillary acidic protein; HO: heme oxygenase; HO2: heme oxygenase 2; HO2$^{-/-}$: HO2 knockout; Hpx: hemopexin; Hpx$^{-/-}$: Hpx knockout; Iba1: ionized calcium-binding adapter protein 1; ICH: intracerebral hemorrhage; PBS: phosphate-buffered saline; PFA: paraformaldehyde; SFHb: stroma-free hemoglobin; WT: wild type.

Competing interests

The authors declare that they have no competing interests.

Authors' contributions

B.M. contributed to the study design, in vivo and in vitro experiments, data analyses, interpretation of results, and writing of the manuscript; J.D., H.P., and B.S. contributed to the Perls' staining, data quantification, in vivo and in vitro experiments, and reviewing of the manuscript; E.T. contributed to the development of the Hpx$^{-/-}$ mice and reviewed the manuscript; S.D. contributed to the study design, interpretation of results, and writing and revision of the manuscript. All authors have read and approved the manuscript for publication.

Acknowledgements

This study was supported in part by grants from the National Institute of Health NS046400 (S.D.) and an American Heart and Stroke Association grant POST2080364 (B.M.).

Author details

[1]Department of Anesthesiology, Center for Translational Research in Neurodegenerative Disease, University of Florida College of Medicine, P.O. Box 100159, Gainesville, FL 32610, USA. [2]Departments of Molecular Biotechnology and Health Sciences, University of Torino, Torino, Italy. [3]Departments of Neuroscience, Neurology, Psychiatry, Psychology and Pharmaceutics, University of Florida College of Medicine, Gainesville, FL 32610, USA.

References

1. Donnan GA, Hankey GJ, Davis SM. Intracerebral haemorrhage: a need for more data and new research directions. Lancet Neurol. 2010;9:133–4.
2. Umbreit J. Methemoglobin–it's not just blue: a concise review. Am J Hematol. 2007;82:134–44.
3. Jeney V, Balla J, Yachie A, Varga Z, Vercellotti GM, Eaton JW, et al. Pro-oxidant and cytotoxic effects of circulating heme. Blood. 2002;100:879–87.
4. Bunn HF, Jandl JH. Exchange of heme among hemoglobins and between hemoglobin and albumin. J Biol Chem. 1968;243:465–75.
5. Pohlman TH, Harlan JM. Adaptive responses of the endothelium to stress. J Surg Res. 2000;89:85–119.
6. Balla J, Jacob HS, Balla G, Nath K, Eaton JW, Vercellotti GM. Endothelial-cell heme uptake from heme proteins: induction of sensitization and desensitization to oxidant damage. Proc Natl Acad Sci U S A. 1993;90:9285–9.
7. Wagener FA, Eggert A, Boerman OC, Oyen WJ, Verhofstad A, Abraham NG, et al. Heme is a potent inducer of inflammation in mice and is counteracted by heme oxygenase. Blood. 2001;98:1802–11.
8. Paoli M, Marles-Wright J, Smith A. Structure-function relationships in heme-proteins. DNA Cell Biol. 2002;21:271–80.
9. Wagner KR, Sharp FR, Ardizzone TD, Lu A, Clark JF. Heme and iron metabolism: role in cerebral hemorrhage. J Cereb Blood Flow Metab. 2003;23:629–52.
10. Grinshtein N, Bamm VV, Tsemakhovich VA, Shaklai N. Mechanism of low-density lipoprotein oxidation by hemoglobin-derived iron. Biochemistry. 2003;42:6977–85.
11. Belcher JD, Beckman JD, Balla G, Balla J, Vercellotti G. Heme degradation and vascular injury. Antioxid Redox Signal. 2010;12:233–48.
12. Aronowski J, Zhao X. Molecular pathophysiology of cerebral hemorrhage: secondary brain injury. Stroke. 2011;42:1781–6.
13. Tolosano E, Altruda F. Hemopexin: structure, function, and regulation. DNA Cell Biol. 2002;21:297–306.
14. Deuel JW, Vallelian F, Schaer CA, Puglia M, Buehler PW, Schaer DJ. Different target specificities of haptoglobin and hemopexin define a sequential protection system against vascular hemoglobin toxicity. Free Radic Biol Med. 2015;89:931.
15. Buehler PW, Abraham B, Vallelian F, Linnemayr C, Pereira CP, Cipollo JF, et al. Haptoglobin preserves the CD163 hemoglobin scavenger pathway by shielding hemoglobin from peroxidative modification. Blood. 2009;113:2578–86.
16. Gutteridge JM, Smith A. Antioxidant protection by haemopexin of haem-stimulated lipid peroxidation. Biochem J. 1988;256:861–5.
17. Hvidberg V, Maniecki MB, Jacobsen C, Hojrup P, Moller HJ, Moestrup SK. Identification of the receptor scavenging hemopexin-heme complexes. Blood. 2005;106:2572–9.
18. Williams KR, Saunders AM, Roses AD, Armati PJ. Uptake and internalization of exogenous apolipoprotein E3 by cultured human central nervous system neurons. Neurobiol Dis. 1998;5:271–9.
19. Borda JT, Alvarez X, Mohan M, Hasegawa A, Bernardino A, Jean S, et al. CD163, a marker of perivascular macrophages, is up-regulated by microglia in simian immunodeficiency virus encephalitis after haptoglobin-hemoglobin complex stimulation and is suggestive of breakdown of the blood-brain barrier. Am J Pathol. 2008;172:725–37.
20. Zhao X, Song S, Sun G, Strong R, Zhang J, Grotta JC, et al. Neuroprotective role of haptoglobin after intracerebral hemorrhage. J Neurosci. 2009;29:15819–27.
21. Li RC, Saleem S, Zhen G, Cao W, Zhuang H, Lee J, et al. Heme-hemopexin complex attenuates neuronal cell death and stroke damage. J Cereb Blood Flow Metab. 2009;29:953–64.
22. Sutherland BA, Rahman RM, Clarkson AN, Shaw OM, Nair SM, Appleton I. Cerebral heme oxygenase 1 and 2 spatial distribution is modulated following injury from hypoxia-ischemia and middle cerebral artery occlusion in rats. Neurosci Res. 2009;65:326–34.
23. Morris CM, Candy JM, Edwardson JA, Bloxham CA, Smith A. Evidence for the localization of haemopexin immunoreactivity in neurones in the human brain. Neurosci Lett. 1993;149:141–4.
24. Dwyer BE, Nishimura RN, Lu SY. Differential expression of heme oxygenase-1 in cultured cortical neurons and astrocytes determined by the aid of a new heme oxygenase antibody. Response to oxidative stress. Brain Res Mol Brain Res. 1995;30:37–47.
25. Fukuda K, Panter SS, Sharp FR, Noble LJ. Induction of heme oxygenase-1 (HO-1) after traumatic brain injury in the rat. Neurosci Lett. 1995;199:127–30.
26. Matz PG, Weinstein PR, Sharp FR. Heme oxygenase-1 and heat shock protein 70 induction in glia and neurons throughout rat brain after experimental intracerebral hemorrhage. Neurosurgery. 1997;40:152–60.
27. Zakhary R, Gaine SP, Dinerman JL, Ruat M, Flavahan NA, Snyder SH. Heme oxygenase 2: endothelial and neuronal localization and role in endothelium-dependent relaxation. Proc Natl Acad Sci U S A. 1996;93:795–8.
28. Zhao H, Wong RJ, Nguyen X, Kalish F, Mizobuchi M, Vreman HJ, et al. Expression and regulation of heme oxygenase isozymes in the developing mouse cortex. Pediatr Res. 2006;60:518–23.
29. Doré S. Decreased activity of the antioxidant heme oxygenase enzyme: implications in ischemia and in Alzheimer's disease. Free Radic Biol Med. 2002;32:1276–82.
30. Kim YS, Doré S. Catalytically inactive heme oxygenase-2 mutant is cytoprotective. Free Radic Biol Med. 2005;39:558–64.
31. Scapagnini G, D'Agata V, Calabrese V, Pascale A, Colombrita C, Alkon D, Cavallaro S: Gene expression profiles of heme oxygenase isoforms in the rat brain. Brain research. 2002;954:51-59.
32. Chang EF, Wong RJ, Vreman HJ, Igarashi T, Galo E, Sharp FR, et al. Heme oxygenase-2 protects against lipid peroxidation-mediated cell loss and

impaired motor recovery after traumatic brain injury. J Neurosci. 2003;23:3689–96.

33. McCoubrey Jr WK, Huang TJ, Maines MD. Heme oxygenase-2 is a hemoprotein and binds heme through heme regulatory motifs that are not involved in heme catalysis. J Biol Chem. 1997;272:12568–74.

34. Yi L, Jenkins PM, Leichert LI, Jakob U, Martens JR, Ragsdale SW. Heme regulatory motifs in heme oxygenase-2 form a thiol/disulfide redox switch that responds to the cellular redox state. J Biol Chem. 2009;284:20556–61.

35. Dore S, Takahashi M, Ferris CD, Zakhary R, Hester LD, Guastella D, et al. Bilirubin, formed by activation of heme oxygenase-2, protects neurons against oxidative stress injury. Proc Natl Acad Sci U S A. 1999;96:2445–50.

36. Dore S, Sampei K, Goto S, Alkayed NJ, Guastella D, Blackshaw S, et al. Heme oxygenase-2 is neuroprotective in cerebral ischemia. Mol Med. 1999;5:656–63.

37. Maines MD. The heme oxygenase system: a regulator of second messenger gases. Annu Rev Pharmacol Toxicol. 1997;37:517–54.

38. Zhao X, Sun G, Zhang J, Strong R, Song W, Gonzales N, et al. Hematoma resolution as a target for intracerebral hemorrhage treatment: role for peroxisome proliferator-activated receptor gamma in microglia/macrophages. Ann Neurol. 2007;61:352–62.

39. Streit WJ. Microglia as neuroprotective, immunocompetent cells of the CNS. Glia. 2002;40:133–9.

40. Neumann J, Gunzer M, Gutzeit HO, Ullrich O, Reymann KG, Dinkel K. Microglia provide neuroprotection after ischemia. FASEB J. 2006;20:714–6.

41. Lalancette-Hebert M, Gowing G, Simard A, Weng YC, Kriz J. Selective ablation of proliferating microglial cells exacerbates ischemic injury in the brain. J Neurosci. 2007;27:2596–605.

42. Meyer-Luehmann M, Spires-Jones TL, Prada C, Garcia-Alloza M, de Calignon A, Rozkalne A, et al. Rapid appearance and local toxicity of amyloid-beta plaques in a mouse model of Alzheimer's disease. Nature. 2008;451:720–4.

43. Nimmerjahn A, Kirchhoff F, Helmchen F. Resting microglial cells are highly dynamic surveillants of brain parenchyma in vivo. Science. 2005;308:1314–8.

44. Tolosano E, Hirsch E, Patrucco E, Camaschella C, Navone R, Silengo L, et al. Defective recovery and severe renal damage after acute hemolysis in hemopexin-deficient mice. Blood. 1999;94:3906–14.

45. Poss KD, Thomas MJ, Ebralidze AK, O'Dell TJ, Tonegawa S. Hippocampal long-term potentiation is normal in heme oxygenase-2 mutant mice. Neuron. 1995;15:867–73.

46. Qu Y, Chen J, Benvenisti-Zarom L, Ma X, Regan RF. Effect of targeted deletion of the heme oxygenase-2 gene on hemoglobin toxicity in the striatum. J Cereb Blood Flow Metab. 2005;25:1466–75.

47. Singh N, Ma B, Leonardo CC, Ahmad AS, Narumiya S, Doré S. Role of PGE(2) EP1 receptor in intracerebral hemorrhage-induced brain injury. Neurotox Res. 2013;24:549–59.

48. Clark W, Gunion-Rinker L, Lessov N, Hazel K. Citicoline treatment for experimental intracerebral hemorrhage in mice. Stroke. 1998;29:2136–40.

49. Schmued LC, Hopkins KJ. Fluoro-Jade B: a high affinity fluorescent marker for the localization of neuronal degeneration. Brain Res. 2000;874:123–30.

50. Kitagawa H, Sasaki C, Sakai K, Mori A, Mitsumoto Y, Mori T, et al. Adenovirus-mediated gene transfer of glial cell line-derived neurotrophic factor prevents ischemic brain injury after transient middle cerebral artery occlusion in rats. J Cereb Blood Flow Metab. 1999;19:1336–44.

51. Knutson M, Wessling-Resnick M. Iron metabolism in the reticuloendothelial system. Crit Rev Biochem Mol Biol. 2003;38:61–88.

52. Li T, Pang S, Yu Y, Wu X, Guo J, Zhang S. Proliferation of parenchymal microglia is the main source of microgliosis after ischaemic stroke. Brain. 2013;136:3578–88.

53. Ohsawa K, Imai Y, Kanazawa H, Sasaki Y, Kohsaka S. Involvement of Iba1 in membrane ruffling and phagocytosis of macrophages/microglia. J Cell Sci. 2000;113(Pt 17):3073–84.

54. Sasaki Y, Ohsawa K, Kanazawa H, Kohsaka S, Imai Y. Iba1 is an actin-cross-linking protein in macrophages/microglia. Biochem Biophys Res Commun. 2001;286:292–7.

55. Qu Y, Chen-Roetling J, Benvenisti-Zarom L, Regan RF. Attenuation of oxidative injury after induction of experimental intracerebral hemorrhage in heme oxygenase-2 knockout mice. J Neurosurg. 2007;106:428–35.

56. Wang J, Doré S. Heme oxygenase 2 deficiency increases brain swelling and inflammation after intracerebral hemorrhage. Neuroscience. 2008;155:1133–41.

57. Morello N, Tonoli E, Logrand F, Fiorito V, Fagoonee S, Turco E, et al. Haemopexin affects iron distribution and ferritin expression in mouse brain. J Cell Mol Med. 2009;13:4192–204.

58. Morello N, Bianchi FT, Marmiroli P, Tonoli E, Rodriguez Menendez V, Silengo L, et al. A role for hemopexin in oligodendrocyte differentiation and myelin formation. PloS one. 2011;6:e20173.

59. Wu J, Hua Y, Keep RF, Nakamura T, Hoff JT, Xi G. Iron and iron-handling proteins in the brain after intracerebral hemorrhage. Stroke. 2003;34:2964–9.

60. Koeppen AH, Dickson AC, McEvoy JA. The cellular reactions to experimental intracerebral hemorrhage. J Neurol Sci. 1995;134(Suppl):102–12.

61. Raivich G, Bohatschek M, Kloss CU, Werner A, Jones LL, Kreutzberg GW. Neuroglial activation repertoire in the injured brain: graded response, molecular mechanisms and cues to physiological function. Brain Res Brain Res Rev. 1999;30:77–105.

62. van Rossum D, Hanisch UK. Microglia. Metab Brain Dis. 2004;19:393–411.

63. Kitamura Y, Yanagisawa D, Inden M, Takata K, Tsuchiya D, Kawasaki T, et al. Recovery of focal brain ischemia-induced behavioral dysfunction by intracerebroventricular injection of microglia. J Pharmacol Sci. 2005;97:289–93.

64. Imai F, Suzuki H, Oda J, Ninomiya T, Ono K, Sano H, et al. Neuroprotective effect of exogenous microglia in global brain ischemia. J Cereb Blood Flow Metab. 2007;27:488–500.

65. Yong VW, Rivest S. Taking advantage of the systemic immune system to cure brain diseases. Neuron. 2009;64:55–60.

66. Yrjanheikki J, Tikka T, Keinanen R, Goldsteins G, Chan PH, Koistinaho J. A tetracycline derivative, minocycline, reduces inflammation and protects against focal cerebral ischemia with a wide therapeutic window. Proc Natl Acad Sci U S A. 1999;96:13496–500.

67. Tikka T, Fiebich BL, Goldsteins G, Keinanen R, Koistinaho J. Minocycline, a tetracycline derivative, is neuroprotective against excitotoxicity by inhibiting activation and proliferation of microglia. J Neurosci. 2001;21:2580–8.

68. Kriz J, Nguyen MD, Julien JP. Minocycline slows disease progression in a mouse model of amyotrophic lateral sclerosis. Neurobiol Dis. 2002;10:268–78.

69. Kriz J, Gowing G, Julien JP. Efficient three-drug cocktail for disease induced by mutant superoxide dismutase. Ann Neurol. 2003;53:429–36.

70. Imai Y, Kohsaka S. Intracellular signaling in M-CSF-induced microglia activation: role of Iba1. Glia. 2002;40:164–74.

71. Kovtunovych G, Eckhaus MA, Ghosh MC, Ollivierre-Wilson H, Rouault TA. Dysfunction of the heme recycling system in heme oxygenase 1-deficient mice: effects on macrophage viability and tissue iron distribution. Blood. 2010;116:6054–62.

Neutrophil to lymphocyte ratio predicts intracranial hemorrhage after endovascular thrombectomy in acute ischemic stroke

Slaven Pikija[1], Laszlo K. Sztriha[2], Monika Killer-Oberpfalzer[3], Friedrich Weymayr[4], Constantin Hecker[1], Christian Ramesmayer[1], Larissa Hauer[5] and Johann Sellner[1,6]* (iD)

Abstract

Background: The development of intracranial hemorrhage (ICH) in acute ischemic stroke is associated with a higher neutrophil to lymphocyte ratio (NLR) in peripheral blood. Here, we studied whether the predictive value of NLR at admission also translates into the occurrence of hemorrhagic complications and poor functional outcome after endovascular treatment (EVT).

Methods: We performed a retrospective analysis of consecutive patients with anterior circulation ischemic stroke who underwent EVT at a tertiary care center from 2012 to 2016. Follow-up scans were examined for non-procedural ICH and scored according to the Heidelberg Bleeding Classification. Demographic, clinical, and laboratory data were correlated with the occurrence of non-procedural ICH.

Results: We identified 187 patients with a median age of 74 years (interquartile range [IQR] 60–81) and a median baseline National Institutes of Health Stroke scale (NIHSS) score of 18 (IQR 13–22). A bridging therapy with recombinant tissue-plasminogen activator (rt-PA) was performed in 133 (71%). Of the 31 patients with non-procedural ICH (16.6%), 13 (41.9%) were symptomatic. Patients with ICH more commonly had a worse outcome at 3 months ($p = 0.049$), and were characterized by a lower body mass index, more frequent presence of tandem occlusions, higher NLR, larger intracranial thrombus, and prolonged rt-PA and groin puncture times. In a multivariate analysis, higher admission NLR was independently associated with ICH (OR 1.09 per unit increase, 95% CI (1.00–1.20, $p = 0.040$). The optimal cutoff value of NLR that best distinguished the development of ICH was 3.89.

Conclusions: NLR is an independent predictor for the development of ICH after EVT. Further studies are needed to investigate the role of the immune system in hemorrhagic complications following EVT, and confirm the value of NLR as a potential biomarker.

Keywords: Ischemic stroke, Inflammation, Intracranial hemorrhage, Thrombectomy, Outcome

Introduction

Stroke resulting from large vessel occlusion is a devastating disease with a mortality rate of up to 80% [1, 2]. Endovascular thrombectomy (EVT) significantly improves outcomes with almost half of the patients achieving functional independence at 90 days [3]. Indeed, benefits of EVT using second-generation devices

over medical therapy alone in five clinical trials of stroke caused by large vessel occlusion were remarkable, and the procedure has been quickly implemented in clinical practice [4]. However, there are peri- and post-interventional complications that need to be considered. Recent EVT trials have reported an occurrence rate of any intracerebral hemorrhage (ICH) of up to 46% [5, 6]. Symptomatic ICH (sICH), however, occurs less frequently, as seen at 4.4% in the meta-analysis of the HERMES collaboration [7]. There is emerging evidence to indicate that reperfusion injury and ICH are facilitated by post-stroke immune responses, and its

* Correspondence: j.sellner@salk.at
[1]Department of Neurology, Christian Doppler Medical Center, Paracelsus Medical University, Ignaz-Harrer-Straße 79, 5020 Salzburg, Austria
[6]Department of Neurology, Klinikum rechts der Isar, Technische Universität München, Munich, Germany
Full list of author information is available at the end of the article

impact on the neurovascular interface. Inflammatory mediators involved in this response include cytokines, chemokines, adhesion molecules, and several immune molecule effectors such as matrix metalloproteinases-9, inducible nitric oxide synthase, nitric oxide, and reactive oxygen species [8, 9]. Of note, neutrophil to lymphocyte ratio (NLR) is seen as a systemic marker of subclinical inflammation, and an increased ratio is of prognostic value in several disorders [10]. Importantly, in-hospital mortality and poor outcome at 90 days in ischemic stroke is associated with a higher NLR on admission [11–13]. A NLR above 5.9 also predicted death and 90 day outcome after endovascular therapy for large vessel ischemic stroke [14]. Moreover, patients with NLR ≥ 4.8 before thrombolysis had a 3.71-fold increased risk for sICH [15]. Here, we hypothesized that NLR predicts non-procedural ICH in patients who undergo EVT for acute stroke caused by large artery occlusion in the anterior circulation.

Subjects and methods

We performed a retrospective review of all consecutive stroke patients admitted to Christian Doppler Medical Center (Salzburg, Austria) from 2012 to 2016. The study protocol was in accordance with the guidance of our hospital's committee for the protection of human subjects (protocol UN 2553). According to Austrian regulations, an informed consent is not required for routinely collected clinical and radiological data as used in this study. A written approval for the retrospective study of patients with acute ischemic stroke was obtained from the local ethics committee (415-EP/73/750-2017).

The inclusion criteria were as follows: ≥ 18 years of age, ICA and/or MCA occlusion confirmed by CT-angiography (CTA) or MR-angiography within 6 h from symptom onset, and EVT was performed with contemporary thrombectomy techniques. Imaging and EVT were conducted according to an in-house protocol regularly updated with published high-quality evidence, as reported previously [11]. A follow-up CT was performed routinely within 24 h from EVT, and thereafter on an individual basis in the case of any clinical deterioration to determine presence of sICH. The hyperdense area of the affected vessel was correlated with CTA to establish the proximal portion of the occlusive hyperdense thrombus, when visible. Manual delineation was used to measure the length (in mm) and area (in mm^3) of hyperdensity in the occluded vessel [16]. The infarct area was manually delineated on each CT slice (4 mm width), which yielded the area in cm^2. The final infarct volume (FIV) in cm^3 was calculated from the measured area and the corresponding slice thickness. Details of scanners, imaging protocols, and methodology for determining the area of hyperdense middle cerebral artery thrombus were reported previously [16]. Leptomeningeal collaterals were

assessed on pre-procedural CT angiography and divided into three categories: 0—absence of collaterals in symptomatic hemisphere, 1—less visibility of collaterals in symptomatic hemisphere, 2—collaterals equal to non-symptomatic hemisphere [17].

A detailed timeline of intravenous thrombolysis (IVT) and endovascular treatment (EVT) was collected alongside the outcome of the recanalization attempt using the Thrombolysis In Cerebral Infarction (TICI) score [18]. Patients were divided into groups of unsuccessful or successful recanalization on the basis of TICI scores of 0, 1, and 2a; or 2b and 3, respectively.

We defined intracranial hemorrhage as per the Heidelberg Bleeding Classification [19]. We did not include patients with procedural ICH in our analysis, i.e., ICH clearly associated with the procedure itself, such as secondary to vessel perforation, arterial dissection, or subarachnoid hemorrhage.

Stroke etiology was established as per the Trial of Org 10172 in Acute Stroke (TOAST) criteria, following extensive workup [20].

Peripheral-venous blood was drawn routinely at the emergency room for assessment of complete blood count (CBC) and included leukocyte, neutrophil, and lymphocyte counts. As part of a standard of care procedure, additional lab tests were performed on the following day in fasting state to evaluate vascular risk factors. The neutrophil count divided by the lymphocyte count yielded the neutrophil to lymphocyte ratio (NLR). Additional variables included demographics, the National Institutes of Health Stroke Scale (NIHSS) score on admission and at discharge, and the modified Rankin Scale (mRS) at 3 months.

Statistical analysis

Depending on the normality of distribution as assessed by the Kolmogorov-Smirnov test, continuous variables were compared using the t test for independent samples, or the Mann-Whitney U test. Categorical variables were compared using Fisher's exact test or the Chi-square test. Binary logistic regression was performed to report odds ratios. All tests used a p value of 0.05 as a threshold for significance. The optimal cut-off value for the continuous NLR was calculated by applying a receiver operating curve analysis to test all possible cutoffs that would discriminate between ICH and no ICH. All statistical analyses were performed using STATA software 13.0 (StataCorp LLC, TX, USA).

Results

Our initial cohort consisted of 204 patients. Eight patients were excluded because they had no follow-up imaging; three of these suffered early hospital death. Additional nine patients were excluded due to absence of laboratory data. Endovascular treatment was performed with stent-retriever devices except for three patients in whom aspiration technique was used.

The final analysis was therefore conducted for 187 patients. The median age of the cohort was 74 years (interquartile range (IQR) 60–81), and 86 (45.9%) were male. The pre-morbid mRS was > 2 in seven (3.7%) patients. The median NIHSS score at presentation was 18 (IQR 13–22). The time to first imaging after symptom onset was a median of 95 min (IQR 65–132). A total of 133 patients (71.1%) received intravenous thrombolysis. There were 37 (19.7%) deaths within the first 3 months from onset. Ninety (51.1%) patients had good outcome at 3 months, defined as a mRS of 0–2. The Alberta Stroke Program Early Computed Tomography Score (ASPECTS) at admission was < 8 in 32 patients (17.1%). The final infarct volume was determined in scans performed within 3 days (70%) and beyond 3 days (30%) from stroke onset. Procedure-related ICH caused by arterial perforation occurred in ten (5.1%) patients. We detected non-procedural ICH in 31 cases (16.6%); these patients also were less likely to experience a good outcome as compared to patients without a procedure-related ICH ($p = 0.049$). The ICH was symptomatic in 13 (8.6% of the entire cohort, and 41.9% of the non-procedural ICHs).

The median NLR was 3.6 (IQR 2.1–5.8). A higher NLR was not associated with the presence of malignancy ($p = 0.662$), chronic renal disease ($p = 0.814$), or heart failure ($p = 0.868$). As compared to patients without an ICH, those having sustained an ICH had higher NLR levels ($p = 0.003$, 5.1 vs. 3.2) and a worse outcome at 3 months as measured with the mRS ($p = 0.013$, 5.3 vs. 4.0). Blood glucose level on admission, leptomeningeal collateral status, and the number of passes during thrombectomy were not different between the groups with or without an ICH. We found, however, that more than three passes of the catheter was associated with sICH (20.4% (> 3 passes) vs. 4.3% (≤ 3 passes); $p = 0.002$). Further characteristics of patients with and without ICH are presented in Table 1.

Patients with a pre-morbid mRS of > 1 were not more frequent in the group that developed ICH ($p = 0.091$). There was a trend for a lower body mass index (BMI) in patients with ICH; however, it did not reach statistical significance (median 24.2 vs. 25.7; $p = 0.058$). The size of the thrombus measured as the area in cm^2 of the hyperdense portion of MCA was significantly larger in patients with ICH ($N = 105$, median 5.06 vs. 3.23 cm^2; $p = 0.039$). Tandem occlusion of the ICA and MCA (ICA cervical occlusion and ICA distal to bifurcation together with MCA occlusion) showed a trend toward an increased risk of ICH (35.5% vs 19.9%; $p = 0.064$). We found a significantly higher NLR in patients with ICH (median 5.1 vs. 3.2; $p = 0.003$). A longer time to thrombolysis and time to first imaging were more common in

patients with ICH (median 135 vs. 105 and median 107 vs. 88 with $p = 0.034$ and $p = 0.045$, respectively). Absence of sufficient reperfusion (TICI score 0-2a) was not significantly different between the two groups (64.5 vs. 35.5%; $p = 0.114$).

In multivariate logistic regression analysis adjusted for age, site of vessel occlusion (ICA ± MCA vs. MCA alone), and intervention time in minutes, NLR was independently associated with ICH (OR 1.09 per unit increase, 95% CI 1.00–1.20; $p = 0.040$). Further details are shown in Table 2.

The area under the curve (AUC) for the ability of the NLR at admission to predict ICH was 0.67 with 67.0% sensitivity and 73.0% specificity (Fig. 1). The optimal cutoff value of NLR that best distinguished the development of ICH was 3.89.

Discussion

In this single-center retrospective study of acute ischemic stroke caused by large vessel occlusion and treated with EVT, we detected non-procedural ICH and sICH rates of 16.6% and 8.6%, respectively. In comparison to large EVT trials, our ICH rates are higher, probably reflecting real-world setting of our study [3]. Most importantly, we could translate previous findings in acute ischemic stroke regarding the predictive value of NLR, a systemic subclinical marker of inflammation, to the development of ICH in EVT-treated ischemic stroke caused by large vessel occlusion. In this regard, we corroborate and expand recent findings by Goyal et al. in that higher admission NLR is an independent predictor of sICH and 3-month mortality [21]. NLR measured at admission in a previous cohort of 143 patients with ischemic stroke and a median NIHSS of 6 predicted 3-month outcome, with a cut-off value for poor outcome of 2.99 [13]. Our study suggested a cut-off for ICH of 3.89 (67.0% sensitivity and 73.0% specificity), whereas the aforementioned study calculated best predictive cut-off values of admission NLR for sICH and 3-month mortality of 6.62 (sensitivity 71% and specificity 76%) and 4.29 (sensitivity 59% and specificity 56%), respectively. We found a median NLR of 3.6 in our cohort, which is much higher than the NLR ratios found in the healthy population. For instance, a large study in healthy Koreans with a median age of 47 years reported a mean NLR ratio of 1.65 [22]. Another study of an adult healthy population reported a median NLR of 1.65 and a range of 0.78–3.53 [23]. This rise of the NLR in acute ischemic stroke is believed to result from an activation of neutrophils (set out to infiltrate brain parenchyma) and a suppression of lymphocytes by systemic stress [24]. The associated increased release of MMP-9, disruptive for the neurovascular unit, is one of the pathophysiological explanations for the development

Table 1 Characteristics of 195 patients who underwent EVT for recanalization of large artery anterior circulation ischemic stroke

	All (N = 187)	ICH (N = 31)	No ICH (N = 156)	p
Age, median (IQR)	74 (60–81)	77 (52–84)	73 (62–80)	0.592
Male sex	86 (45.9)	12 (38.7)	19 (61.3)	0.433
Hypertension	119 (63.6)	20 (64.5)	99 (63.5)	1.000
Diabetes mellitus	24 (12.9)	3 (9.7)	21 (13.5)	0.771
Atrial fibrillation	112 (59.9)	15 (48.4)	16 (51.6)	0.165
Cancer	8 (4.4)	1 (3.2)	7 (4.6)	1.000
Chronic kidney failure	11 (6.1)	1 (9.1)	10 (6.6)	0.694
Chronic heart failure	25 (13.9)	6 (24)	20 (12.8)	0.371
Admission values				
Pre-morbid mRS > 1	7 (3.7)	3 (9.7)	4 (2.6)	0.091
Body mass index (N = 156)	25.4 (23.1–29.0)	24.2 (21.9–27.8)	25.7 (23.4–29.0)	0.058
NIHSS	18 (13–22)	18 (14–23)	18 (13–22)	0.311
Occlusion site				0.064
M1	145 (77.5)	20 (64.5)	125 (80.1)	
ACI + M1/M2	22 (22.5)	11 (35.5)	31 (19.9)	
ASPECTS	8 (8–9)	8 (7–9)	9 (8–9)	0.226
Serum glucose	118 (107–142)	123 (112–150)	118 (106–142)	0.290
Neutrophil to lymphocyte ratio	3.6 (2.1–5.8)	5.1 (2.9–8.4)	3.2 (1.9–5.2)	0.003
Hyperdense thrombus area (N = 105)	25.7 (15.3–45.2)	34.0 (25.1–52.7)	22.3 (13.6–41.8)	0.039
Stroke etiology				0.075
Cardioembolic and unknown	153 (81.8)	29 (93.5)	124 (75.4)	
Large artery atherosclerotic + other etiology	34 (18.2)	2 (6.4)	32 (20.5)	
Procedure related				
Intravenous thrombolysis	133 (71.5)	21 (67.7)	112 (72.3)	0.664
Time to first imaging, min	95 (65–132)	107 (83–155)	88.5 (64–128)	0.045
Time to needle	112 (85–150)	135 (110–167)	105 (82–140)	0.034
Time to groin puncture	189 (148–233)	205 (180–252)	186 (144–227)	0.073
Number of passes > 3	76 (50.0)	16 (59.3)	60 (48.0)	0.396
Intervention time	52 (25–93)	70 (35–116)	50 (21–85)	0.059
ICA Stenting	15 (28.3)	2 (22.2)	13 (29.5)	1.000
TICI 2b or 3	141 (75.8)	20 (64.5)	11 (35.5)	0.114

Numbers are medians with interquartile range in parentheses or number (percentage)

EVT endovascular treatment, *NIHSS* National Institutes of Health Stroke scale, *mRS* modified Rankin scale, *ASPECTS* Alberta Stroke Program Early Computed Tomography Score, *ICA* internal carotid artery, *MCA* middle cerebral artery, *TICI* thrombolysis in cerebral infarction

of ICH and poor outcome in patients with high NLR. The role of neutrophils becomes even more complex as pro-inflammatory N1 neutrophils are implicated in brain edema and neurotoxicity, whereas anti-inflammatory N2 neutrophils were found to limit this excessive immune response promoting neuronal survival and successful brain remodeling [25]. There is a paucity of studies, however, investigating factors associated with hemorrhagic transformation in general, and particularly in the setting of EVT. A recent study performed in an Asian population of 632 patients treated with EVT for anterior circulation stroke showed a high occurrence of sICH of 16% [7]. The occurrence of sICH was independently associated with a baseline NLR ratio of > 0.83, pretreatment ASPECTS of < 6, delayed recanalization treatment, multiple device passes, stroke of cardioembolic type, and poor collateral circulation. These findings are likely to be influenced by the significant number of intra-arterial use of rt-PA or tirofiban in that study. In addition, the reported NLR is well under normal values, therefore its interpretation should warrant some caution. Maestrini et al. studied baseline NLR in 846 patients (median NIHSS 10) treated with rt-PA, and found an independent

Table 2 Results of multivariate logistic regression analysis of predictors for intracranial hemorrhage in 187 patients with endovascular treatment due to large artery occlusion of the anterior circulation

Variables	Values	Odds ratio (95% confidence interval)	p
Age	Years	0.99 (0.96–1.02)	0.628
Occlusion site	M1 vs. ICA ± M1/2	1.73 (0.70–4.27)	0.232
Intervention time	By 1 min increase	1.00 (0.99–1.01)	0.192
Neutrophil/lymphocyte ratio	By 1 unit increase	1.09 (1.00–1.20)	0.040

M1 M1 segment of middle cerebral artery, *ICA* internal carotid artery

association with sICH (6.4%), death, and worse outcome at 3 months [15]. They calculated a NLR ≥ 4.80 (sensitivity 66.7%, specificity 71.3%) as the discriminative threshold.

We could not confirm systemic rt-PA treatment as a risk factor for ICH in our EVT-treated cohort. We had a rt-PA rate of 71%, and a door to needle time of a median of 112 min (IQR 85–150). A study by Guo et al. analyzed 189 patients with acute ischemic stroke, a third of whom were also treated with EVT [26]. Interestingly, NLR measured at admission was not predictive of ICH or sICH. The main finding of that, however, was an independent association of NLR obtained at 12–18 h post-treatment with ICH and sICH, with NLR > 10.59 leading to a 8.50-fold greater risk of ICH, and a 7.93-fold increased risk for sICH, although the confidence intervals were wide (2.69–26.89 and 2.25–27.99, respectively). In our sample, NLR at admission had lower sensitivity and specificity for predicting ICH (67% and 73%, respectively), and the cut-off value was significantly lower. Furthermore, only 13 (7%) of our

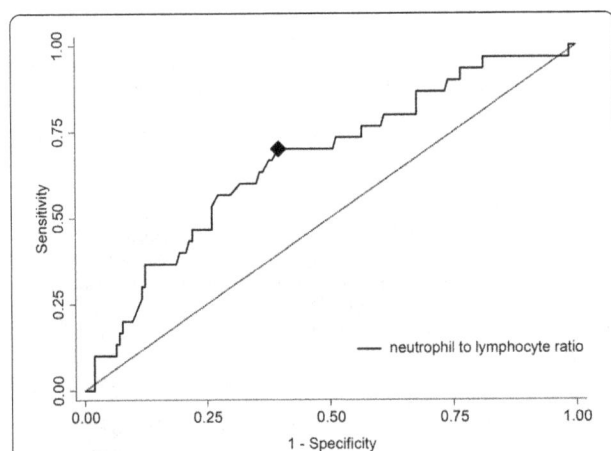

Fig. 1 Discriminative ability presented as receiver operating curve of neutrophil to lymphocyte ratio (NLR) to predict intracranial hemorrhage. Area under curve: 0.67. Diamond representing cut-off NLR value of 3.89

patients were above the proposed cut-of value of Guo et al. The differences between the two studies include the time of NLR determination and treatment approaches, with all our patients receiving EVT that is superior to rt-PA alone. Xue et al. [11] and Fang et al. [27] reported a correlation between NIHSS and NLR determined at admission in 280 and 1731 stroke patients, respectively, but the treatment modalities were not reported. We could not confirm these findings since NLR was not correlated with stroke severity at admission in our cohort. The discrepancy most probably is due to the fact that Xue et al. recruited patients experiencing stroke within 6 days before admission, and Fang et al. within 48 prior to admission. In addition, Xue et al. found association of NLR with primary unfavorable outcome, similar to our cohort, and increased risk for recurrent stroke with a hazard ratio of 1.499 (95% CI 1.161–1.935, p = 0.002). Fang et al. observed that patients with an NLR ≥ 3.2 had a 2.55-fold risk of in-hospital mortality. Neither of these studies however reported on the incidence of ICH or sICH.

Reports describing an association of BMI with stroke outcome have been controversial. In the setting of rt-PA treatment, BMI had no prognostic significance for sICH or the 3-month outcome [28]. Another study suggested underweight state as risk factor for unfavorable outcome [29].Using standard groups of BMI categories (underweight < 18.5 kg/m^2, reference 18.5–24.9 kg/m^2, overweight 25.0–29.9 kg/m^2, and obese > 30.0 kg/m^2), our patients in the underweight group (N = 9) had a 33.3% chance for ICH, whereas this risk was the smallest for the overweight group at only 5% (N = 59). The association of BMI with ICH is most likely multifactorial, and not necessarily causative. Tandem occlusions are known predictors for sICH with up to 22.0% of patients affected after EVT [30]. Larger clot burden could impair penumbral perfusion and damage the vessel wall itself, leading to vessel disruption and intracerebral hematoma [31]. Leptomeningeal collaterals were shown to protect against ICH, but in our study the absence of collaterals was not associated with ICH or sICH [32]. The reason for this is not clear since the collateral status had a significant influence on final infarct volume and 3-month outcome. We had a rate of 5.1% for procedure-related ICH, which is in a similar range reported in the REVASCAT trial (4.9%). In four other trials, however, the rate of arterial perforation ranged from 0 to 2.9% [33].

There are some limitations to our study. There is retrospective bias inherent to the study design, and also there were prolonged times to imaging and rt-PA in patients who developed ICH. Future studies should also take immunologically relevant comorbidities such as sarcopenia and rheumatoid arthritis into account.

Conclusions

We found NLR at admission to be an independent predictor of non-procedural ICH in acute ischemic stroke caused by large vessel occlusion when treated with EVT. Our findings in a moderate-sized retrospective cohort highlight the need to better understand post-stroke immune response and confirm the value of NLR as a potential biomarker of a subgroup at risk for ICH.

Abbreviations

ASPECTS: Alberta stroke programme early CT score; BMI: Body mass index; CT: Computed tomography; EVT: Endovascular therapy; ICH: Intracerebral hemorrhage; NIHSS: National Institute of Health Stroke Scale; NLR: Neutrophil to lymphocyte ratio; rt-PA: Recombinant tissue-plasminogen activator

Acknowledgements

The authors thank Prof. Eugen Trinka for his continuous support.

Funding

None.

Authors' contributions

SP and JS planned and conceived the study. SP and CR collected the data. SP, LKS, MKO, CH, FW, and JS interpreted the data. SP, LKS, LH, and JS wrote and critically revised the manuscript. All authors have read and approved the final manuscript.

Competing interests

The authors declare that they have no competing interests.

Author details

[1]Department of Neurology, Christian Doppler Medical Center, Paracelsus Medical University, Ignaz-Harrer-Straße 79, 5020 Salzburg, Austria. [2]Department of Neurology, King's College Hospital, Denmark Hill, London, UK. [3]Research Institute for Neurointervention, Christian Doppler Medical Center, Paracelsus Medical University, Salzburg, Austria. [4]Division of Neuroradiology, Christian Doppler Medical Center, Paracelsus Medical University, Salzburg, Austria. [5]Department of Psychiatry, Psychotherapy and Psychosomatics, Christian Doppler Medical Center, Paracelsus Medical University, Salzburg, Austria. [6]Department of Neurology, Klinikum rechts der Isar, Technische Universität München, Munich, Germany.

References

1. Broderick JP, Berkhemer OA, Palesch YY, Dippel DW, Foster LD, Roos YB, van der Lugt A, Tomsick TA, Majoie CB, van Zwam WH, et al. Endovascular therapy is effective and safe for patients with severe ischemic stroke: pooled analysis of interventional management of stroke III and multicenter randomized clinical trial of endovascular therapy for acute ischemic stroke in the Netherlands data. Stroke. 2015;46:3416–22.

2. Berkhemer OA, Majoie CB, Dippel DW, Investigators MC. Endovascular therapy for ischemic stroke. N Engl J Med. 2015;372:2363.

3. Badhiwala JH, Nassiri F, Alhazzani W, Selim MH, Farrokhyar F, Spears J, Kulkarni AV, Singh S, Alqahtani A, Rochwerg B, et al. Endovascular thrombectomy for acute ischemic stroke: a meta-analysis. JAMA. 2015; 314:1832–43.

4. Saver JL, Goyal M, van der Lugt A, Menon BK, Majoie CB, Dippel DW, Campbell BC, Nogueira RG, Demchuk AM, Tomasello A, et al. Time to treatment with endovascular thrombectomy and outcomes from ischemic stroke: a meta-analysis. JAMA. 2016;316:1279–88.

5. Bracard S, Ducrocq X, Mas JL, Soudant M, Oppenheim C, Moulin T, Guillemin F, Investigators T. Mechanical thrombectomy after intravenous alteplase versus alteplase alone after stroke (THRACE): a randomised controlled trial. Lancet Neurol. 2016;15:1138–47.

6. Goyal M, Demchuk AM, Menon BK, Eesa M, Rempel JL, Thornton J, Roy D, Jovin TG, Willinsky RA, Sapkota BL, et al. Randomized assessment of rapid endovascular treatment of ischemic stroke. N Engl J Med. 2015;372:1019–30.

7. Hao Y, Yang D, Wang H, Zi W, Zhang M, Geng Y, Zhou Z, Wang W, Xu H, Tian X, et al. Predictors for symptomatic intracranial hemorrhage after endovascular treatment of acute ischemic stroke. Stroke. 2017;48:1203–9.

8. Choi JH, Pile-Spellman J. Reperfusion changes after stroke and practical approaches for neuroprotection. Neuroimaging Clin N Am. 2018;28:663–82.

9. Suzuki Y, Nagai N, Umemura K. A review of the mechanisms of blood-brain barrier permeability by tissue-type plasminogen activator treatment for cerebral ischemia. Front Cell Neurosci. 2016;10:2.

10. Dentali F, Conte G, Guasti L. Neutrophil-to-lymphocyte ratio: a new prognostic factor even in patients with heart failure. Pol Arch Med Wewn. 2016;126:116–7.

11. Xue J, Huang W, Chen X, Li Q, Cai Z, Yu T, Shao B. Neutrophil-to-lymphocyte ratio is a prognostic marker in acute ischemic stroke. J Stroke Cerebrovasc Dis. 2017;26:650–7.

12. Yu S, Arima H, Bertmar C, Clarke S, Herkes G, Krause M. Neutrophil to lymphocyte ratio and early clinical outcomes in patients with acute ischemic stroke. J Neurol Sci. 2018;387:115–8.

13. Qun S, Tang Y, Sun J, Liu Z, Wu J, Zhang J, Guo J, Xu Z, Zhang D, Chen Z, et al. Neutrophil-to-lymphocyte ratio predicts 3-month outcome of acute ischemic stroke. Neurotox Res. 2017;31:444–52.

14. Brooks SD, Spears C, Cummings C, VanGilder RL, Stinehart KR, Gutmann L, Domico J, Culp S, Carpenter J, Rai A, Barr TL. Admission neutrophil-lymphocyte ratio predicts 90 day outcome after endovascular stroke therapy. J Neurointerv Surg. 2014;6:578–83.

15. Maestrini I, Strbian D, Gautier S, Haapaniemi E, Moulin S, Sairanen T, Dequatre-Ponchelle N, Sibolt G, Cordonnier C, Melkas S, et al. Higher neutrophil counts before thrombolysis for cerebral ischemia predict worse outcomes. Neurology. 2015;85:1408–16.

16. Pikija S, Trkulja V, Mutzenbach JS, McCoy MR, Ganger P, Sellner J. Fibrinogen consumption is related to intracranial clot burden in acute ischemic stroke: a retrospective hyperdense artery study. J Transl Med. 2016;14:250.

17. Pikija S, Sztriha LK, Killer-Oberpfalzer M, Weymayr F, Hecker C, Ramesmayer C, Hauer L, Sellner J. Contribution of serum lipid profiles to outcome after endovascular thrombectomy for anterior circulation ischemic stroke. Mol Neurobiol; 2018. https://doi.org/10.1007/s12035-018-1391-3.

18. Higashida RT, Furlan AJ, Roberts H, Tomsick T, Connors B, Barr J, Dillon W, Warach S, Broderick J, Tilley B, et al. Trial design and reporting standards for intra-arterial cerebral thrombolysis for acute ischemic stroke. Stroke. 2003;34:e109–37.

19. von Kummer R, Broderick JP, Campbell BC, Demchuk A, Goyal M, Hill MD, Treurniet KM, Majoie CB, Marquering HA, Mazya MV, et al. The Heidelberg bleeding classification: classification of bleeding events after ischemic stroke and reperfusion therapy. Stroke. 2015;46:2981–6.

20. Adams HP Jr, Bendixen BH, Kappelle LJ, Biller J, Love BB, Gordon DL, Marsh EE 3rd. Classification of subtype of acute ischemic stroke. Definitions for use in a multicenter clinical trial. TOAST. Trial of org 10172 in acute stroke treatment. Stroke. 1993;24:35–41.

21. Goyal N, Tsivgoulis G, Chang JJ, Malhotra K, Pandhi A, Ishfaq MF, Alsbrook D, Arthur AS, Elijovich L, Alexandrov AV. Admission neutrophil-to-lymphocyte ratio as a prognostic biomarker of outcomes in large vessel occlusion strokes. Stroke. 2018;49(8):1985–198. https://doi.org/10.1161/STROKEAHA.118.021477.

22. Lee JS, Kim NY, Na SH, Youn YH, Shin CS. Reference values of neutrophil-lymphocyte ratio, lymphocyte-monocyte ratio, platelet-lymphocyte ratio,

Neutrophil to lymphocyte ratio predicts intracranial hemorrhage after endovascular thrombectomy in acute...

151

and mean platelet volume in healthy adults in South Korea. Medicine (Baltimore). 2018;97:e11138.

23. Forget P, Khalifa C, Defour JP, Latinne D, Van Pel MC, De Kock M. What is the normal value of the neutrophil-to-lymphocyte ratio? BMC Res Notes. 2017;10:12.

24. Gokhan S, Ozhasenekler A, Mansur Durgun H, Akil E, Ustundag M, Orak M. Neutrophil lymphocyte ratios in stroke subtypes and transient ischemic attack. Eur Rev Med Pharmacol Sci. 2013;17:653–7.

25. Hermann DM, Kleinschnitz C, Gunzer M. Implications of polymorphonuclear neutrophils for ischemic stroke and intracerebral hemorrhage: predictive value, pathophysiological consequences and utility as therapeutic target. J Neuroimmunol. 2018;321:138–43.

26. Guo Z, Yu S, Xiao L, Chen X, Ye R, Zheng P, Dai Q, Sun W, Zhou C, Wang S, et al. Dynamic change of neutrophil to lymphocyte ratio and hemorrhagic transformation after thrombolysis in stroke. J Neuroinflammation. 2016;13:199.

27. Fang YN, Tong MS, Sung PH, Chen YL, Chen CH, Tsai NW, Huang CJ, Chang YT, Chen SF, Chang WN, et al. Higher neutrophil counts and neutrophil-to-lymphocyte ratio predict prognostic outcomes in patients after non-atrial fibrillation-caused ischemic stroke. Biom J. 2017;40:154–62.

28. Gensicke H, Wicht A, Bill O, Zini A, Costa P, Kagi G, Stark R, Seiffge DJ, Traenka C, Peters N, et al. Impact of body mass index on outcome in stroke patients treated with intravenous thrombolysis. Eur J Neurol. 2016; 23:1705–12.

29. Sun W, Huang Y, Xian Y, Zhu S, Jia Z, Liu R, Li F, Wei JW, Wang JG, Liu M, Anderson CS. Association of body mass index with mortality and functional outcome after acute ischemic stroke. Sci Rep. 2017;7:2507.

30. Heck DV, Brown MD. Carotid stenting and intracranial thrombectomy for treatment of acute stroke due to tandem occlusions with aggressive antiplatelet therapy may be associated with a high incidence of intracranial hemorrhage. J Neurointerv Surg. 2015;7:170–5.

31. Puetz V, Dzialowski I, Hill MD, Subramaniam S, Sylaja PN, Krol A, O'Reilly C, Hudon ME, Hu WY, Coutts SB, et al. Intracranial thrombus extent predicts clinical outcome, final infarct size and hemorrhagic transformation in ischemic stroke: the clot burden score. Int J Stroke. 2008;3:230–6.

32. Bang OY, Saver JL, Kim SJ, Kim GM, Chung CS, Ovbiagele B, Lee KH, Liebeskind DS, Collaborators UC-SS. Collateral flow averts hemorrhagic transformation after endovascular therapy for acute ischemic stroke. Stroke. 2011;42:2235–9.

33. Balami JS, White PM, McMeekin PJ, Ford GA, Buchan AM. Complications of endovascular treatment for acute ischemic stroke: prevention and management. Int J Stroke. 2018;13:348–61.

Treatment with TO901317, a synthetic liver X receptor agonist, reduces brain damage and attenuates neuroinflammation in experimental intracerebral hemorrhage

Chun-Hu Wu[1,2†], Chien-Cheng Chen[3†], Chai-You Lai[1,2], Tai-Ho Hung[4], Chao-Chang Lin[3], Min Chao[5] and Szu-Fu Chen[1,3*]

Abstract

Background: Intracerebral hemorrhage (ICH) induces a series of inflammatory processes that contribute to neuronal damage and neurological deterioration. Liver X receptors (LXRs) are nuclear receptors that negatively regulate transcriptional processes involved in inflammatory responses, but their role in the pathology following ICH remains unclear. The present study investigated the neuroprotective effects and anti-inflammatory actions of TO901317, a synthetic LXR agonist, in a model of collagenase-induced ICH and in microglial cultures.

Methods: Mice subjected to collagenase-induced ICH injury were injected with either TO901317 (30 mg/kg) or vehicle 10 min after ICH and subsequently daily for 2 days. Behavioral studies, histology analysis, and assessments of hematoma volumes, brain water content, and blood-brain barrier (BBB) permeability were performed. The protein expression of LXR-α, LXR-β, ATP binding cassette transporter-1 (ABCA-1), and inflammatory molecules was analyzed. The anti-inflammatory mechanism of TO901317 was investigated in cultured microglia that were stimulated with either lipopolysaccharide (LPS) or thrombin.

Results: ICH induced an increase in LXR-α protein levels in the hemorrhagic hemisphere at 6 h whereas LXR-β expression remained unaffected. Both LXR-α and LXR-β were expressed in neurons and microglia in the peri-ICH region and but rarely in astrocytes. TO901317 significantly attenuated functional deficits and brain damage up to 28 days post-ICH. TO901317 also reduced neuronal death, BBB disruption, and brain edema at day 4 post-ICH. These changes were associated with marked reductions in microglial activation, neutrophil infiltration, and expression levels of inflammatory mediators at 4 and 7 days. However, TO901317 had no effect on matrix metalloproteinase-9 activity. In BV2 microglial cultures, TO901317 attenuated LPS- and thrombin-stimulated nitric oxide production and reduced LPS-induced p38, JNK, MAPK, and nuclear factor-kappa B (NF-κB) signaling. Moreover, delaying administration of TO901317 to 3 h post-ICH reduced brain tissue damage and neuronal death.

Conclusions: Our results suggest that enhancing LXR activation may provide a potential therapy for ICH by modulating the cytotoxic functions of microglia.

Keywords: Liver X receptors, Microglia, Inflammation, Intracerebral hemorrhage, Neuronal damage, TO901317

* Correspondence: szufuchen@yahoo.com.tw
†Equal contributors
[1]Department of Physiology and Biophysics, National Defense Medical Center, Taipei, Taiwan, Republic of China
[3]Department of Physical Medicine and Rehabilitation, Cheng Hsin General Hospital, Taipei, Taiwan, Republic of China
Full list of author information is available at the end of the article

Background

Intracerebral hemorrhage (ICH) accounts for approximately 15 % of all strokes with high mortality and morbidity [1]. ICH induces brain damage due to initial tissue disruption from hematoma compression and subsequent development of excitotoxicity, oxidative damage, and inflammation [2, 3]. Of these, cerebral inflammation is considered to be a key pathological factor of ICH-induced brain damage and correlates with deterioration and poor outcomes in patients [4]. Suppression of inflammatory responses has also been reported to improve both histological and functional outcomes and to reduce brain edema in animal studies [5–8]. Inflammation after ICH involves infiltration of peripheral inflammatory cells, activation of microglia, and overproduction of inflammatory mediators, such as cytokines, chemokines, and matrix metalloproteases (MMPs) via nuclear factor-kappa B (NF-κB) signaling [9]. These inflammatory events may induce blood-brain barrier (BBB) disruption and brain edema, which ultimately lead to neuronal death and neurological deterioration [9]. Thus, defining the signals that control cerebral inflammatory responses has important implications for modulating disease processes following ICH.

Liver X receptors (LXRs) are nuclear receptors that regulate lipid metabolism at the transcriptional level [10]. Two members of the LXR superfamily have been identified, LXR-α and LXR-β, both of which are present in the nervous system and which have highly similar DNA or ligand-binding domains [10, 11]. LXRs can be activated by natural ligands, such as oxysterols [12] or by synthetic agonists [13]. The activation of LXRs regulates the expression of several genes that are involved in cholesterol metabolism [10]. In addition, LXRs negatively regulate transcriptional processes that are involved in inflammatory responses [10]. Previous in vitro studies have shown that LXR agonists attenuate inflammation by inhibiting NF-κB activity, and the expression of inflammatory mediators, such as inducible nitric oxide synthase (iNOS), cyclooxygenase-2 (COX-2), and proinflammatory cytokines and chemokines in microglia and astrocytes [14–16]. The anti-inflammatory activities of LXRs have also been observed in animal models of Alzheimer's disease [17], Parkinson's disease [18], spinal cord injury [19], and cerebral ischemia [20, 21]. LXR agonists also exert neuroprotection [20, 22, 23] and attenuate functional deficits [20, 22, 24] in experimental cerebral ischemia. However, no information is available concerning the possible therapeutic efficacy and anti-inflammatory activity of LXR activation after hemorrhagic stroke.

The aim of the present study was to determine the neuroprotective effect of LXR activation using a synthetic agonist, TO901317, in a mouse model of ICH.

We also examined whether LXR activation attenuated ICH-induced microglial activation in both cell and animal models.

Methods

Animals

All animal protocols were carried out according to the Guide for the Care and Use of Laboratory Animals published by the US National Institutes of Health (NIH Publication No. 85-23, revised 1996), and were approved by the Animal Research Committee at Cheng Hsin General Hospital. Adult male C57BL/6J mice (age 8–10 weeks, weight 23–28 g) were kept at a constant temperature (21–25 °C) under a 12-h light/dark cycle with a humidity of approximately 45–50 %. Water and pellet chow were provided ad libitum.

Experimental protocol

Mice were randomized into different treatment groups by using computer-generated random numbers. All outcome measurements and analyses described below were performed in a blinded manner. Four studies were conducted (Fig. 1). The first study examined the temporal profile and cellular localization of LXR expression after ICH. Assessment included western blots ($n = 7$/group) and double immunofluorescence labeling ($n = 6$/group). The second study evaluated the neuroprotective effect of the synthetic LXR agonist TO901317, which has been widely used in experimental studies and activates both LXR isoforms with similar potency [25]. TO901317 (30 mg/kg, Cayman Chemical, Ann Arbor, MI, USA) dissolved in either 30 % dimethyl sulfoxide (DMSO) (100 μL) or a corresponding volume of vehicle (30 % DMSO) was administered intraperitoneally (ip) 10 min after ICH and subsequently daily for 2 days (10 min, 24 h, and 48 h). Testing was as follows: (1) behavioral tests ($n = 13$/group); (2) metabolic characteristics and histology ($n = 5$–7/group); (3) hemoglobin assay, brain water content, and Evans Blue dye extravasation ($n = 6$–8/group); and (4) western blot analysis ($n = 6$–8/group). The dose and route of TO901317 were selected based on previous work on experimental cerebral ischemia [20, 21, 23] and on our pilot study, in which concentrations of 20, 30, and 40 mg/kg were tested. TO901317 at 30 and 40 mg/kg, but not at 20 mg/kg, reduced ICH-induced behavioral deficits with equivalent efficacy (Additional file 1: Figure S1). The three-dose regimen was chosen because inflammatory-related signals peak between 1 and 3 days after collagenase-induced ICH and decline thereafter [26, 27].

The third study investigated the anti-inflammatory effect of TO901317. Assessments included matrix metalloproteinase-9 (MMP-9) zymography and western blot analysis, enzyme-linked immunosorbent assay

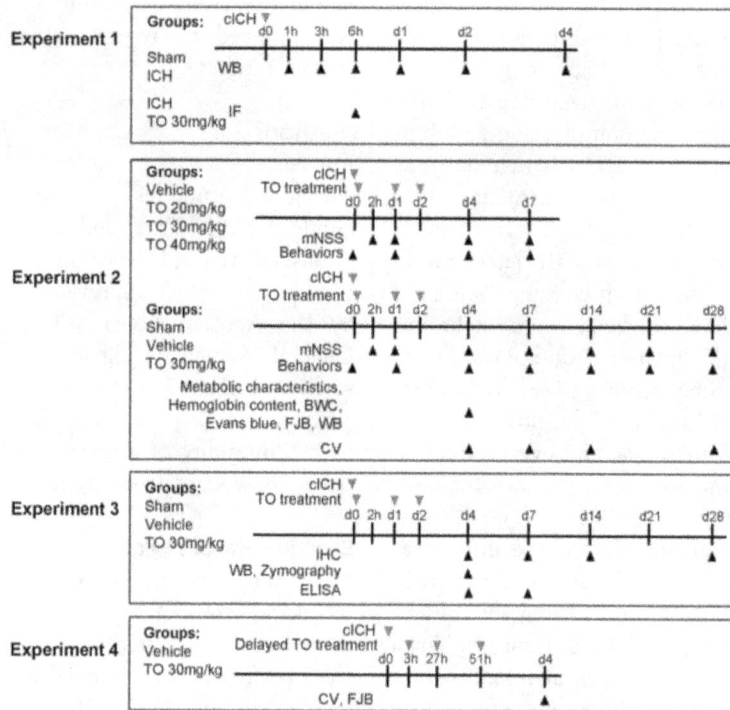

Fig. 1 Experimental design and animal group classification. *cICH* collagenase-induced intracerebral hemorrhage, *IF* immunofluorescence staining, *TO* TO901317, *mNSS* modified neurological severity score, *BWC* brain water content, *FJB* Fluoro-Jade B staining, *WB* western blot, *CV* cresyl violet, *IHC* immunohistochemal staining, *ELISA* enzyme-linked immunosorbent assay

(ELISA), and immunohistochemistry ($n = 5$–7/group). The fourth study examined the delayed therapeutic potential of TO901317 for ICH. Either TO901317 or vehicle was administered ip at 3 h following ICH and subsequently daily for 2 days (3, 27, and 51 h), and protective effects were assessed using cresyl violet staining and Fluoro-Jade B (FJB) histology ($n = 7$/group).

Intracerebral hemorrhage model

ICH model was performed as previously described [28]. Briefly, mice were placed into a stereotaxic frame after anesthesia with sodium pentobarbital (65 mg/kg, ip; Rhone Merieux, Harlow, UK). After retracting the scalp, a 30-gauge needle attached to a Hamilton syringe was implanted through a 1-mm-diameter burr hole into the right striatum (stereotaxic coordinates: 0.8 mm anterior and 2.5 mm lateral to bregma, 2.5 mm in depth). Bacterial collagenase (type VII-S; Sigma, St. Louis, MO, USA; 0.15 U in 0.5 μL of saline) was infused into the brain at a rate of 0.05 μL/min over 10 min with an infusion pump to induce intracerebral hemorrhage, and the needle was left in place for an additional 20 min to prevent reflux. After removal of the needle, the craniotomy was sealed with dental cement and the scalp was sutured closed. Mice were maintained at a 37.0 ± 0.5 °C body temperature using a heated pad throughout the surgery and recovery period. Sham-operated mice received an equal volume of normal saline in the same manner.

Metabolic characteristics assessment

Mice were anesthetized with an overdose of sodium pentobarbital (200 mg/kg, ip), and right atrial puncture was performed to collect venous blood. The collected blood was centrifuged (3500 g for 5 min), and the serum was stored on ice until analysis. Serum blood urea nitrogen (BUN), creatinine (CRE), alanine aminotransferase (ALT), triglyceride (TG), and cholesterol (CHO) were measured by a chemistry autoanalyzer (Synchron Clinical System LX20; Beckman Coulter, Fullerton, CA, USA) to assess renal, liver, and cholesterol metabolisms.

Behavioral testing

Behavioral recovery was assessed using modified neurological severity score (mNSS) test, rotarod test, and beam walking test. Animals were pre-trained for 3 days for both rotarod and beam walking tests.

Modified neurological severity score

The mNSS included motor, sensory, reflex, and balance tests [29]. A higher score represented a more severe injury. Neurological function was graded on a scale of 0–18 (normal score, 0; maximal deficit score, 18).

Rotarod test

An accelerating rotarod was used to measure motor function and balance in mice [30]. The rotarod speed was slowly increased from 6 to 42 rpm within 7 min, and the time for mice to fall off was recorded.

Beam walking test

The test was used to evaluate fine motor coordination and function by measuring the ability of the animals to traverse an elevated narrow beam as described previously [30].

For the rotarod and beam walking tests, three measurements per trial were recorded 1 h before ICH (baseline) and at 1, 4, 7, 14, 21, and 28 days after ICH.

Hemoglobin assay

The hemoglobin contents of ICH brains were quantified using a spectrophotometric assay as previously described [28]. Mice were transcardially perfused and both ipsilateral and contralateral striatum regions were collected following ICH. Distilled water (300 μL) was added to each hemisphere, followed by homogenization for 30 s, sonication on ice for 1 min, and centrifugation at 13,000 rpm for 30 min. Drabkin reagent (80 μL; Sigma) was added to a 20-μL aliquot of supernatant (which contained the hemoglobin) and allowed to stand for 15 min at room temperature. Optical density was then measured at a wavelength of 545 nm to assess the concentration of cyanmethemoglobin. To generate a standard curve, blood was obtained by cardiac punctures in anesthetized control mice. Incremental volumes of this blood (0, 0.5, 1.0, 2.0, 4.0, and 8.0 μL) were then added to 300 μL of tissue lysate from a normal hemispheric sample.

Brain water content

Brain water content was used as a measure of brain edema, which occurred because of BBB breakdown post-ICH. Following terminal anesthesia, mice were decapitated after ICH. The brains were immediately removed and divided into five parts, consisting of the ipsilateral and contralateral cortexes (CX), ipsilateral and contralateral basal ganglia (BG), and the cerebellum (which served as an internal control). Brain samples were immediately weighed on an electric analytical balance to obtain the wet weight and then dried at 100 °C for 24 h to obtain the dry weight. The water content of each sample was calculated using the following formula: [(wet weight – dry weight)/wet weight] × 100 %.

Blood-brain barrier permeability

A 2 % solution of Evans Blue dye in normal saline (4 mL/kg of body weight) was injected into the tail vein and was allowed to circulate for 1 h. The mice were then transcardially perfused with phosphate-buffered saline (PBS) following terminal anesthesia, and samples from both hemispheres were homogenized in 1000 μL of trichloroacetic acid, sonicated, and centrifuged (15 min, 4500 rpm, 4 °C). The absorbance of each supernatant for Evans Blue dye was measured at 620 nm using a spectrophotometer. Evans Blue dye concentrations were calculated and expressed as micrograms per gram of brain tissue against a standard curve.

Tissue processing and histology

Following terminal anesthesia, mice were transcardially perfused with PBS and then 4 % paraformaldehyde after ICH or sham surgery. Brains were removed, post-fixed in 4 % paraformaldehyde overnight, cryoprotected with 30 % sucrose, and then sectioned coronally (10 μm) over the entire region of injury.

Hemorrhagic injury and hemispheric enlargement analysis

Injury volume, hemispheric atrophy, striatal atrophy, and hemispheric enlargement ratios were quantified using coronal sections stained with cresyl violet at 20 rostral-caudal levels that were spaced 200 μm apart. Sections were analyzed using ImageJ software version 1.48 (ImageJ, National Institutes of Health, Bethesda, MD, USA). Volume measurement was computed by a summation of the areas multiplied by the interslice distance (200 mm). Hemispheric or striatal atrophy was assessed using the following formula: ([Contralateral hemisphere or striatal volume – ipsilateral hemisphere or striatal volume]/contralateral hemisphere or striatal volume) × 100 %. Hemispheric enlargement was assessed using the following formula: ([ipsilateral hemisphere volume – contralateral hemisphere volume]/contralateral hemisphere volume) × 100 %. Analysis was performed by two experimenters who were blinded to all animal groups. Inter-rater reliability was within 10 %.

Double immunofluorescence

To assess the cellular localization of LXR-α and LXR-β, double immunofluorescence labeling was performed by simultaneous incubation of either mouse anti-LXR-α (1:200; Abcam, Cambridge, MA, USA) or rabbit anti-LXR-β (1:50; Santa Cruz Biotechnology, Santa Cruz, CA, USA) with mouse anti-neuronal nuclei antigen (NeuN; a neuronal marker; 1:100; Millipore, Billerica, MA, USA), rabbit anti-microtubule-associated protein 2 (MAP2; a neuronal marker; 1:200; Millipore), rat anti-glial fibrillary acidic protein (GFAP; an astrocyte marker; 1:500; Invitrogen, Camarillo, CA, USA), rabbit anti-ionized calcium-binding adaptor molecule 1 (Iba-1; a microglia/macrophage marker; 1:400; Wako, Richmond, VA, USA), or rat anti-F4/80 (a microglia/macrophage marker; 1:400; Serotec, Düsseldorf, Germany) overnight at 4 °C. Sections were then washed, incubated with Alexa Fluor 488- or Alexa Fluor 594-conjugated secondary antibodies

(1:400; Molecular Probes, Eugene, OR, USA) for 2 h, observed under a fluorescence microscope (Olympus BX-51; Olympus, Tokyo, Japan), and photographed.

Immunohistochemistry

Immunohistochemical analyses were carried out as previously described [31]. After quenching of endogenous peroxidase activity and blocking of nonspecific binding, sections were allowed to react with the primary antibodies (rabbit anti-myeloperoxidase [MPO; a neutrophil marker; 1:1000; Dako, Carpinteria, CA, USA], rabbit anti-Iba-1 [a microglia/macrophage marker; 1:1000; Wako], or rat anti-CD45 [a marker for microglia and all blood-born leukocytes, including macrophages, monocytes, neutrophils, and T cells; 1:100; BD Biosciences Pharmigen, San Jose, CA, USA]) at 4 °C overnight. Further colorimetric detection was processed according to the instructions of a Vectastain Elite ABC Kit (Vector Laboratories, Burlingame, CA, USA) with the use of diaminobenzidine as a peroxidase substrate. The specificity of the staining reaction was assessed in several control procedures, including omission of the primary antibody and substitution of the primary antibody with non-immune rabbit serum.

Fluoro-Jade B histochemistry

FJB is a polyanionic fluorescein derivative that binds with high sensitivity and specificity to degenerating neurons. Briefly, sections were rehydrated in graded ethanol solutions (75, 50, and 25 %, 5 min each) and distilled water, incubated in 0.06 % $KMnO_4$ for 10 min, rinsed in distilled water for 2 min, incubated in a 0.0004 % solution of FJB (Chemicon, Temecula, CA, USA) for 30 min, and observed under a fluorescence microscope (Olympus) at 450–490 nm.

Quantification of FJB, Iba-1, MPO, and CD45 staining

For each animal, FJB, Iba-1, MPO, and CD45 staining or double immunofluoresence for cellular markers and LXRs were quantified on three consecutive sections from the hemorrhagic core at the level of 0.24 mm from the bregma. The number of positive cells was counted in an area of 920×860 μm^2 in 10–12 non-overlapping fields immediately adjacent to the hematoma using a magnification of ×200 as previously described [28, 32]. Iba-1-positive resting microglia/macrophages were defined as resting if they contained relatively small cell bodies (<7.5 μm in diameter) with long slender processes [33]. Microglia were defined as activated when a cell body increased in size compared to resting microglia with short, thick processes and intense immunointensity. Activated microglia/macrophages were defined based on a combination of morphological criteria and a cell body diameter cutoff of 7.5 μm. The total number of FJB-,

Iba-1-, and MPO-positive cells was expressed as the mean number per field of view. Quantification of LXRs in neurons or microglia was expressed as (LXR-stained neurons or microglia/neurons or microglia) × 100 %. Analysis was performed by two experimenters who were blinded to all animal groups. Inter-rater reliability was within 10 %.

Western blot

Samples were collected and western blot was performed as previously described [28]. A 2-mm-thick coronal section from the ipsilateral hemisphere was collected following ICH or sham surgery. Equal amounts of protein (35 to 50 μg protein in 20 μL for tissue samples and 20 μg protein in 20 μL for cell lysates) were separated by sodium dodecyl sulfate-polyacrylamide gels, transferred to Immobilon-P membranes (Millipore), blocked using 5 % milk in PBS containing 0.1 % Tween-20, and probed overnight at 4 °C with primary antibodies including mouse anti-LXR-α (1:1000; Abcam), rabbit anti-LXR-β (1:1000; Santa Cruz), mouse anti-ATP binding cassette transporter-1 (ABCA-1; 1:1000; Abcam), mouse anti-iNOS (1:200; Sigma), rabbit anti-COX-2 (1:1000; Cayman), rabbit anti-NF-κB p65 (1:1000; Santa Cruz), rabbit phospho-p38 (1:1000; Cell Signaling, Danvers, MA, USA), rabbit total p38 (1:2000; Cell Signaling), rabbit phospho-Jun amino-terminal kinases (JNK; Thr183/Tyr185, 1:1000; Cell Signaling), rabbit total JNK (1:2000; Cell Signaling), rabbit phospho-extracellular signal-regulated kinases p44/42 (Erk p44/42; Thr202/Tyr204, 1:1000; Cell Signaling), and rabbit total Erk (1:2000; Cell Signaling). The membranes were then incubated with horseradish peroxidase-linked anti-rabbit or anti-mouse secondary antibodies (Santa Cruz Biotechnology; 1:1000) for 1 h at 4 °C. Protein band intensities were quantified using ImageJ software, and the relative intensity of protein signals was normalized to the corresponding β-actin intensity.

Gelatin zymography

Zymography was performed as previously described [28]. Briefly, protein samples were equally loaded and separated by a 10 % Tris-glycine gel with 0.1 % gelatin as a substrate. After separation, the gel was washed in distilled water twice for 30 min, re-natured for 1 h with 2.5 % Triton X-100 buffer at room temperature, and incubated for 48 h with developing buffer (0.05 M Tris-HCl, pH 7.5; 0.2 mol/L NaCl; 5 mmol/L $CaCl_2$; 0.05 % Brij-35; and 0.2 mmol/L NaN_3) at 37 °C. Following this, the gel was stained with 0.05 % Coomassie R-250 dye (Sigma) for 30 min and appropriately de-stained. Gelatinolytic activity (MMP-9, 92 kDa) was determined as by the appearance of clear bands at the appropriate molecular weights.

Enzyme-linked immunosorbent assay and nitrite assay

Protein samples were collected as in western blotting following ICH or sham surgery. Monocyte chemoattractant protein-1 (MCP-1), macrophage inflammatory protein-2 (MIP-2), interleukin (IL)-6, and interleukin-1β (IL-1β) were measured in brain homogenates or cell lysates using a commercially available ELISA kit (R&D Systems, Minneapolis, MN, USA). All samples and standards were assayed in duplicate according to the manufacturer's instructions. Nitric oxide (NO) production was assessed by measuring the nitrite levels of the culture supernatants with Griess reagent (Sigma).

Microglial culture

The mouse microglial BV2 cell line was cultured in Dulbecco's modified Eagle's media (DMEM; Gibco/BRL, Bethesda, MD, USA) supplemented with 10 % heat-inactivated fetal bovine serum (FBS; Gibco/BRL), 100 U/mL penicillin and 100 μg/mL streptomycin in a humidified atmosphere of 5 % CO_2 at 37 °C. BV2 microglia were stimulated with either 0.1 μg/mL lipopolysaccharide (LPS) or 10 U/mL thrombin in the absence or presence of varying concentrations of TO901317 for 24 h. The experiments were repeated four times with different batches of cultures.

Statistical analyses

All data are presented as the mean and standard error of the mean (mean ± SEM). One-way or two-way analysis of variance (ANOVA) followed by post hoc Bonferroni evaluation was used for multiple groups to determine significant differences. Student's t test was used to test the differences between two groups. Statistical significance was set at $P < 0.05$.

Results

Increased LXR-α protein expression in mice after ICH

We first examined the temporal profiles and cellular localizations of LXRs following ICH in mice. ICH induced an increase in LXR-α protein levels in the hemorrhagic hemisphere at 6 h (284 % of the sham level; $P = 0.019$), 1 day (272 %; $P = 0.038$) and 4 days (277 %; $P = 0.029$), whereas LXR-β expression remained mostly unaffected (Fig. 2a, b). Because LXR-α expression peaked at 6 h after collagenase-induced ICH, we investigated the cellular localizations of LXRs at this time point. Dual-label immunofluorescence demonstrated that both LXR-α and LXR-β were mainly expressed in neurons and microglia in the peri-ICH region and rarely in astrocytes (Fig. 2c, d). Quantification results showed that in the vehicle-treated ICH group, 44.1 ± 1.5 % of neurons were positive for LXR-α and 67.1 ± 1.9 % of neurons were positive for LXR-β. For microglia/macrophages, 26.2 ± 1.2 % were positive for LXR-α and 24.4 ± 2.2 % were positive for

LXR-β. Similarly, in the TO901317-treated group, 42.0 ± 1.2 % of neurons were positive for LXR-α and 64.1 ± 0.7 % of neurons were positive for LXR-β. For microglia/macrophages, 26.1 ± 1.2 % were positive for LXR-α and 24.8 ± 0.6 % were positive for LXR-β. There was no difference between the vehicle and TO901317-treated groups for the ratios of LXR-positive neurons or microglia.

TO901317 improved long-term neurobehavioral function but did not alter hemorrhage size in mice after ICH

To investigate the protective efficacy of LXR activation in ICH, TO901317 was employed to activate LXR following ICH. We first assessed the safety of TO901317 in mice on the 4th day post-ICH, at which point one dose of either vehicle or TO901317 was administered daily for 3 days. Treatment with TO901317 did not alter plasma concentrations of BUN and CRE, which are indicators of renal function, ALT, an indicator of hepatic function, or TG and CHO, which are indicators of cholesterol metabolism (Table 1). Similarly, no significant between-group differences were found in body weight change at 28 days (Fig. 3a) or in brain hemoglobin content, an indicator of hemorrhage size, at 4 days (Fig. 3b). We then assessed the protective effects of TO901317 on behavioral recovery following ICH using three different behavioral tests. The extent of global neurological deficit was evaluated by mNSS. At 2 h after injury, there was no difference in mNSS between vehicle-treated and TO901317-treated groups, indicating that injury severity was initially similar regardless of treatment (Fig. 3c). Significant improvement in neurological function was observed from 4 to 28 days in the TO901317 group compared with the vehicle group (all $P < 0.05$; Fig. 3c). Rotarod and beam walking tests were employed to evaluate motor and coordination functions. The TO901317 group had better rotarod performance compared to that of the vehicle group at 4, 14, 21, and 28 days (all $P < 0.01$; Fig. 3d). Likewise, beam walk latencies were shorter in the TO901317 group from 1 to 14 days (all $P < 0.05$; Fig. 3e).

TO901317 ameliorated brain tissue loss and neuronal damage in mice after ICH

To determine whether the above changes in behavioral function reflected in a reduction of brain tissue damage and neuronal death, histological outcomes were evaluated. ICH induced pronounced loss of tissue in the hemorrhagic hemisphere and striatum at day 28 post-ICH (Fig. 4a). However, TO901317 significantly reduced the degree of hemispheric atrophy (2.5 ± 1.5 % versus 10.4 ± 0.7 %, $P < 0.001$; Fig. 4a) and striatal atrophy compared to vehicle (11.6 ± 2.6 % versus 31.9 ± 4.0 %, $P = 0.0029$) at 28 days. We further

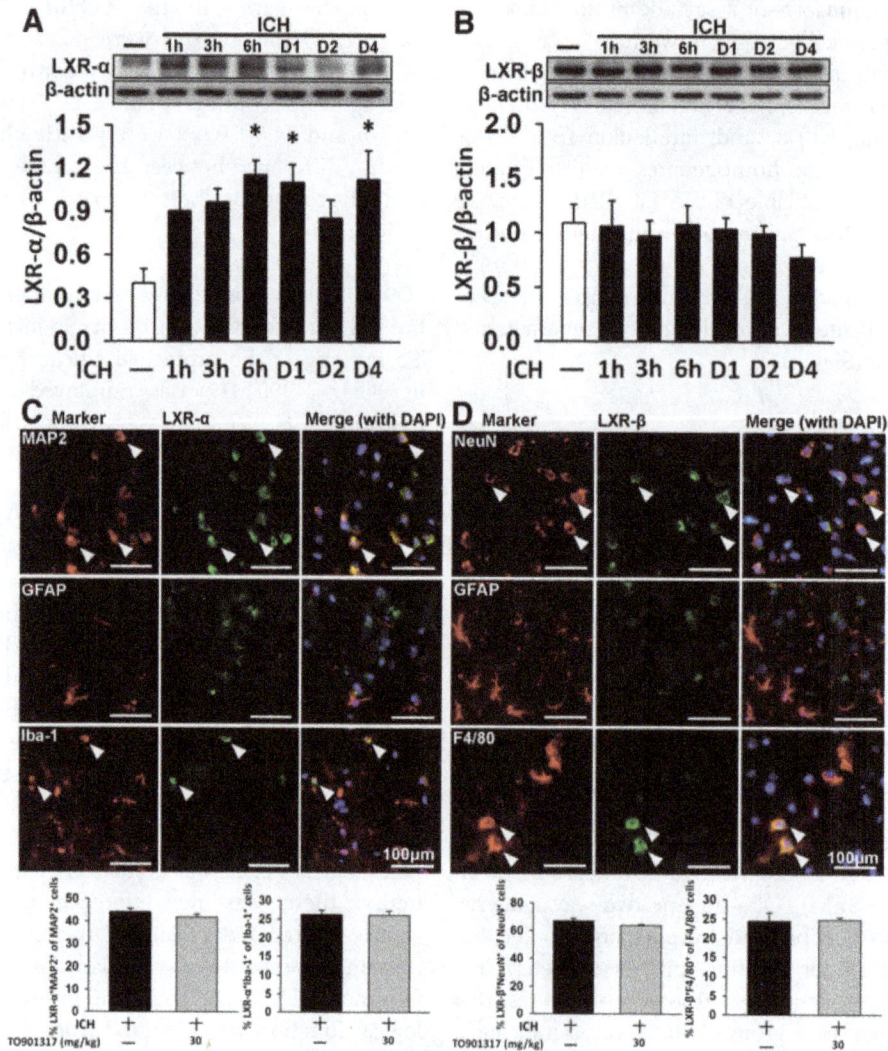

Fig. 2 Expression and cellular distribution of LXR-α and LXR-β receptor isoforms in mouse brains subjected to ICH. Representative immunoblots and quantitative data of **a** the LXR-α and **b** LXR-β protein levels in the ipsilateral (hemorrhagic) hemispheres from ICH or sham-operated mice after collagenase injection. Bar graphs of densitometric analysis of bands show a significant increase in LXR-α protein levels in the ipsilateral hemispheres of ICH mice at 6 h, 1 day, and 4 days post-ICH, compared with the sham-operated mice. LXR-β expression remained unaffected after ICH. Values are mean ± SEM; *$P < 0.05$ versus sham group ($n = 7$ mice/group, one-way ANOVA). **c** LXR-α and **d** LXR-β in the peri-hematomal area observed by immunofluorescence labeling. LXRs are shown in *green*, and immunolabeling of MAP 2 or NeuN (neurons), Iba-1 or F4/80 (microglia), or GFAP (astrocytes) is shown in *red*. Yellow labeling (*white arrows*) indicates co-localization. Both LXR-α and LXR-β were mainly expressed in neurons and microglia and rarely in astrocytes. Sections were stained with DAPI (*blue*) to show all nuclei. The scale bar is 100 μm. Values are mean ± SEM ($n = 6$ mice/group, Student's t test)

evaluated whether TO901317 attenuated brain tissue damage and neuronal injury during the earlier stage of ICH. Consistent with the protective effect at 28 days, TO901317 treatment significantly reduced hemorrhagic injury volume to 69 % of the vehicle group (9.5 ± 1.3 mm^3 versus 13.9 ± 1.3 mm^3, $P = 0.047$; Fig. 4b) at 4 days. Hemispheric enlargement, an indicator of brain edema, was also significantly smaller in TO901317-treated mice (4.1 ± 0.8 %) than in vehicle-treated mice (8.5 ± 1.4 %, $P = 0.02$; Fig. 4b) at 4 days. Moreover, TO901317

significantly attenuated hemorrhagic injury volume at both 7 (0.9 ± 0.2 mm^3 versus 3.5 ± 0.6 mm^3, $P < 0.001$; Fig. 4c) and 14 days (0.4 ± 0.2 mm^3 versus 1.8 ± 0.6 mm^3, $P = 0.0426$; Fig. 4d). At 7 and 14 days after ICH, tissue loss was primary in the ipsilateral striatum, and the total hemispheric atrophy was more evident at 28 days. TO901317 significantly reduced the degree of striatal atrophy at 7 (2.7 ± 1.5 % versus 7.9 ± 0.6 %, $P = 0.0133$; Fig. 4c) and 14 days (6.7 ± 2.5 % versus 19.8 ± 2.6 %, $P = 0.0066$; Fig. 4d). In parallel with the effect of brain tissue

Table 1 Metabolic characteristics of the mice treated with vehicle and TO901317 30 mg/kg

	ICH day 4		
	Vehicle	TO901317 30 mg/kg	Reference range
BUN (mg/dL)	20.60 ± 2.45	18.48 ± 3.92	8–33
CRE (mg/dL)	0.06 ± 0.02	0.05 ± 0.02	0.2–0.9
ALT (mg/dL)	25.00 ± 4.53	29.20 ± 4.47	17–77
TG (mg/dL)	78.00 ± 18.02	62.20 ± 28.79	60–160
CHO (mg/dL)	74.60 ± 12.46	73.40 ± 19.57	90–170

Values are expressed as means ± SEM. $n = 5$ mice/group [31, 57]
ICH intracerebral hemorrhage, *BUN* blood urea nitrogen, *CRE* creatinine, *ALT* alanine aminotransferase, *TG* triglyceride, *CHO* cholesterol

protection, TO901317 significantly attenuated the number of FJB-positive degenerative neurons around the hematoma when compared to vehicle administration at 4 days post-ICH (54.3 ± 4.3 versus 111.3 ± 7.6 cells/field, $P < 0.001$; Fig. 4e).

TO901317 attenuated brain edema and BBB permeability in mice after ICH

We next explored whether TO901317 influenced ICH-induced brain edema and BBB breakdown as both are consequences of inflammatory responses following hemorrhagic stroke [34]. Brain water content was significantly increased in the ipsilateral hemisphere in the vehicle group compared with the contralateral counterpart (82.0 ± 0.5 % versus 78.4 ± 0.6 %; $P < 0.001$) at 4 days post-ICH, which was significantly decreased with TO901317 treatment (79.2 ± 0.3 % versus 82.0 ± 0.5 %, $P < 0.001$; Fig. 4f). To further examine the effects of TO901317 on BBB permeability, we used Evans Blue dye as a marker for albumin extravasation. ICH resulted in significantly increased Evans Blue extravasation in the hemorrhagic hemisphere compared to the contralateral side at 4 days post-ICH (19.2 ± 0.7 versus 4.9 ± 0.4 µg/g, $P < 0.001$; Fig. 4g). However, TO901317 administration resulted in attenuated levels of extracted Evans Blue compared to vehicle-treated mice at 4 days (13.5 ± 1.0 versus 19.2 ± 0.7 µg/g, $P < 0.001$; Fig. 4g).

TO901317 activated the LXR target gene ABCA-1 in mice after ICH

To determine whether TO901317 acted through LXR, we examined the expression levels of LXRs and their target gene ABCA-1 in ICH following the administration of TO901317. ICH induced a significant increase in LXR-α protein expression compared to the sham control at day 4, whereas LXR-β expression remained unchanged (Fig. 5a, b). Both LXR-α and LXR-β protein levels were unaltered in the ICH mice after TO901317 treatment compared with vehicle treatment. However, the protein level of ABCA-1, a representative LXR-regulated gene, was significantly elevated following TO901317 administration at day 4 post-ICH ($P = 0.019$; Fig. 5c). These results suggest that brain LXRs were activated in a ligand-dependent manner after ICH.

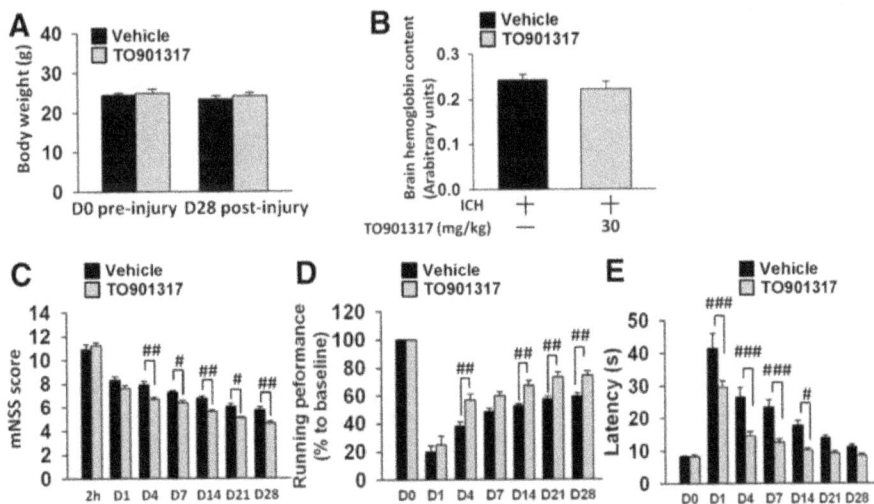

Fig. 3 TO901317 improved neurobehavioral function but did not alter body weight or hemorrhage size after ICH. **a** There were no significant differences in body weight between the control (vehicle-treated) and 30 mg/kg TO901317-treated groups before or at 28 days after ICH. **b** Hemoglobin levels in vehicle-treated and TO901317-treated mice were not significantly different at 4 days post-ICH. Treatment with 30 mg/kg TO901317 (compared with vehicle) significantly **c** reduced the modified neurological severity score (mNSS) from 4 to 28 days (all $P < 0.05$), **d** improved the rotarod performance at 4, 14, 21, and 28 days (all $P < 0.01$), and **e** reduced the beam walk traversing time from 1 to 14 days (all $P < 0.05$) post-ICH. Values are mean ± SEM; #$P < 0.05$, ##$P < 0.01$, and ###$P < 0.001$ versus vehicle group ($n = 13$ mice/group, Student's *t* test for body weight; $n = 8$ mice/group, Student's *t* test for hemoglobin assay; $n = 13$ mice/group, repeated measures two-way ANOVA for behavioral tests)

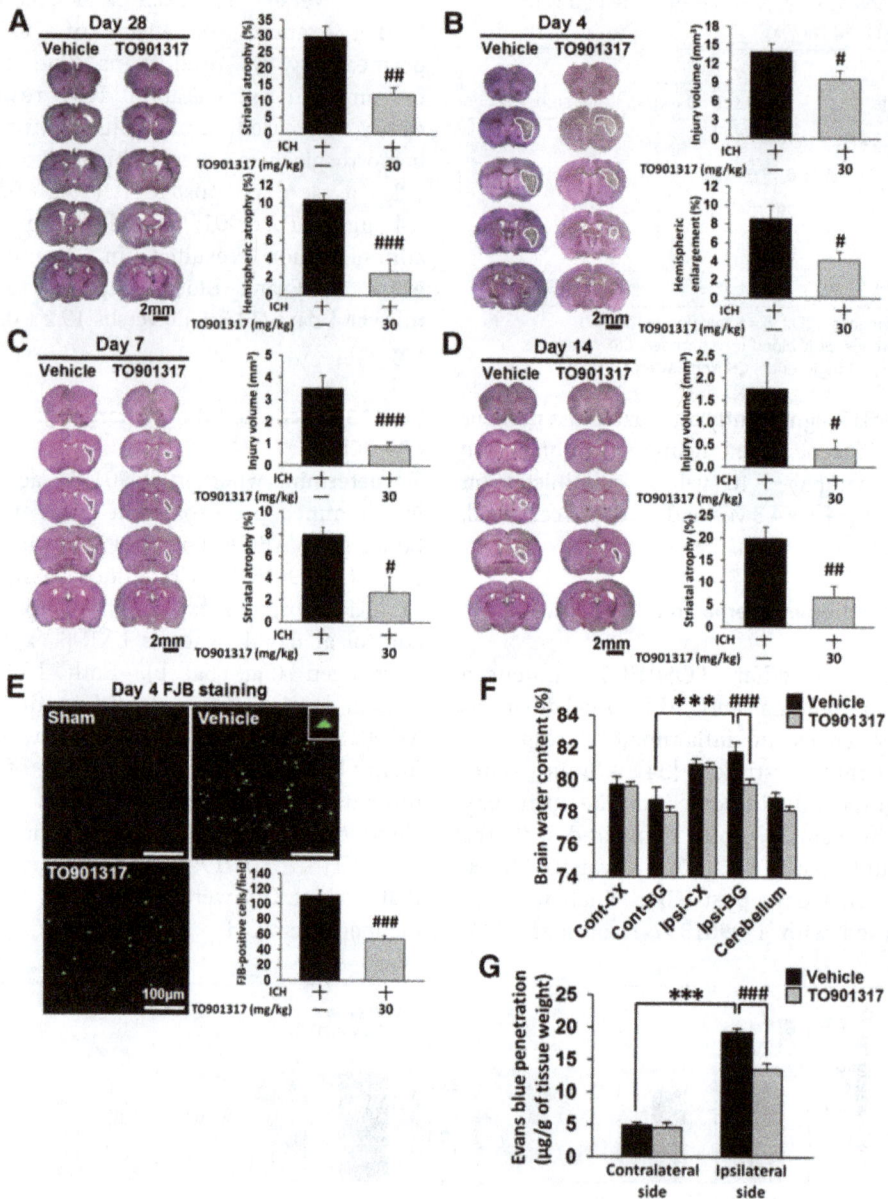

Fig. 4 TO901317 attenuated brain tissue and neuronal damage reduced brain edema and BBB disruption after ICH. Representative cresyl violet-stained brain sections of vehicle-treated and 30 mg/kg TO901317-treated mice at **a** 28, **b** 4, **c** 7, and **d** 14 days post-ICH. Analysis of lesion volumes demonstrates that 30 mg/kg TO901317 significantly reduced hemispheric and striatal atrophy at 28 days and significantly reduced hemorrhagic injury volume and hemispheric enlargement at 4 days. TO901317 also attenuated hemorrhagic injury volume and striatal atrophy at 7 and 14 days. The scale bar is 2 mm. **e** Representative FJB-stained sections of a sham-injured, a vehicle-treated, and a 30 mg/kg TO901317-treated mouse at 4 days post-ICH. The *inset* is a representative FJB-positive cell at higher magnification. Quantification analysis shows that TO901317 significantly reduced the number of degenerating neurons at 4 days post-ICH. The scale bar is 100 μm. **f** Brain water content in the ipsilateral basal ganglion of vehicle-treated mice was significantly higher than in the contralateral basal ganglion at 4 days post-ICH. In the ipsilateral basal ganglion, brain water content of 30 mg/kg TO901317-treated mice was significantly lower than in vehicle-treated mice. *Cont-BG* contralateral basal ganglia, *Cont-CX* contralateral cortex, *Ipsi-BG* ipsilateral basal ganglia, *Ipsi-CX* ipsilateral cortex. **g** TO901317 (30 mg/kg) significantly decreased leakage of Evans Blue dye into the brain in the ipsilateral hemisphere compared with the vehicle-treated mice. Values are mean ± SEM; $^{***}P < 0.001$ versus contralateral hemisphere, $^{\#}P < 0.05$, $^{\#\#}P < 0.01$, and $^{\#\#\#}P < 0.001$ versus vehicle group ($n = 6$–8 mice/group, Student's t test)

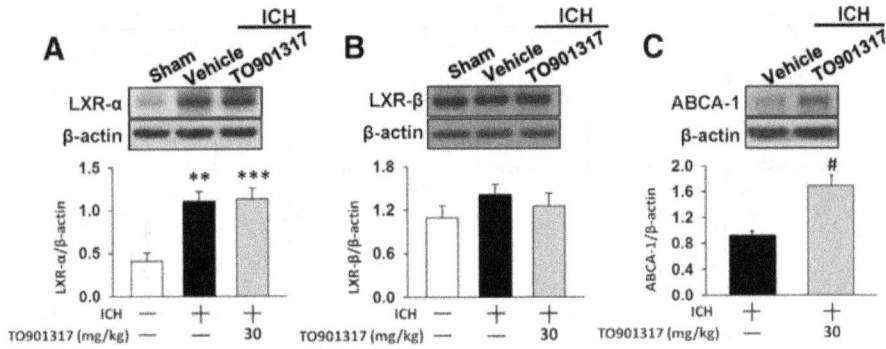

Fig. 5 TO901317 did not affect LXR expression but increased the LXR target gene, ABCA-1 protein expression post-ICH. Representative immunoblots of **a** LXR-α, **b** LXR-β, and **c** ABCA-1 proteins in the ipsilateral hemisphere of sham-injured, vehicle-treated, and 30 mg/kg TO901317-treated mice at 4 days post-ICH. Bar graphs of densitometric analysis of bands show that TO901317 did not affect either LXR-α or LXR-β protein expression but increased the LXR target gene, ABCA-1 protein expression. Values are mean ± SEM; $^{**}P < 0.01$, and $^{***}P < 0.001$ versus sham group, $^{#}P < 0.05$ versus vehicle group ($n = 5$–7 mice/group, one-way ANOVA for LXRs and Student's t test for ABCA-1 western blot).

TO901317 attenuated neutrophil infiltration, microglial activation, and macrophage infiltration but did not affect MMP-9 activity in mice after ICH

We next evaluated degrees of neutrophil infiltration and microglial activation to determine the anti-inflammatory activity of TO901317. ICH resulted in an accumulation of neutrophils in the peri-hematoma area at 4 days (34.0 ± 2.1 cells/field) and 7 days (38.5 ± 5.6 cells/field), and TO901317 treatment significantly reduced this response (21.4 ± 1.6 cells/field at 4 days, $P < 0.001$; 11.4 ± 2.2 cells/field at 7 days, $P = 0.0011$; Fig. 6a). The infiltrated neutrophils were nearly absent in the peri-hematoma area at 14 days. The number of total microglia/macrophages (Iba-1-positive) cells in the hemorrhagic brain also significantly increased compared with the sham group (38.8 ± 2.2 cells/field) in the peri-hematoma area at both 4 days (69.2 ± 1.6 cells/field) and 7 days (87.9 ± 3.7 cells/field; Fig. 6b). On the other hand, animals who received TO901317 treatment showed significant reductions in the total number of Iba-1-positive cells at both 4 days (54.1 ± 3.5 cells/field, $P = 0.002$) and 7 days (66.1 ± 4.9 cells/field, $P = 0.005$) following ICH. There was no difference between the vehicle and TO901317-treated groups at 14 days (35.1 ± 3.8 versus 33.7 ± 3.1 cells/field, $P = 0.785$). There was also a large number of activated microglia/macrophages in the peri-hematoma area at 4 and 7 days after ICH, which was scant at 14 days. TO901317 significantly reduced the number of activated Iba-1-positive cells at 4 days (28.6 ± 3.1 cells/field versus 43.1 ± 4.0 cells/field, $P = 0.013$, Fig. 6b) and 7 days (22.2 ± 3.2 cells/field versus 43.8 ± 1.9 cells/field, $P < 0.001$). However, TO901317 treatment did not affect the number of resting microglia at both 4 and 7 days. We then used CD45 staining, an antigen associated with microglia and all leukocytes, including macrophages, monocytes, neutrophils, and T cells, to identify inflammatory cells. The expression of CD45 is low in resting microglia and increases during microglial activation, whereas CD45 expression is high in blood-born monocytes [35, 36]. Similarly, TO901317 treatment significantly reduced the number of CD45-positive cells in the peri-hematoma area at 4 days (22.6 ± 1.7 cells/field versus 30.6 ± 0.5 cells/field, $P = 0.0043$; Fig. 6c) and 7 days (21.5 ± 1.0 cells/field versus 25.7 ± 1.3 cells/field, $P = 0.0256$) compared with the control group. Both activated Iba-1- and CD45-positive cells were scant at 14 days following ICH. We further analyzed MMP-9 activity, which mediates BBB breakdown by degrading the basal lamina and contributes to the pathophysiology of ICH. MMP-9 activity was significantly increased at 4 days post-ICH, but there was no difference in MMP-9 activity between vehicle-treated and TO901317-treated mice (Fig. 6d).

TO901317 reduced expression of inflammatory mediators in mice after ICH

We then assessed whether TO901317 influenced the expression of inflammatory mediators following ICH. ICH induced an increase in MCP-1, MIP-2, and interleukin-6 (IL-6) protein expression in hemorrhagic hemispheres at 4 and 7 days, but treatment with TO901317 significantly reduced the MCP-1, MIP-2, and IL-6 levels at both 4 days (MCP-1: 33.1 ± 2.7 versus 52.1 ± 4.2 pg/mg protein, $P = 0.001$; MIP-2: 5.5 ± 1.9 versus 13.4 ± 1.8 pg/mg protein, $P = 0.009$; IL-6: 8.6 ± 2.5 versus 23.9 ± 2.8 pg/mg protein, $P < 0.001$; Fig. 7a, b, c) and 7 days (MCP-1: 23.7 ± 1.6 versus 41.8 ± 4.9 pg/mg protein, $P = 0.003$; MIP-2: 5.0 ± 2.5 versus 11.8 ± 1.8 pg/mg protein, $P = 0.003$; IL-6: 9.3 ± 1.2 versus 24.3 ± 1.4 pg/mg protein, $P < 0.001$; Fig. 7a, b, c). Similarly, ICH-induced increases in iNOS and COX-2 levels were significantly attenuated by TO901317 treatment. Protein levels of iNOS and COX-2 in TO901317-treated hemorrhagic hemispheres were 35 % ($P = 0.02$) and 42 % ($P = 0.035$) of the vehicle groups, respectively (Fig. 7d, e).

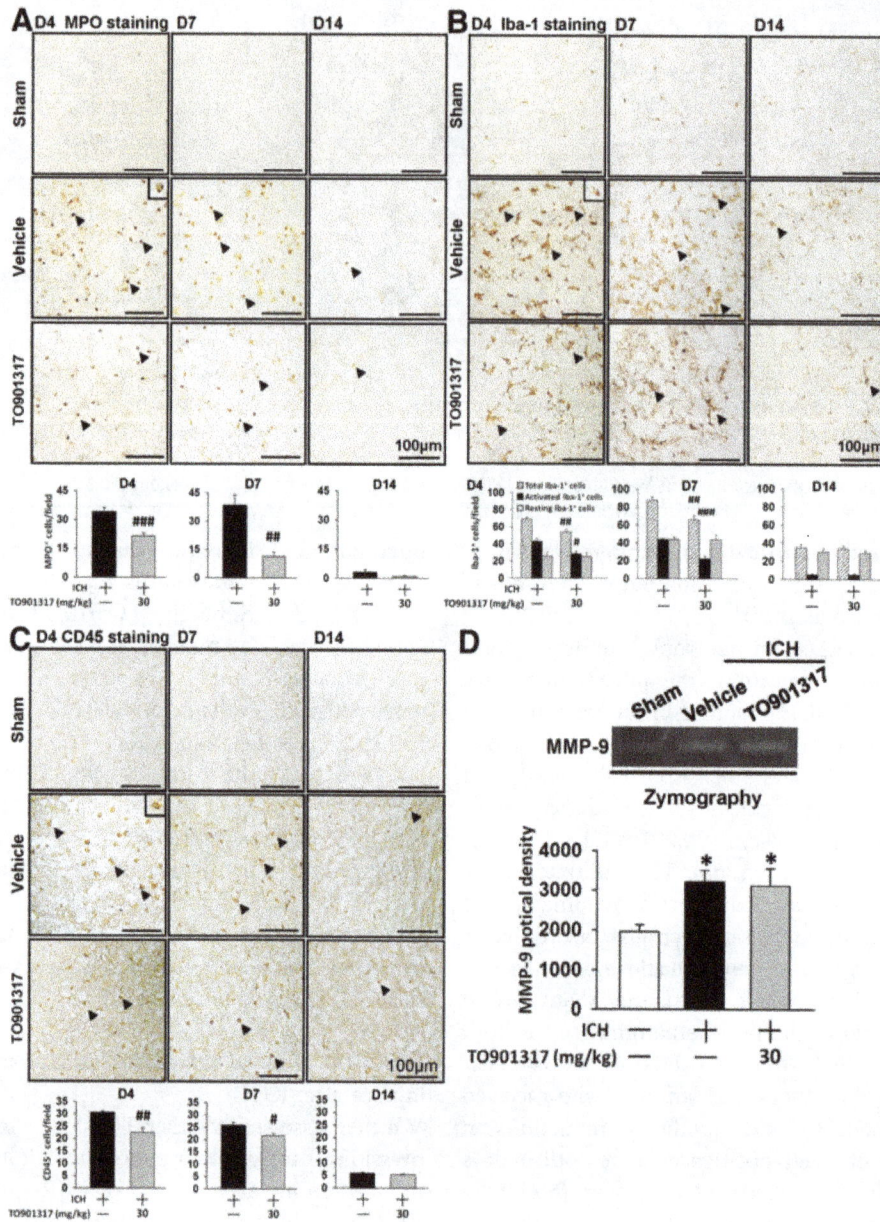

Fig. 6 TO901317 reduced neutrophil infiltration and microglial activation but had no effect on MMP-9 activity. Representative **a** MPO-stained, **b** Iba-1-stained, and **c** CD45-stained brain sections from sham-injured, vehicle-treated, and 30 mg/kg TO901317-treated mice at 4, 7 and 14 days post-ICH. Cell count analysis shows that TO901317-treated mice had significantly fewer MPO-positive, total Iba-1-positive, activated Iba-1-positive, and CD45-positive cells than vehicle-treated mice in the peri-hematoma area at 4 and 7 days post-ICH. The number of MPO-positive, Iba-1-positive, and CD45 positive cells is expressed as the mean number per field of view (0.8 mm²). The scale bar is 100 μm. **d** Representative zymography of MMP-9 activity from a sham-injured control, a vehicle-treated, and a 30 mg/kg TO901317-treated mouse at 1 day post-ICH. There was no difference in MMP-9 activity between vehicle-treated and TO901317-treated mice. Values are mean ± SEM; $^*P < 0.05$ versus sham group, $^#P < 0.05$, $^{##}P < 0.01$, and $^{###}P < 0.001$ versus vehicle group ($n = 6$–7 mice/group, Student's t test for MPO, Iba-1, and CD45 immunohistochemistry; $n = 6$ mice/group, one-way ANOVA for MMP-9 zymography)

TO901317 attenuated LPS- and thrombin-induced pro-inflammatory responses in cultured microglia

Our in vivo results demonstrated that TO901317 preserved neuronal function and reduced microglia activation after ICH; thus, we next used mouse BV2 microglial cells to elucidate the underlying molecular mechanisms.

We used LPS, a strong immunostimulant, and thrombin, a component of coagulation cascade that is rapidly released following ICH, to activate microglia. The exposure of BV2 microglial cells to LPS for 24 h led to an increase in NO release in the culture supernatant, but co-treatment with 1, 5, 10, or 50 μM TO901317 for 24 h

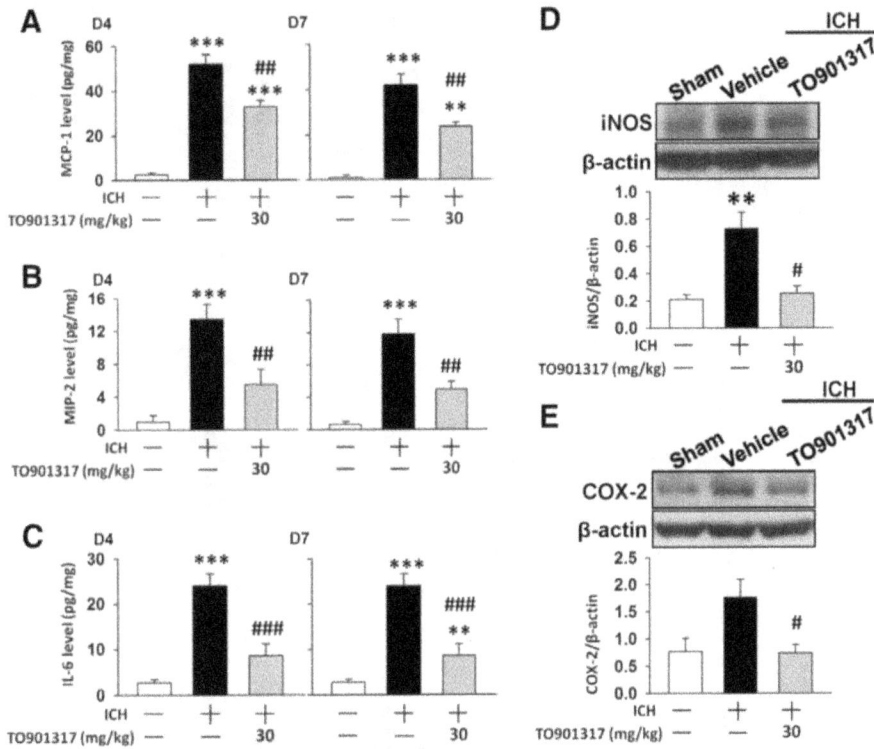

Fig. 7 TO901317 reduced expression of inflammatory mediators in mice after ICH. Bar graphs of **a** MCP-1, **b** MIP-2, and **c** IL-6 protein concentrations, as assessed by ELISA in ipsilateral hemispheres of sham control, vehicle-treated, and 30 mg/kg TO901317-treated mice at 4 and 7 days post-ICH. TO901317-treated mice exhibited significantly reduced MCP-1, MIP-2, and IL-6 protein levels compared with vehicle-treated mice at 4 and 7 days. Representative immunoblots of **d** iNOS and **e** COX-2 proteins in ipsilateral hemispheres of sham control, vehicle-treated, and 30 mg/kg TO901317-treated mice at 4 days post-ICH. Bar graphs of densitometric analysis of bands show a significant decrease of iNOS and COX-2 protein levels in ipsilateral hemispheres of TO901317-treated mice, compared with vehicle-treated mice. Values are presented as means ± SEM; $^{**}P < 0.01$ and $^{***}P < 0.001$ versus sham control; $^{#}P < 0.05$, $^{##}P < 0.01$, $^{###}P < 0.001$ versus vehicle group ($n = 6$–7 mice/group, one-way ANOVA)

significantly reduced LPS-induced NO production to 58, 57, 48, and 60 % of that observed for the vehicle control group, respectively, and 10 μM TO901317 provided the highest degree of anti-inflammatory action (all $P < 0.001$; Fig. 8a). Therefore, a dosage of 10 μM was employed for subsequent biochemical studies. Similar results were observed after thrombin stimulation (all $P < 0.001$; Fig. 8b). Treatment with 10 μM TO901317 also significantly attenuated LPS-induced production of IL-1β (11.0 ± 1.3 versus 24.0 ± 0.7 pg/mg; $P < 0.001$; Fig. 8c), IL-6 (13.0 ± 0.2 versus 25.8 ± 0.6 pg/mg; $P < 0.001$; Fig. 8c), and MIP-2 (9.2 ± 0.1 versus 29.4 ± 0.3 pg/mg; $P < 0.001$; Fig. 8c) as measured in the supernatants of microglial cultures.

We further investigated whether TO901317 influenced the activation of NF-κB, a major transcription factor that regulates pro-inflammatory gene expression and can be activated by mitogen-activated protein kinases (MAPKs), a family of serine/threonine protein kinases that mediate microglial activation [37]. Nuclear NF-κB p65 levels were low in the control group under basal (unstimulated) conditions. Activation of NF-κB, as indicated by nuclear translocation of p65, was observed at 1, 3, 6, and

24 h following LPS stimulation (all $P < 0.001$; Fig. 8d). Co-treatment with 10 μM TO901317 significantly attenuated the LPS-induced increased nuclear levels of NF-κB at 1 h (69 % of vehicle level, $P = 0.004$), 3 h (73 % of vehicle level, $P = 0.042$), and 6 h (61 % of vehicle level, $P = 0.011$) after LPS stimulation (Fig. 8d).

Previous report studies have shown that MAPKs play critical roles in harmful microglial activation during acute brain injury [37]. Therefore, we evaluated the inhibitory effects of TO901317 on LPS-induced activation of MAPKs, including p38, JNK, and Erk. Stimulation of microglia with LPS resulted in rapid activation of p38, JNK, and Erk. Co-treatment with 10 μM TO901317 significantly reduced LPS-induced p38 and JNK phosphorylation at 3 and 6 h (all $P < 0.05$; Fig. 8d). However, there was no difference in the phosphorylation of Erk between TO901317-treated and vehicle-treated groups (all $P > 0.05$; Fig. 8d). Together, these results suggest that TO901317 may inhibit reactive microglial activation and subsequently attenuate the production of pro-inflammatory mediators by suppressing p38 and JNK signaling pathways and NF-κB activation.

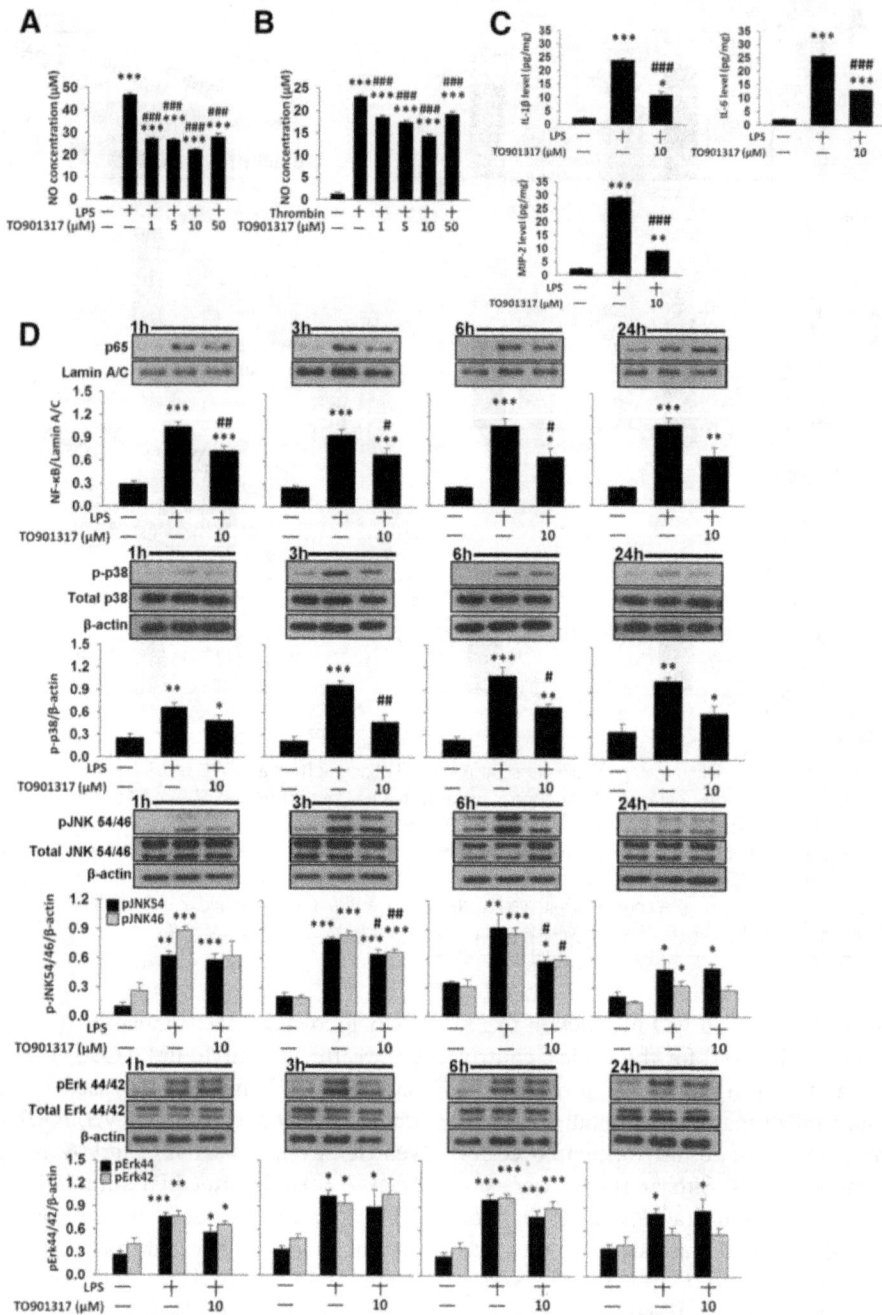

Fig. 8 TO901317 inhibited LPS- and thrombin-induced inflammatory responses in cultured microglia. In BV2 microglia, co-treatment of 1, 5, 10, or 50 μM TO901317 with LPS or thrombin for 24 h significantly attenuated **a** LPS- or **b** thrombin-induced release of NO from the supernatant of microglial cultures. **c** Co-treatment of 10 μM TO901317 with LPS for 24 h significantly reduced LPS-induced release of IL-1β, IL-6, and MIP-2 from the supernatant of BV2 microglial cultures. **d** Representative immunoblots and bar graphs show that co-treatment of 10 μM TO901317 with LPS significantly reduced LPS-induced p65 nuclear translocation at 1, 3, and 6 h, p38 and JNK phosphorylation at 3 and 6 h but did not affect Erk phosphorylation in BV2 microglia. Values are presented as mean ± SEM of four independent experiments. $^{*}P < 0.05$, $^{**}P < 0.01$, and $^{***}P < 0.001$ versus normal control; $^{#}P < 0.05$, $^{##}P < 0.01$, and $^{###}P < 0.001$ versus LPS or thrombin stimulation alone (one-way ANOVA)

Delayed administration of TO901317 reduced brain damage and neuronal death

To determine whether TO901317 still exerts neuroprotective effects when administered at later time points after ICH, TO901317 treatment was delayed by 3 h post-injury.

TO901317 treatment at 3 h significantly reduced injury volume (9.3 ± 0.9 mm^3 versus 14.0 ± 1.1 mm^3; $P < 0.001$; Fig. 9a) and hemispheric enlargement, an indicator of brain edema (5.3 ± 1.0 % versus 10.5 ± 1.2 %, $P = 0.0068$; Fig. 9a) at 4 days. The number of FJB-positive neurons

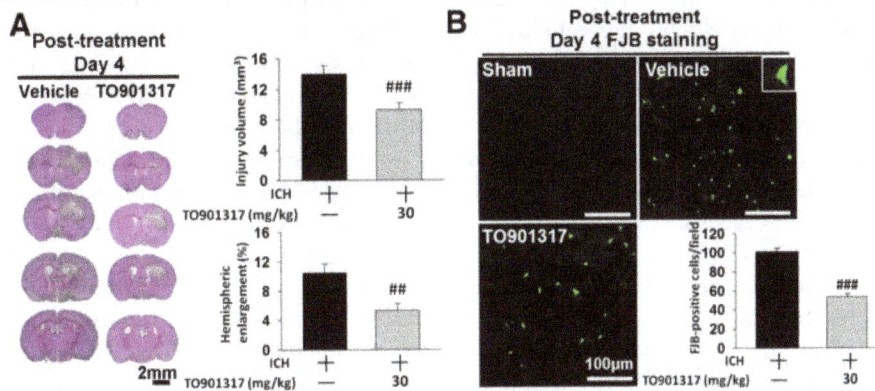

Fig. 9 Delayed TO901317 treatment attenuated injury volume, hemispheric enlargement, and neuronal death after ICH. **a** Representative cresyl violet-stained brain sections of a vehicle-treated and a delayed 30 mg/kg TO901317-treated mouse at 4 days post-ICH. Analysis of lesion volumes demonstrates that treatment with 30 mg/kg TO901317 at 3 h post-ICH significantly reduced hemorrhagic injury volume and hemispheric enlargement at 4 days. The scale bar is 2 mm. **b** Representative FJB-stained sections of a sham-injured, a vehicle-treated, and a delayed 30 mg/kg TO901317-treated mouse at 4 days post-ICH. The *inset* is a representative FJB-positive cell at higher magnification. Quantification analysis shows that treatment with 30 mg/kg TO901317 at 3 h post-ICH significantly reduced the number of degenerating neurons at 4 days post-ICH. The scale bar is 100 μm. Values are presented as means ± SEM; $^{##}P < 0.01$ and $^{###}P < 0.001$ versus vehicle group ($n = 7$ mice/group, Student's t test)

around the peri-hematoma area was also reduced (53.9 ± 3.1 versus 100.9 ± 4.0 cells/field; $P < 0.001$; Fig. 9b) compared to the vehicle at day 4 post-injury. The neuroprotective effects of TO901317 treatment either immediately after or at 3 h after ICH were similar; injury volume, hemispheric enlargement, and neuronal damage were attenuated by 31, 52, and 51 % when administered immediately post-ICH (Fig. 4) and by 34, 50, and 47 % when treatment started at 3 h post-injury, respectively (Fig. 9).

Discussion

In this study, we provide the first evidence that activation of LXRs with the synthetic ligand TO901317 improved behavioral outcomes and attenuated brain edema in mice subjected to ICH. Brain tissue damage, neuronal death, and BBB disruption were also reduced following TO901317 treatment. This neuroprotection was observed in conjunction with a reduction of microglial activation, neutrophil infiltration, and expression of inflammatory molecules. Mechanistically, TO901317 attenuated LPS- and thrombin-stimulated NO production in BV2 microglia, which was associated with reduced activation of p38, JNK, MAPK, and NF-κB signaling in LPS-stimulated microglia. Notably, TO901317 was still neuroprotective when using a more clinically relevant treatment time window. Our results suggest that enhancing LXR activation may provide a potential therapy for ICH by modulating the cytotoxic functions of microglia.

We found that LXR-α is selectively upregulated by ICH, although both LXR-α and LXR-β subtypes were detected in the normal brain. Our findings are in agreement with previous reports showing that LXR-α is the form that is predominantly induced in response to a deleterious stimulus such as cerebral ischemia [20] or myocardial ischemia/reperfusion injury [38]. While previous evidence has demonstrated that both LXR-α and LXR-β mediate anti-inflammatory action [39], LXR-α is more responsive in controlling the production of inflammatory molecules compared to LXR-β [40]. On the other hand, whereas LXR-α is expressed predominantly in liver, kidney, intestine, and tissue macrophages, LXR-β is highly expressed in the brain [10, 11]. The importance of LXR-β in brain function is supported by previous studies showing that LXR-β deficiency is associated with central nervous system pathologies and brain development abnormalities [18, 41–43]. For example, LXR-β expression is essential to the formation of the cerebral cortex via its role in guiding the migration of later-born neurons during corticogenesis [41] and is also involved in white matter development and myelination [43]. LXR-β knockout mice exhibit degeneration of motor neurons in the spinal cord and of dopaminergic neurons in the substantia nigra [42]. Furthermore, LXR-β deletion aggravates the loss of dopaminergic neurons in the substantia nigra in an animal model of Parkinson's disease [18]. Therefore, the specific roles of the individual LXR subtypes in ICH require further clarification.

We showed that TO901317 reduced activation of microglia and ICH-induced upregulation of inflammatory molecules (e.g., MCP-1, MIP-2, IL-6, COX-2, and iNOS) in hemorrhagic brain. In parallel with these in vivo results, TO901317 suppressed LPS- and thrombin-induced production of inflammatory mediators and LPS-induced activation of p38, JNK, and NF-κB pathways in BV2 microglia. Our results suggest a direct effect of LXRs on microglial activation and p38 phosphorylation. Most importantly, we demonstrated that the LXR ligand attenuated inflammation in microglia that were activated by thrombin, which is rapidly produced following ICH and contributes to ICH-induced brain damage [2]. Our findings are in line with previous studies showing that LXR activation suppresses inflammatory responses in animal models of CNS diseases [17–20, 22] and in cultured microglia stimulated with LPS or IL-1β [14–16]. LXRs have been reported to deactivate microglia from an amoeboid, active form to a ramified, resting configuration [44]. Following ICH, microglia are activated and then mediate neuroinflammatory responses via producing multiple inflammatory molecules [9], which can activate receptor-dependent apoptotic pathways and contribute to neuronal damage [45]. Experimental evidence has further shown that blocking microglial activation protects against ICH-induced brain damage [46, 47]. In our study, TO901317 reduced neuronal damage at 4 days post-ICH and diminished neurological deficits and decreased brain atrophy at 28 days following ICH. These findings correlated with a reduction of microglia activation in hemorrhagic brain. Thus, it seems very likely that LXR activation may limit brain damage following ICH, in part by blocking microglial activation and attenuating the production of pro-inflammatory mediators.

Our results demonstrated that TO901317 reduced neutrophil infiltration and BBB disruption but did not affect MMP-9 activity. This reduction of infiltrating neutrophils is consistent with previous studies in which TO90317 decreased neutrophil recruitment significantly in damaged spinal cord [19] and lung tissue [48]. The protective effect of TO901317 on neutrophil infiltration may be attributed to a reduction of pro-inflammatory chemokines, which are involved in BBB disruption and the migration of peripheral immune cells into hemorrhagic brain [9]. It is also possible that TO901317 exerts a direct effect on neutrophil responses because a recent study reports that LXR signaling controls peripheral neutrophil homeostasis via regulation of neutrophil clearance and cytokine expression [49]. In contrast with previous reports showing that pharmacological activation of LXRs reduced MMP-9 protein expression following cerebral ischemia [20] and suppressed MMP-9 mRNA and protein expression in macrophages [39], we found that MMP-9 activity was not altered by TO901317 after ICH. One possible explanation for this disparity is that because MMP-9 gene expression is regulated by both NF-κB and activator protein-1 (AP-1) activities [50], antagonism of NF-κB signaling by TO901317 may not be able to suppress AP-1-dependent MMP-9 activity. Another explanation is the time point that was examined. We measured MMP-9 activity at day 4, which is not the peak time point of MMP-9 activation after ICH. Cerebral MMP-9 levels were reported to peak in a bimodal pattern after ICH, with the first peak occurring during days 1–3 and

the second peak occurring around day 7 [51]. Indeed, our findings are consistent with previous neuroprotective studies showing that minocycline significantly reduced neuroinflammation and BBB disruption but did not affect MMP-9 levels [27, 52].

Apart from these anti-inflammatory actions, LXRs may provide neuroprotection via other mechanisms. For example, LXR activation by GW3965, a synthetic LXR agonist, suppressed brain beta-amyloid (Aβ) accumulation in a model of mild traumatic brain injury (TBI) in which cerebral inflammation is not significant [53]. This result suggests that the beneficial effects of LXR agonists on mild TBI recovery may be independent from their anti-inflammatory effects. Other studies further show that LXR agonists modulate the deposition and clearance of Aβ metabolism and attenuate Alzheimer's pathology both in vivo and in vitro [15, 54, 55]. In addition to regulating Aβ metabolism, the LXR agonist TO901317 promoted synaptic plasticity and axonal regeneration following experimental cerebral ischemia and increased neurite outgrowth by increasing PI3K signaling in hypoxic cortical neurons [21]. The activation of LXR signaling also protected cultured neurons from oxidative damage-induced toxicity [56]. Furthermore, TO901317 was reported to promote angiogenesis and vascular maturation through eNOS following cerebral ischemia [24]. Whether LXRs exert direct actions on neurons or vessels following ICH warrants further investigation.

Conclusions

In conclusion, we demonstrated that activation of LXRs by T0901317 reduced functional deficits and brain tissue damage and attenuated neuroinflammation following ICH. T0901317 also reduced activation of p38, JNK, MAPK, and NF-κB signaling in cultured microglia. Considering the extended therapeutic window of T0901317 and its long-lasting effects, our results suggest that pharmacological enhancement of LXRs may have a role as a therapeutic intervention in ICH.

Additional file

Additional file 1: Figure S1. Effects of 3 different doses of TO901317 on collagenase-induced ICH in mice. (**A**) In all treatment groups, the mNSSs were significantly lower than the vehicle group at 4 and 7 days post-ICH. (**B**) There was no significant difference between the 20 mg/kg TO901317-treated and vehicle-treated groups at all tested time points in the rotarod test. Treatment with 30 mg/kg and 40 mg/kg TO901317 significantly improved rotarod performance compared with the vehicle-treated group at all tested time points following ICH. (**C**) There was no significant difference between the 20 mg/kg TO901317-treated and vehicle-treated groups at all tested time points in the beam walk test. Beam walk latencies were significantly shorter for both the 30 mg/kg and 40 mg/kg groups than the vehicle group at all tested time points following ICH. Values are presented as mean ± SEM; #$P < 0.05$, ##$P < 0.01$, and ###$P < 0.001$ versus vehicle group ($n = 12$ mice/group, repeated measures two-way ANOVA) (TIFF 1107 kb)

Abbreviations
ABCA-1: ATP binding cassette transporter-1; ALT: alanine aminotransferase; ANOVA: analysis of variance; BBB: blood-brain barrier; BUN: blood urea nitrogen; COX-2: cyclooxygenase-2; DMEM: Dulbecco's modified Eagle's media; DMSO: dimethyl sulfoxide; Erk: extracellular signal-regulated kinases; ELISA: enzyme-linked immunosorbent assay; FJB: Fluoro-Jade B; GFAP: glial fibrillary acidic protein; Iba-1: anti-ionized calcium-binding adaptor molecule 1; IL-1β: interleukin-1β; IL-6: interleukin-6; iNOS: inducible nitric oxide synthase; JNK: Jun amino-terminal kinases; LPS: lipopolysaccharide; LXR: liver X receptor; MAP2: microtubule-associated protein 2; MCP-1: monocyte chemoattractant protein-1; MIP-2: macrophage inflammatory protein; MMP-9: matrix metalloproteinase-9; mNSS: modified neurological severity score; MPO: myeloperoxidase; NF-κB: nuclear factor-kappa B; NO: nitric oxide; PBS: phosphate-buffered saline; SEM: standard error of the mean.

Competing interests
The authors declare that they have no competing interests.

Authors' contributions
CHW and SFC participated in the design and coordination of the study, performed the experiments, analyzed the data, and contributed to the writing of the manuscript. CCC, THH, and CCL participated in the design and coordination of the study as well as helped to draft the manuscript. CYL and MC performed experiments and analyzed data. All authors read and approved the final manuscript.

Acknowledgements
This work was supported by grants from the Ministry of Science and Technology of Taiwan, R.O.C. (NSC 101-2314-B-350-001-MY3) and the Cheng Hsin General Hospital (CH-104 29 to S.-F.C. and CH-104 30 to C.-C. C).

Author details
[1]Department of Physiology and Biophysics, National Defense Medical Center, Taipei, Taiwan, Republic of China. [2]Graduate Institute of Life Sciences, National Defense Medical Center, Taipei, Taiwan, Republic of China. [3]Department of Physical Medicine and Rehabilitation, Cheng Hsin General Hospital, Taipei, Taiwan, Republic of China. [4]Department of Obstetrics and Gynecology, Chang Gung Memorial Hospital at Taipei and College of Medicine, Chang Gung University, Taipei, Taiwan, Republic of China. [5]School of Medicine, National Defense Medical Center, Taipei, Taiwan, Republic of China.

References
1. Xi G, Keep RF, Hoff JT. Mechanisms of brain injury after intracerebral haemorrhage. Lancet Neurol. 2006;5:53–63.
2. Keep RF, Hua Y, Xi G. Intracerebral haemorrhage: mechanisms of injury and therapeutic targets. Lancet Neurol. 2012;11:720–31.
3. MacLellan CL, Paquette R, Colbourne F. A critical appraisal of experimental intracerebral hemorrhage research. J Cereb Blood Flow Metab. 2012;32:612–27.
4. Fang HY, Ko WJ, Lin CY. Inducible heat shock protein 70, interleukin-18, and tumor necrosis factor alpha correlate with outcomes in spontaneous intracerebral hemorrhage. J Clin Neurosci. 2007;14:435–41.
5. Hou J, Manaenko A, Hakon J, Hansen-Schwartz J, Tang J, Zhang JH. Liraglutide, a long-acting GLP-1 mimetic, and its metabolite attenuate inflammation after intracerebral hemorrhage. J Cereb Blood Flow Metab. 2012;32:2201–10.
6. Lei B, Dawson HN, Roulhac-Wilson B, Wang H, Laskowitz DT, James ML. Tumor necrosis factor alpha antagonism improves neurological recovery in murine intracerebral hemorrhage. J Neuroinflammation. 2013;10:103.
7. Rolland WB, Lekic T, Krafft PR, Hasegawa Y, Altay O, Hartman R, et al. Fingolimod reduces cerebral lymphocyte infiltration in experimental models of rodent intracerebral hemorrhage. Exp Neurol. 2013;241:45–55.
8. Wang YC, Wang PF, Fang H, Chen J, Xiong XY, Yang QW. Toll-like receptor 4 antagonist attenuates intracerebral hemorrhage-induced brain injury. Stroke. 2013;44:2545–52.
9. Zhou Y, Wang Y, Wang J, Anne Stetler R, Yang QW. Inflammation in intracerebral hemorrhage: from mechanisms to clinical translation. Prog Neurobiol. 2014;115C:25–44.
10. Zelcer N, Tontonoz P. Liver X receptors as integrators of metabolic and inflammatory signaling. J Clin Invest. 2006;116:607–14.
11. Im SS, Osborne TF. Liver x receptors in atherosclerosis and inflammation. Circ Res. 2011;108:996–1001.
12. Beyea MM, Heslop CL, Sawyez CG, Edwards JY, Markle JG, Hegele RA, et al. Selective up-regulation of LXR-regulated genes ABCA1, ABCG1, and APOE in macrophages through increased endogenous synthesis of 24(S),25-epoxycholesterol. J Biol Chem. 2007;282:5207–16.
13. Hong C, Tontonoz P. Liver X receptors in lipid metabolism: opportunities for drug discovery. Nat Rev Drug Discov. 2014;13:433–44.
14. Kim OS, Lee CS, Joe EH, Jou I. Oxidized low density lipoprotein suppresses lipopolysaccharide-induced inflammatory responses in microglia: oxidative stress acts through control of inflammation. Biochem Biophys Res Commun. 2006;342:9–18.
15. Zelcer N, Khanlou N, Clare R, Jiang Q, Reed-Geaghan EG, Landreth GE, et al. Attenuation of neuroinflammation and Alzheimer's disease pathology by liver x receptors. Proc Natl Acad Sci U S A. 2007;104:10601–6.
16. Zhang-Gandhi CX, Drew PD. Liver X receptor and retinoid X receptor agonists inhibit inflammatory responses of microglia and astrocytes. J Neuroimmunol. 2007;183:50–9.
17. Cui W, Sun Y, Wang Z, Xu C, Peng Y, Li R. Liver X receptor activation attenuates inflammatory response and protects cholinergic neurons in APP/PS1 transgenic mice. Neuroscience. 2012;210:200–10.
18. Dai YB, Tan XJ, Wu WF, Warner M, Gustafsson JA. Liver X receptor beta protects dopaminergic neurons in a mouse model of Parkinson disease. Proc Natl Acad Sci U S A. 2012;109:13112–7.
19. Paterniti I, Genovese T, Mazzon E, Crisafulli C, Di Paola R, Galuppo M, et al. Liver X receptor agonist treatment regulates inflammatory response after spinal cord trauma. J Neurochem. 2010;112:611–24.
20. Morales JR, Ballesteros I, Deniz JM, Hurtado O, Vivancos J, Nombela F, et al. Activation of liver X receptors promotes neuroprotection and reduces brain inflammation in experimental stroke. Circulation. 2008;118:1450–9.
21. Chen J, Zacharek A, Cui X, Shehadah A, Jiang H, Roberts C, et al. Treatment of stroke with a synthetic liver X receptor agonist, TO901317, promotes synaptic plasticity and axonal regeneration in mice. J Cereb Blood Flow Metab. 2010;30:102–9.
22. Cheng O, Ostrowski RP, Liu W, Zhang JH. Activation of liver X receptor reduces global ischemic brain injury by reduction of nuclear factor-kappaB. Neuroscience. 2010;166:1101–9.
23. Sironi L, Mitro N, Cimino M, Gelosa P, Guerrini U, Tremoli E, et al. Treatment with LXR agonists after focal cerebral ischemia prevents brain damage. FEBS Lett. 2008;582:3396–400.
24. Chen J, Cui X, Zacharek A, Roberts C, Chopp M. eNOS mediates TO90317 treatment-induced angiogenesis and functional outcome after stroke in mice. Stroke. 2009;40:2532–8.
25. Beltowski J. Liver X receptors (LXR) as therapeutic targets in dyslipidemia. Cardiovasc Ther. 2008;26:297–316.
26. Chen M, Li X, Zhang X, He X, Lai L, Liu Y, et al. The inhibitory effect of mesenchymal stem cell on blood-brain barrier disruption following intracerebral hemorrhage in rats: contribution of TSG-6. J Neuroinflammation. 2015;12:61.
27. Wasserman JK, Zhu X, Schlichter LC. Evolution of the inflammatory response in the brain following intracerebral hemorrhage and effects of delayed minocycline treatment. Brain Res. 2007;1180:140–54.
28. Chang CF, Chen SF, Lee TS, Lee HF, Shyue SK. Caveolin-1 deletion reduces early brain injury after experimental intracerebral hemorrhage. Am J Pathol. 2011;178:1749–61.
29. Chen SF, Hsu CW, Huang WH, Wang JY. Post-injury baicalein improves histological and functional outcomes and reduces inflammatory cytokines after experimental traumatic brain injury. Br J Pharmacol. 2008;155:1279–96.
30. Chen SF, Tsai HJ, Hung TH, Chen CC, Lee CY, Wu CH, et al. Salidroside improves behavioral and histological outcomes and reduces apoptosis via PI3K/Akt signaling after experimental traumatic brain injury. PLoS ONE. 2012;7, e45763.
31. Wu CH, Hung TH, Chen CC, Ke CH, Lee CY, Wang PY, et al. Post-injury treatment with 7,8-dihydroxyflavone, a TrkB receptor agonist, protects against experimental traumatic brain injury via PI3K/Akt signaling. PLoS ONE. 2014;9, e113397.

32. Chen CC, Hung TH, Lee CY, Wang LF, Wu CH, Ke CH, et al. Berberine protects against neuronal damage via suppression of glia-mediated inflammation in traumatic brain injury. PLoS ONE. 2014;9, e115694.

33. Batchelor PE, Liberatore GT, Wong JY, Porritt MJ, Frerichs F, Donnan GA, et al. Activated macrophages and microglia induce dopaminergic sprouting in the injured striatum and express brain-derived neurotrophic factor and glial cell line-derived neurotrophic factor. J Neurosci. 1999;19:1708–16.

34. Wasserman JK, Schlichter LC. Minocycline protects the blood-brain barrier and reduces edema following intracerebral hemorrhage in the rat. Exp Neuro. 2007;207(2):227-37.

35. Sedgwick JD, Schwender S, Imrich H, Dorries R, Butcher GW, ter Meulen V. Isolation and direct characterization of resident microglial cells from the normal and inflamed central nervous system. Proc Natl Acad Sci U S A. 1991;88:7438–42.

36. Ford AL, Goodsall AL, Hickey WF, Sedgwick JD. Normal adult ramified microglia separated from other central nervous system macrophages by flow cytometric sorting. Phenotypic differences defined and direct ex vivo antigen presentation to myelin basic protein-reactive CD4+ T cells compared. J Immunol. 1995;154:4309–21.

37. Koistinaho M, Koistinaho J. Role of p38 and p44/42 mitogen-activated protein kinases in microglia. Glia. 2002;40:175–83.

38. He Q, Pu J, Yuan A, Lau WB, Gao E, Koch WJ, et al. Activation of liver-X-receptor alpha but not liver-X-receptor beta protects against myocardial ischemia/reperfusion injury. Circ Heart Fail. 2014;7:1032–41.

39. Castrillo A, Joseph SB, Marathe C, Mangelsdorf DJ, Tontonoz P. Liver X receptor-dependent repression of matrix metalloproteinase-9 expression in macrophages. J Biol Chem. 2003;278:10443–9.

40. Wang YY, Dahle MK, Steffensen KR, Reinholt FP, Collins JL, Thiemermann C, et al. Liver X receptor agonist GW3965 dose-dependently regulates lps-mediated liver injury and modulates posttranscriptional TNF-alpha production and p38 mitogen-activated protein kinase activation in liver macrophages. Shock. 2009;32:548–53.

41. Fan X, Kim HJ, Bouton D, Warner M, Gustafsson JA. Expression of liver X receptor beta is essential for formation of superficial cortical layers and migration of later-born neurons. Proc Natl Acad Sci U S A. 2008;105:13445–50.

42. Kim HJ, Fan X, Gabbi C, Yakimchuk K, Parini P, Warner M, et al. Liver X receptor beta (LXRbeta): a link between beta-sitosterol and amyotrophic lateral sclerosis-Parkinson's dementia. Proc Natl Acad Sci U S A. 2008;105:2094–9.

43. Xu P, Xu H, Tang X, Xu L, Wang Y, Guo L, et al. Liver X receptor beta is essential for the differentiation of radial glial cells to oligodendrocytes in the dorsal cortex. Mol Psychiatry. 2014;19:947–57.

44. Repa JJ, Li H, Frank-Cannon TC, Valasek MA, Turley SD, Tansey MG, et al. Liver X receptor activation enhances cholesterol loss from the brain, decreases neuroinflammation, and increases survival of the NPC1 mouse. J Neurosci. 2007;27:14470–80.

45. Haase G, Pettmann B, Raoul C, Henderson CE. Signaling by death receptors in the nervous system. Curr Opin Neurobiol. 2008;18:284–91.

46. Wang J, Tsirka SE. Tuftsin fragment 1-3 is beneficial when delivered after the induction of intracerebral hemorrhage. Stroke. 2005;36:613–8.

47. Wu J, Yang S, Xi G, Song S, Fu G, Keep RF, et al. Microglial activation and brain injury after intracerebral hemorrhage. Acta Neurochir Suppl. 2008;105:59–65.

48. Solan PD, Piraino G, Hake PW, Denenberg A, O'Connor M, Lentsch A, et al. Liver X receptor alpha activation with the synthetic ligand T0901317 reduces lung injury and inflammation after hemorrhage and resuscitation via inhibition of the nuclear factor kappaB pathway. Shock. 2011;35:367–74.

49. Hong C, Kidani Y, A-Gonzalez N, Phung T, Ito A, Rong X, et al. Coordinate regulation of neutrophil homeostasis by liver X receptors in mice. J Clin Invest. 2012;122:337–47.

50. Woo MS, Park JS, Choi IY, Kim WK, Kim HS. Inhibition of MMP-3 or -9 suppresses lipopolysaccharide-induced expression of proinflammatory cytokines and iNOS in microglia. J Neurochem. 2008;106:770–80.

51. Chang JJ, Emanuel BA, Mack WJ, Tsivgoulis G, Alexandrov AV. Matrix metalloproteinase-9: dual role and temporal profile in intracerebral hemorrhage. J Stroke Cerebrovasc Dis. 2014;23:2498–505.

52. Power C, Henry S, Del Bigio MR, Larsen PH, Corbett D, Imai Y, et al. Intracerebral hemorrhage induces macrophage activation and matrix metalloproteinases. Ann Neurol. 2003;53:731–42.

53. Namjoshi DR, Martin G, Donkin J, Wilkinson A, Stukas S, Fan J, et al. The liver X receptor agonist GW3965 improves recovery from mild repetitive traumatic brain injury in mice partly through apolipoprotein E. PLoS ONE. 2013;8, e53529.

54. Koldamova RP, Lefterov IM, Staufenbiel M, Wolfe D, Huang S, Glorioso JC, et al. The liver X receptor ligand T0901317 decreases amyloid beta production in vitro and in a mouse model of Alzheimer's disease. J Biol Chem. 2005;280:4079–88.

55. Riddell DR, Zhou H, Comery TA, Kouranova E, Lo CF, Warwick HK, et al. The LXR agonist TO901317 selectively lowers hippocampal Abeta42 and improves memory in the Tg2576 mouse model of Alzheimer's disease. Mol Cell Neurosci. 2007;34:621–8.

56. Okabe A, Urano Y, Itoh S, Suda N, Kotani R, Nishimura Y, et al. Adaptive responses induced by 24S-hydroxycholesterol through liver X receptor pathway reduce 7-ketocholesterol-caused neuronal cell death. Redox Biol. 2013;2:28–35.

57. Gad SC. Animal models in toxicology. 2nd ed. Boca Raton: CRC/Taylor & Francis; 2007.

Heme oxygenase-1-mediated neuroprotection in subarachnoid hemorrhage via intracerebroventricular deferoxamine

Robert H. LeBlanc III[1], Ruiya Chen[1], Magdy H. Selim[1] and Khalid A. Hanafy[1,2*]

Abstract

Background: Subarachnoid hemorrhage (SAH) is a devastating disease that affects over 30,000 Americans per year. Previous animal studies have explored the therapeutic effects of deferoxamine (DFX) via its iron-chelating properties after SAH, but none have assessed the necessity of microglial/macrophage heme oxygenase-1 (HO-1 or Hmox1) in DFX neuroprotection, nor has the efficacy of an intracerebroventricular (ICV) administration route been fully examined. We explored the therapeutic efficacy of systemic and ICV DFX in a SAH mouse model and its effect on microglial/macrophage HO-1.

Methods: Wild-type (WT) mice were split into the following treatment groups: SAH sham + vehicle, SAH + vehicle, SAH + intraperitoneal (IP) DFX, and SAH + ICV DFX. For each experimental group, neuronal damage, cognitive outcome, vasospasm, cerebral and hematogenous myeloid cell populations, cerebral IL-6 concentration, and mitochondrial superoxide anion production were measured. HO-1 co-localization to microglia was measured using confocal images. Trans-wells with WT or HO-1$^{-/-}$ microglia and hippocampal neurons were treated with vehicle, red blood cells (RBCs), or RBCs with DFX; neuronal damage, TNF-α concentration, and microglial HO-1 expression were measured. HO-1 conditional knockouts were used to study myeloid, neuronal, and astrocyte HO-1 involvement in DFX-induced neuroprotection and cognitive recovery.

Results: DFX treatment after SAH decreased cortical damage and improved cognitive outcome after SAH yet had no effect on vasospasm; ICV DFX was most neuroprotective. ICV DFX treatment after SAH decreased cerebral IL-6 concentration and trended towards decreased mitochondrial superoxide anion production. ICV DFX treatment after SAH effected an increase in HO-1 co-localization to microglia. DFX treatment of WT microglia with RBCs in the trans-wells showed decreased neuronal damage; this effect was abolished in HO-1$^{-/-}$ microglia. ICV DFX after SAH decreased neuronal damage and improved cognition in $Hmox1^{fl/fl}$ control and $Nes^{Cre}{:}Hmox1^{fl/fl}$ mice, but not $LyzM^{Cre}{:}Hmox1^{fl/fl}$ mice.

Conclusions: DFX neuroprotection is independent of vasospasm. ICV DFX treatment provides superior neuroprotection in a mouse model of SAH. Mechanisms of DFX neuroprotection after SAH may involve microglial/macrophage HO-1 expression. Monitoring patient HO-1 expression during DFX treatment for hemorrhagic stroke may help clinicians identify patients that are more likely to respond to treatment.

Keywords: Deferoxamine, Heme oxygenase, Immunology, Intracerebroventricular, Microglia, Subarachnoid hemorrhage, Vasospasm-independent

* Correspondence: khanafy@bidmc.harvard.edu
[1]Department of Neurology, Beth Israel Deaconess Medical Center, Harvard Medical School, 3 Blackfan Circle, Boston, MA 02140, USA
[2]Division of Neurointensive Care Medicine, Beth Israel Deaconess Medical Center, Harvard Medical School, 3 Blackfan Circle, Boston, MA 02140, USA

Background

Over 30,000 Americans will fall victim to an aneurysmal subarachnoid hemorrhage (SAH) this year; nearly half of these patients will die within 6 months [1, 2]. Of those SAH survivors, approximately 50 % will develop severe cognitive and functional deficits [3, 4]. Although the majority of research in SAH has focused on the treatment of vasospasm, only nimodipine has been shown to improve outcome [5, 6]. Multiple clinical trials have demonstrated that even when vasospasm was effectively treated, morbidity and mortality were not ameliorated [7–9]. These studies suggest that neurological injury can be vasospasm-independent. Further research aimed at mitigating this heme-induced cerebral inflammatory response is required [10].

In SAH, the heme from blood spilled into the subarachnoid space is metabolized by heme oxygenase (HO), generating excess free iron [11]. This iron is hypothesized to enable cell membrane damage via free radicals [12] with studies showing a causal relationship between unbound iron and brain injury following SAH [13]. Deferoxamine (DFX), an iron-chelating agent, has been shown to be neuroprotective in various hemorrhagic models via several mechanisms [12, 14]. Previous studies using a rat model of SAH showed decreased brain edema, oxidative stress, and neuronal apoptosis after DFX treatment [15, 16]. However, none of these studies assess the necessity of heme oxygenase-1 (HO-1 or Hmox1) in DFX neuroprotection nor has the efficacy of intracerebroventricular administration been fully examined. Our lab previously showed microglia to be critical in red blood cell-induced neuroinflammation [10], and most recently, we found microglial HO-1 to be neuroprotective after SAH in a mouse model [17]. We hypothesized that microglial/macrophage HO-1 is critical for DFX neuroprotection and that intracerebroventricular administration would provide superior neuroprotection in a mouse model of SAH.

We undertook the current set of experiments to first compare the effects of systemic versus intracerebroventricular injection of DFX on neuronal damage, vasospasm, proinflammatory and oxidative biomarkers, and immune cell populations in a mouse model of SAH; second, to see if microglial/macrophage HO-1 is sufficient for DFX neuroprotection; and third, to compare the effects of cell-specific HO-1 knockouts on DFX neuroprotection and cognitive outcome. Our study provides a platform for the potential translation of DFX treatment into the SAH patient population.

Methods

Animal information and anesthesia

All experimental procedures were approved by the Institutional Animal Care and Use Committee

(IACUC) of Beth Israel Deaconess Medical Center (BIDMC). The facility is accredited by the Association for Assessment and Accreditation of Lab Animal Care and fully complied with all Federal, State and Local Law. Animals were housed at BIDMC and fed a standard rodent diet ad libitum with 24-h access to either water and/or hydrogel while kept on a 12-h light/12-h dark cycle. All surgical manipulations were performed under general anesthesia with ketamine (10 mg/kg) and xylazine (4 mg/kg), and buprenorphine (50 µg/kg) was systemically administered. All mice used were male on a C57BL/6 background (The Jackson Laboratory). Cell-specific HO-1 knockout in myeloid cells ($LyzM^{Cre}$:$Hmox1^{fl/fl}$) and astrocytes and neurons (Nes^{Cre}:$Hmox1^{fl/fl}$) was achieved as previously described by our lab [17]. All mice had similar fur color and were approximately the same size and weight. The average mouse weight was 25 g (0.025 kg) with a weight range of 24 g (0.024 kg) to 27 g (0.027 kg). Wild-type (WT) mice were randomly assigned between the following four treatment groups equally: WT subarachnoid hemorrhage (SAH) sham + intraperitoneal (IP) normal saline (NS) + intracerebroventricular (ICV) NS (SAH sham + vehicle), WT SAH + IP NS + ICV NS (SAH + vehicle), WT SAH + IP deferoxamine (DFX) + ICV NS (SAH + IP DFX), and WT SAH + IP NS + ICV DFX (SAH + ICV DFX). Lab personnel performing surgical procedures were not the same as those performing cognitive assays to allow for appropriate blinding.

SAH

The method used to induce SAH has been previously tested and validated in a mouse model [18]. After the mice were anesthetized with xylazine (10 mg/kg) and ketamine (12 mg/kg), SAH was performed as previously described by our lab using a standard stereotaxic instrument set-up (KOPF Instruments, Tujunga, CA, USA) [17]. To open the skin overlying the anterior skull, a midline incision was performed. Then, a burr hole was drilled into the anterior skull, 4.5 mm anterior to the bregma. Sixty microliters of autologous blood from a C57BL/6 wild-type blood donor mouse was injected over a 10-s period with a 27-gauge needle at a 40° caudal angle into the drilled burr hole. The needle was left in place for 5 min to prevent backflow of blood.

Intracerebroventricular injection of deferoxamine

After the mice were anesthetized, intracerebroventricular injection was performed using a standard stereotaxic instrument set-up (KOPF Instruments, Tujunga, CA, USA). One burr hole was drilled 0.22 mm posterior to the bregma, 1 mm lateral, and 2.25 mm in depth to enter the ventricle. On SAH POD1, 24 h after the induced SAH, a single, non-repeated injection of 8 mg/kg of DFX was administered using pre-measured capillaries. Dosing was chosen based on dose-tolerance data generated by our lab (Table 1).

Intraperitoneal injection of deferoxamine

Starting on SAH POD1, 24-h after the induced SAH, the mice were given systemic injections of 200 mg/kg of DFX every morning, 30 min prior to cognitive test, until euthanization on SAH POD7. Dosage was chosen based on a previous publication testing systemic deferoxamine treatment in another mouse model of hemorrhagic stroke [19].

TUNEL

All in vivo imaging was taken on SAH sham or SAH post-operative day (POD) 7 due to our lab's previous publication showing SAH POD7 to have the most significant hippocampal cell damage [10]. Brain sections and HT-22 cells were stained with terminal deoxynucleotidyl transferase dUTP nick end labeling (TUNEL; Roche Life Science, Indianapolis, IN, USA). Slides were covered using Vectashield mounting medium with DAPI (Vector Laboratories, Burlingame, CA, USA) for nuclear counterstaining. HT-22 cells were counterstained with Hoechst 33258 (Sigma-Aldrich, Natick, MA, USA). Lab personnel interpreting TUNEL stains were not aware of the groups to which they were assigned.

H&E

Coronal brain sections were stained with hematoxylin and eosin (H&E) (Poly Scientific R&D Corp., Bay Shore, NY, USA). The middle cerebral artery (MCA) lumen radius/wall thickness ratio was quantified using ImageJ software (NIH). Lab personnel interpreting H&E stains were not aware of the groups to which they were assigned.

Confocal imaging

Eight-micrometer coronal brain sections from each experimental group were post-fixed and permeabilized,

Table 1 Intracerebroventricular deferoxamine dose-tolerance chart

ICV dose	Total mice tested	Tolerance
0.8 mg/kg (~0.02 mg per mouse)	3	Well tolerated
8 mg/kg[a] (~0.2 mg per mouse)	3	Well tolerated
80 mg/kg (~2 mg per mouse)	2	Immediately died

Wild-type mice were injected with a one-time intracerebroventricular (ICV) dose of deferoxamine diluted in normal saline, to test how well each dose would be tolerated
[a]The highest dose tolerated was chosen for all experimental procedures

followed by being blocked with 10 % donkey serum. The sections were then stained with the following primary antibodies: goat anti-Iba1 (1:500) and rabbit anti-HO-1 (1:500) to identify HO-1 expression and HO-1 co-localization to microglia. The sections were then stained with the following secondary antibodies: donkey anti-goat 488 (1:250) and donkey anti-rabbit 594 (1:250). The sections were then counterstained with nuclei marker DAPI and sealed. The sections were viewed and images were taken on a Zeiss confocal microscope. Layers of images from the most anterior to the most posterior portion were taken, and a Z-stack image was created. ImageJ software was used for co-localization cell counting as well as co-localization heat maps. Co-localization percentage per high-powered field for each experimental group's confocal Z-stacked images was obtained by dividing the total number of yellow-positive by the total number of DAPI-positive cells. Co-localization histograms were generated using the coloc-2 feature of ImageJ software. In brief, the program combines the green HO-1 single channel-1 saturation pixels with the red Iba-1/microglia single channel-2 saturation pixels to calculate the level at which they overlap. The x-axis represents channel-1 pixel intensity, while the y-axis represents channel-2 pixel intensity. Blue represents the lowest population frequency possible while yellow represents the highest. The lower the slope for each heat map, the more HO-1 staining there is per Iba-1/microglia staining.

ELISA

Whole brain lysates were equally loaded onto a 96-well plate and cerebral IL-6 concentration was determined using ELISA Max Biolegend kit per manufacturer's instructions. Media from microglia-neuron trans-well experiments were equally loaded onto a 96-well plate and culture TNF-α concentration was determined using ELISA Max Biolegend kit per manufacturer's instructions (Biolegend, San Diego, CA, USA).

Flow cytometry

All flow cytometry acquisition was performed on a FACSCalibur (BD Biosciences, San Jose, CA, USA), and analysis was completed using FlowJo software (FlowJo, LLC, Ashland, OR, USA). Cells were isolated from whole brain or blood and re-suspended in FACS buffer (1 % bovine albumin, 2 mM ethylenediaminetetraacetic acid (EDTA), and 0.05 % NaN$_3$ in phosphate-buffered saline (PBS)). To block unspecific sites, the cells were first stained with CD16/32 Trustain (1:100; Biolegend, San Diego, CA, USA). The cells were then washed with FACS buffer and stained with the following fluorescent-tagged antibodies: PE-Gr-1 and PeCy7-CD11b (1:100; Biolegend, San Diego, CA, USA). To identify the myeloid cell populations in the blood and brain, CD45$^+$ cells were gated off of a CD45/SSC-H dot plot. Then, using a Gr-1/CD11b dot plot, macrophages were identified as CD11b^{hi}/Gr-1^{lo} while neutrophils were CD11b^{hi}Gr-1^{hi} (Additional file 1: Figure S1). To measure the total mitochondrial superoxide anion production, whole brain cell lysates were incubated with MitoSOX red mitochondrial superoxide indicator per manufacturer's instructions (5 µM; Life Technologies/Thermo-Fisher, Cambridge, MA, USA) and cells positive in the FL-2 channel were reported. Appropriate unstained controls for each channel were used to determine stained cell populations.

Primary microglia and neuronal HT-22 cells—trans-wells
Microglia cells were isolated from the brains of neonatal mice using the Neural Tissue Dissociation Kit (P) (Miltenyi Biotec, Cambridge, MA, USA). The resulting mixed glia culture, containing astrocytes and microglia, was cultivated in media containing macrophage-colony stimulating factor (M-CSF). After 1 week of cultivation, the microglia were collected and grown on 3-µm cell culture inserts (EMD Millipore, Billerica, MA, USA). Murine hippocampal neuronal HT-22 cells were grown on six-well plates in normal media without M-CSF. For trans-well assays, the inserts with microglia were placed on top of the HT-22 neuron wells; microglia and HT-22 neuronal cells shared media during experiments. A total of 200 µl of whole blood was collected from the submandibular vein of a wild-type donor mouse and placed into 10 ml of PBS to keep the blood from clotting. The whole blood in PBS was then centrifuged at 2000 rpm for 5 min. The plasma, leukocyte, and platelet layers were aspirated, leaving an erythrocyte pellet. The erythrocytes were washed in an additional 10 ml of PBS and centrifuged at 2000 rpm for 5 min. The supernatant was aspirated and the erythrocyte pellet was resuspended in 2 ml of PBS; 100 µl of this RBC suspension in PBS was added to the top microglia-containing chamber of the microglia-neuron trans-well; after 1-h of blood exposure, DFX (100 µM) or vehicle was added to the microglia chamber, and an additional hour of incubation was completed.

Western blot
Primary microglial cell lysates were equally loaded onto a polyacrylamide gel and transferred to an immune-blot PVDF membrane (Bio-Rad, Hercules, CA, USA). Membranes were blocked with 5 % milk and stained with rabbit HO-1 antibody (1:1000, Abcam, Cambridge, MA, USA) and mouse vinculin antibody (1:1000, Sigma-Aldrich, Natick, MA, USA).

Morris water maze
Cognitive performance was assessed using the Morris water maze as previously described, with minor modifications made by our lab [17]. In brief, after 7 days of acquisition, SAH sham or SAH was performed. On the day of SAH sham or SAH surgical procedure, the mice were not tested on the Morris water maze. The mice resumed testing on the Morris water maze on POD1. The mice to be treated with DFX were then either given daily IP DFX injections starting on POD1 and ending on POD7 or a one-time ICV injection of DFX on POD1. Additionally, mice that received daily IP DFX injections also got a one-time ICV injection of NS on POD1, and the mice that received a one-time ICV DFX injection also got daily IP NS injections from POD1 to POD7. SAH sham or SAH mice that were not treated with DFX, each received daily IP NS from POD1 to POD7 and a one-time injection of ICV NS on POD1 (Table 2). Spatial memory testing, measured by time to reach goal platform and consisting of 1-trial in the morning per animal per day, was started on SAH POD1 and continued for 7-days. On SAH POD4, the goal platform was moved to the opposite side of the maze (spatial reversal), while visual cue locations were unchanged. An investigator blinded to treatment groups performed the maze procedures.

Statistical analysis
Multiple experimental groups were compared using repeated-measures two-way ANOVA with Bonferroni's post hoc test for in vivo TUNEL staining and HO-1/Iba1 co-localization of multiple brain regions, and the results are presented as the mean ± SD (GraphPad Prism). Morris water maze data was presented as the mean ± SEM (GraphPad Prism) and analyzed using repeated-measures two-way ANOVA with Bonferroni's post hoc test. For all other statistical comparisons, multiple experimental groups were compared using one-way ANOVA with Bonferroni's post hoc test, and the results are presented as the mean ± SD (GraphPad Prism). Differences were considered significant at $P < 0.05$.

Study approval
All procedures involving animals were approved by the IACUC and the Radiation Safety Office (RSO) of Beth Israel Deaconess Medical Center.

Results
Intracerebroventricular deferoxamine injection dose-tolerance in wild-type mice
In order to determine the dose of DFX to be injected into the intracerebroventricular (ICV) space, a dose-tolerance chart was generated using WT mice (Table 1). Since 8 mg/kg was the highest dose tested that was well

Table 2 Wild-type experimental mouse groups

Mouse group	Abbreviation	Explanation
WT SAH sham + IP NS + ICV NS	SAH sham + vehicle	Mice received subarachnoid hemorrhage (SAH), sham surgical procedure, daily intraperoteneal (IP) injections of normal saline (NS) starting on post-operative day (POD) 1 and ending on POD7, and a one-time intracerebroventricular (ICV) injection of NS on POD1.
WT SAH + IP NS + ICV NS	SAH + vehicle	Mice received SAH surgical procedure, daily IP injections of NS starting on POD1 and ending on POD7, and a one-time ICV injection of NS on POD1.
WT SAH + IP DFX + ICV NS	SAH + IP DFX	Mice received SAH surgical procedure, daily IP injections of deferoxamine (DFX) starting on POD1 and ending on POD7, and a one-time ICV injection of NS on POD1.
WT SAH + IP NS + ICV DFX	SAH + ICV DFX	Mice received SAH surgical procedure, daily IP injections of NS starting on POD1 and ending on POD7, and a one-time ICV injection of DFX on POD1.

Wild-type (WT) mice were randomly assigned between the four treatment groups listed in the table. Each mouse was exposed to all surgical procedures and injections as specified in the explanation. The abbreviation listed in the table was used throughout the results including figures and figure legends for simplicity.

tolerated by the mice, this dose was chosen for further experimental procedures.

Degree of deferoxamine neuroprotection and cognitive improvement after SAH depends on drug administration route and is vasospasm-independent

All mice used had similar size and weight and appeared otherwise healthy prior to any surgical procedure. The WT mice were randomly assigned between the following four treatment groups: subarachnoid hemorrhage (SAH) sham + vehicle, SAH + vehicle, SAH + intraperoteneal (IP) DFX, and SAH + ICV DFX (Table 2). Neuronal damage and vasospasm were assessed for all of the treatment groups on POD7, based on our previous work [10]; cognitive outcome was assessed on POD1–7 using the Morris water maze (Fig. 1a–g). The SAH + vehicle mice had significantly increased cortical and hippocampal cellular damage compared to the SAH sham + vehicle mice, while the SAH + IP DFX mice and SAH + ICV DFX mice had markedly decreased cortical and hippocampal damage as compared to the SAH mice (ANOVA $P < 0.05$; $P < 0.05$ between groups; $n = 5$; Fig. 1b, c). The one-time ICV DFX injection decreased cortical and hippocampal damage to a greater extent than daily IP DFX injections ($P < 0.05$ versus SAH + IP DFX; Fig. 1b, c). Differences in cognitive outcome arose between the treatment groups on POD4, 5, and 7. The SAH + ICV DFX treatment group resulted in better cognitive performance than the SAH + vehicle and SAH + IP DFX groups on POD4 and the SAH + vehicle group on POD5. Additionally, both DFX treatment groups after SAH improved cognitive function when compared to the SAH + vehicle group on POD7 (ANOVA $P < 0.05$; $P < 0.05$ between groups; $n = 5$; Fig. 1d). Although the SAH + group had a significantly lower lumen radius to wall thickness (LR/WT) of the middle

cerebral artery (MCA) than the SAH sham + vehicle group, DFX treatment had no effect on this SAH-induced MCA vasospasm (ANOVA $P < 0.05$; $P < 0.05$ SAH sham + vehicle versus SAH + vehicle; $n = 5$; Fig. 1f, g).

Next, we determined whether or not DFX had an effect on cerebral and hematogenous myeloid cell populations; it did not ($n = 4$; Fig. 2a, b). Subsequently, we measured the effects of DFX on cerebral inflammatory milieu after SAH on POD7 by quantifying interleukin (IL)-6 and mitochondrial superoxide anion in whole brain lysates. In the SAH + vehicle group, cerebral IL-6 production was increased as compared to control (ANOVA $P < 0.05$; $P < 0.05$ versus SAH sham + vehicle; $n = 4$; Fig. 2c); ICV DFX treatment markedly decreased the concentration of cerebral IL-6 after SAH while IP DFX did not ($P < 0.05$ versus SAH + vehicle; $n = 4$; Fig. 2c). Additionally, the SAH + vehicle group had increased mitochondrial superoxide anion production as compared to the control (ANOVA $P < 0.05$; $P < 0.05$ versus SAH sham + vehicle; $n = 4$; Fig. 2d, e), and while not statistically significant, there was a trend towards decreased mitochondrial superoxide anion in the SAH + ICV DFX treatment group as compared to the SAH + vehicle group ($n = 4$; Fig. 2d, e).

Microglial HO-1 is sufficient for deferoxamine neuroprotection in an in vitro model

To determine if DFX treatment of microglia was sufficient to reduce neuronal damage, we performed in vitro trans-well assays with WT microglia and hippocampal neuronal HT-22 cells. WT microglia incubated with red blood cells (RBCs) for 2 h demonstrated marked neuronal damage by the trans-well assay (ANOVA $P < 0.05$; $P < 0.05$ versus control; $n = 3$; Fig. 3a, b). Additionally, there was a trend towards increased TNF-α production in the trans-well assays incubated with RBCs (ANOVA

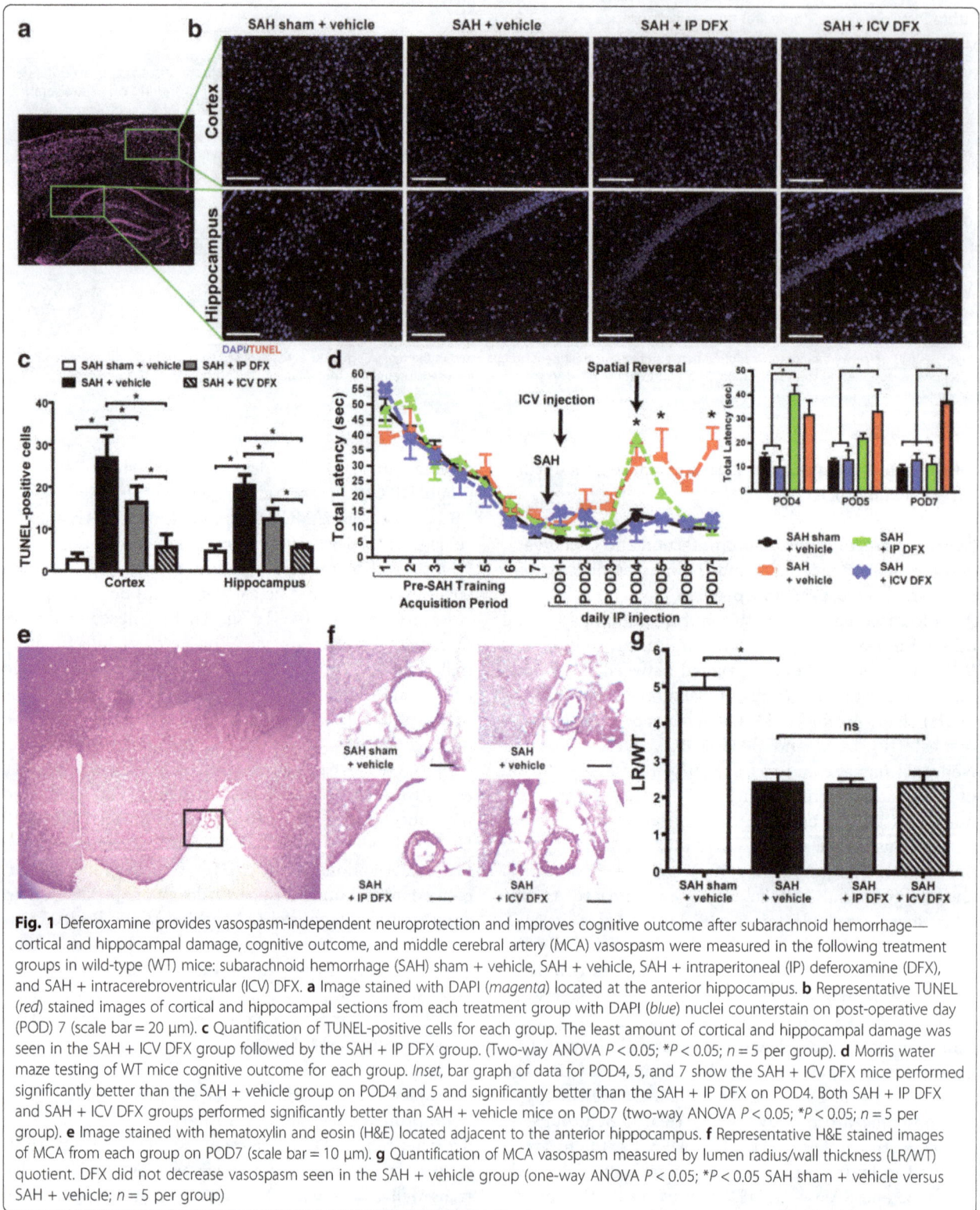

Fig. 1 Deferoxamine provides vasospasm-independent neuroprotection and improves cognitive outcome after subarachnoid hemorrhage—cortical and hippocampal damage, cognitive outcome, and middle cerebral artery (MCA) vasospasm were measured in the following treatment groups in wild-type (WT) mice: subarachnoid hemorrhage (SAH) sham + vehicle, SAH + vehicle, SAH + intraperitoneal (IP) deferoxamine (DFX), and SAH + intracerebroventricular (ICV) DFX. **a** Image stained with DAPI (*magenta*) located at the anterior hippocampus. **b** Representative TUNEL (*red*) stained images of cortical and hippocampal sections from each treatment group with DAPI (*blue*) nuclei counterstain on post-operative day (POD) 7 (scale bar = 20 μm). **c** Quantification of TUNEL-positive cells for each group. The least amount of cortical and hippocampal damage was seen in the SAH + ICV DFX group followed by the SAH + IP DFX group. (Two-way ANOVA $P < 0.05$; *$P < 0.05$; $n = 5$ per group). **d** Morris water maze testing of WT mice cognitive outcome for each group. *Inset*, bar graph of data for POD4, 5, and 7 show the SAH + ICV DFX mice performed significantly better than the SAH + vehicle group on POD4 and 5 and significantly better than the SAH + IP DFX on POD4. Both SAH + IP DFX and SAH + ICV DFX groups performed significantly better than SAH + vehicle mice on POD7 (two-way ANOVA $P < 0.05$; *$P < 0.05$; $n = 5$ per group). **e** Image stained with hematoxylin and eosin (H&E) located adjacent to the anterior hippocampus. **f** Representative H&E stained images of MCA from each group on POD7 (scale bar = 10 μm). **g** Quantification of MCA vasospasm measured by lumen radius/wall thickness (LR/WT) quotient. DFX did not decrease vasospasm seen in the SAH + vehicle group (one-way ANOVA $P < 0.05$; *$P < 0.05$ SAH sham + vehicle versus SAH + vehicle; $n = 5$ per group)

$P < 0.05$; $n = 3$; Fig. 3b). RBC-induced neuronal damage was significantly reduced when DFX was added 1 h after RBC exposure began, for a total RBC exposure of 2 h ($P < 0.05$ versus RBC only exposure; $n = 3$; Fig. 3a, b).

Further, there was a trend towards decreased TNF-α production in the trans-well assays treated with DFX after RBC exposure ($n = 3$; Fig. 3b). To determine if the HO-1 pathway in microglia was involved, we repeated the trans-

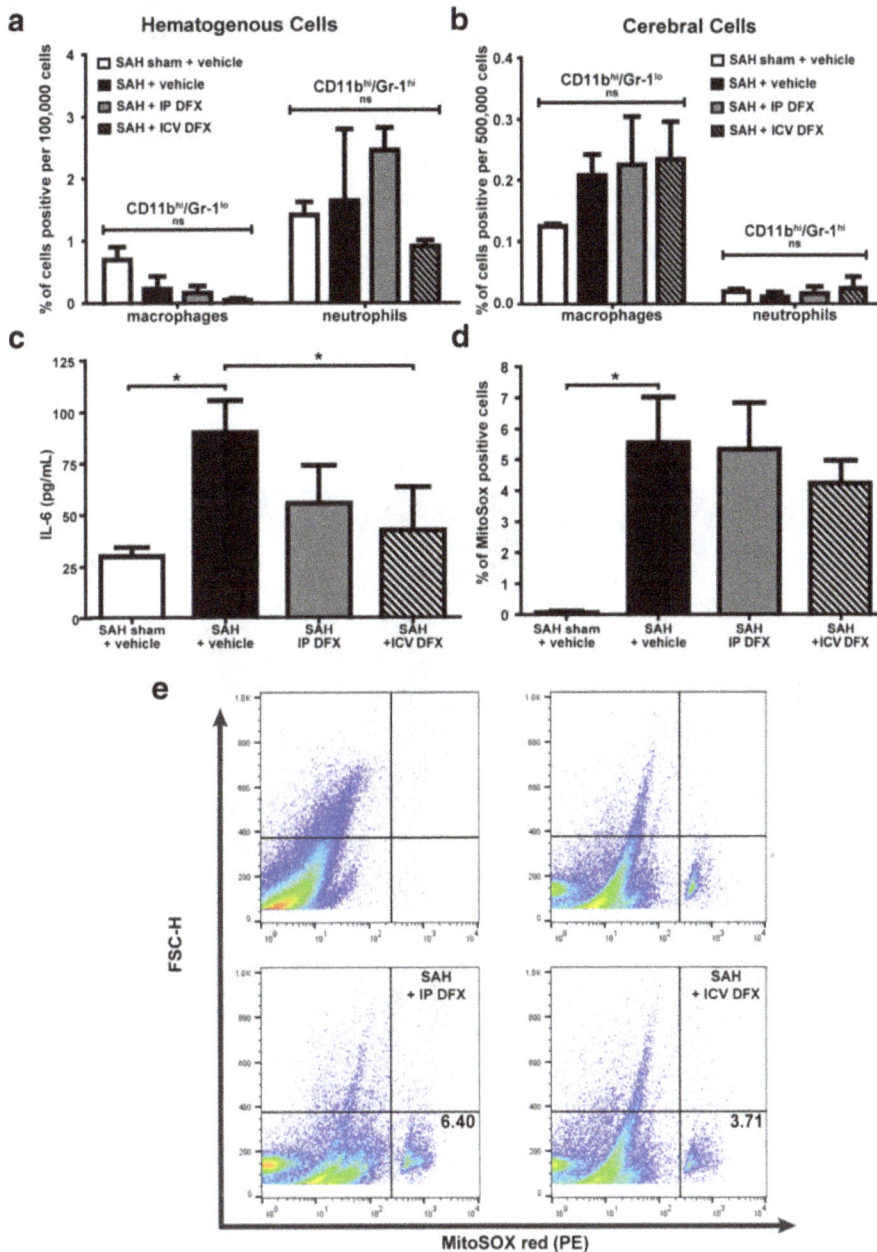

Fig. 2 ICV DFX reduces cerebral inflammatory milieu after SAH—hematogenous and cerebral myeloid cell populations, cerebral IL-6 concentration, and cerebral mitochondrial superoxide anion were measured in the following treatment groups on POD7 in WT mice: SAH sham + vehicle, SAH + vehicle, SAH + IP DFX, and SAH + ICV DFX. **a** Flow cytometry of hematogenous cell populations show no significant change between any of the groups (one-way ANOVA; $n = 4$ per group). **b** Flow cytometry of cerebral myeloid cell populations show a trend towards increase in the microglia/macrophage populations of the SAH + vehicle group versus the SAH sham + vehicle group; but no significant changes between any of the other groups (one-way ANOVA; $n = 4$ per group). **c** Cerebral IL-6 concentration as measured by ELISA was significantly increased in the SAH + vehicle group (*$P < 0.05$ versus the SAH sham + vehicle group) and markedly decreased in the SAH + ICV DFX group (*$P < 0.05$ versus the SAH + vehicle group) (one-way ANOVA $P < 0.05$; $n = 4$ per group). **d** Cerebral mitochondrial superoxide anion (MitoSox) positive cells measured by flow cytometry did not show significant decrease in the SAH + ICV DFX group versus the SAH + vehicle group and the SAH + IP DFX group (one-way ANOVA $P < 0.05$; $n = 4$ per group). **e** Representative flow cytometry dot plots from each group. The Q3 percentage (shown) represents the percentage of cells positive for MitoSOX red

well experiment using HO-1$^{-/-}$ microglia. In the trans-well assays with HO-1$^{-/-}$ microglia, neuronal damage and TNF-α production was notably increased in trans-wells exposed to RBCs for 2 h (ANOVA $P < 0.05$; $P < 0.05$ versus

control; $n = 3$; Fig. 3c, d). But unlike the WT microglia trans-wells, RBC-induced neuronal damage was *not* significantly reduced in neurons underlying HO-1$^{-/-}$ microglia when DFX was added ($n = 3$; Fig. 3c, d). Further,

TNF-α concentrations remained markedly elevated in assays with HO-1$^{-/-}$ microglia after DFX addition to the RBC-treated trans-wells ($n = 3$; Fig. 3d).

Next, we sought to determine why the loss of microglial HO-1 diminished the neuroprotective effects of DFX. First, we measured the HO-1 protein expression in primary microglial lysates exposed to vehicle, RBCs, or RBCs with DFX. There was increased HO-1 protein expression in the microglia treated with RBCs and DFX as compared to vehicle (ANOVA $P < 0.05$; $P < 0.05$ versus control; $n = 3$; Fig. 3e, f).

Intracerebroventricular deferoxamine increases in vivo microglia and HO-1 co-localization

We wanted to validate the results we observed in our in vitro model, in vivo. That is, we wanted to examine whether ICV DFX increased microglial HO-1 expression in our in vivo SAH model. To see if DFX caused an increase in microglia and HO-1 co-localization, we took Z-stacked confocal images of brain sections adjacent to the anterior hippocampus, stained for microglia (Iba-1 positive) and HO-1 of all four of our in vivo experimental groups (Table 2). HO-1 co-localization to microglial

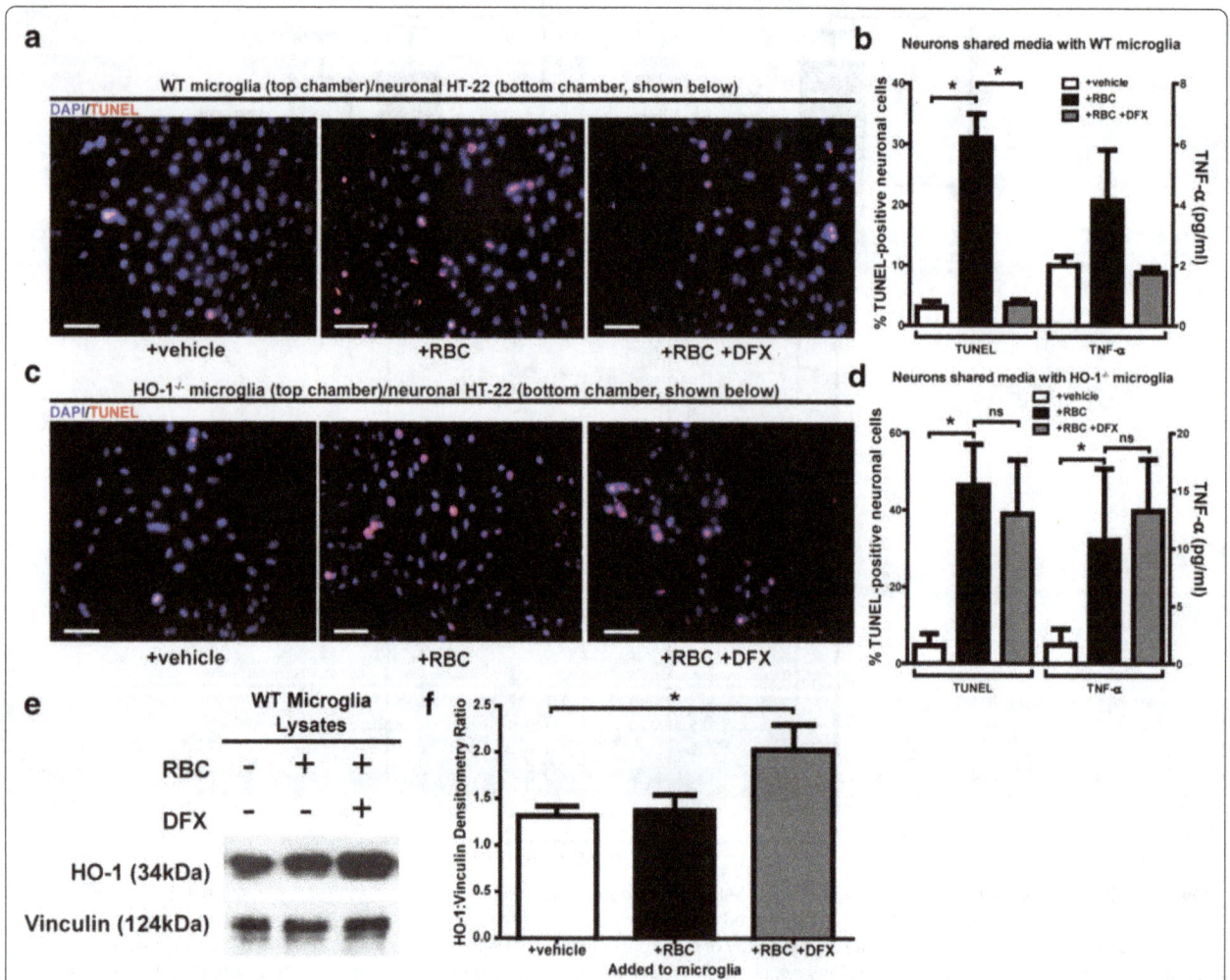

Fig. 3 Microglial HO-1 has a role in deferoxamine protection from red blood cell (RBC)-induced neuronal damage—Trans-wells with WT or HO-1$^{-/-}$ primary microglia were plated with hippocampal neurons (HT-22) and treated with vehicle, red blood cells (RBCs), or RBCs with DFX. **a** Representative TUNEL (*red*) stained images of neurons from each WT primary microglia trans-well with DAPI (*blue*) nuclei counterstain (all scale bars = 20 μm). **b** Quantification of TUNEL-positive neurons and TNF-α concentration from each WT primary microglia trans-well; RBC exposure significantly increased neuronal damage while DFX significantly reduced this RBC-induced damage (one-way ANOVA $P < 0.05$; *$P < 0.05$; $n = 3$ per group). Trend towards increased TNF-α production in the trans-well assays incubated with RBCs (one-way ANOVA $P < 0.05$; $n = 3$; **b**); trend towards decreased TNF-α production in the trans-well assays treated with DFX after RBC exposure ($n = 3$; **b**). **c** TUNEL stained images of neurons from each HO-1$^{-/-}$ primary microglia trans-well with DAPI nuclei counterstain. **d** Quantification of TUNEL-positive neurons and TNF-α concentration from each HO-1$^{-/-}$ primary microglia trans-well; RBC exposure significantly increased neuronal damage as well as TNF-α production, and DFX did not reduce this RBC-induced damage or TNF-α concentration (one-way ANOVA $P < 0.05$; *$P < 0.05$; $n = 3$ per group). **e** Western blot of primary microglial lysates from each group. **f** Quantification of bands from Western blot of primary microglial lysate; showed that HO-1 protein expression significantly increased in WT primary microglia culture exposed to RBCs with DFX (one-way ANOVA $P < 0.05$; *$P < 0.05$; $n = 3$ per group)

cells on these in vivo sections from lowest to highest was as follows: SAH sham + vehicle, SAH + vehicle, SAH + IP DFX, and SAH + ICV DFX (ANOVA $P < 0.05$; $P < 0.05$ between groups; $n = 3$; Fig. 4a–c).

Microglial/macrophage HO-1 is critical to intracerebroventricular deferoxamine neuroprotection and cognitive improvement after SAH

We performed SAH on $LyzM^{Cre}:Hmox1^{fl/fl}$ mice lacking microglial, neutrophil, and all other myeloid HO-1 as well as in $Nes^{Cre}:Hmox1^{fl/fl}$ mice lacking neuronal and astrocyte HO-1 and $Hmox1^{fl/fl}$ control mice and measured the amount of HO-1 co-localization to microglia in each. $LyzM^{Cre}:Hmox1^{fl/fl}$ SAH mice showed the least HO-1/Iba-1 co-localization percentage in both the cortex and hippocampus as compared to $Hmox1^{fl/fl}$ and $Nes^{Cre}:Hmox1^{fl/fl}$ SAH mice on POD7 (two-way ANOVA $P < 0.05$; $P < 0.05$ between groups; $n = 4$; Fig. 5a, b). We then performed SAH and subsequent ICV DFX treatment on $LyzM^{Cre}:Hmox1^{fl/fl}$, $Nes^{Cre}:Hmox1^{fl/fl}$, and $Hmox1^{fl/fl}$ control mice. ICV DFX-treated $LyzM^{Cre}:Hmox1^{fl/fl}$ mice after SAH showed significant cortical and hippocampal damage on POD7 as compared to ICV DFX treated $Hmox1^{fl/fl}$ SAH controls, while ICV DFX treated $Nes^{Cre}:Hmox1^{fl/fl}$ mice after SAH did *not* (ANOVA $P < 0.05$; $P < 0.05$ between groups; $n = 4$; Fig. 5c, d). Cognitive protection of ICV DFX after SAH was tested on $Hmox1^{fl/fl}$, $LyzM^{Cre}:Hmox1^{fl/fl}$, and $Nes^{Cre}:Hmox1^{fl/fl}$ mice. The $LyzM^{Cre}:Hmox1^{fl/fl}$ mice performed markedly worse than the $Hmox1^{fl/fl}$ control mice (ANOVA $P < 0.05$; $P < 0.05$ between groups for POD5 and 7; $n = 4$ Fig. 5e) while $Nes^{Cre}:Hmox1^{fl/fl}$ mice performed just as well as $Hmox1^{fl/fl}$ control mice and significantly better than $LyzM^{Cre}:Hmox1^{fl/fl}$ mice ($P < 0.05$; $P < 0.05$ between groups for POD5 and 7; $n = 4$ Fig. 5e).

Discussion

In a mouse model of SAH, we found that DFX exerted neuroprotective effects by non-canonical mechanisms. (1) DFX improved cognitive outcomes and reduced cerebral damage, independent of vasospasm. (2) ICV DFX was the most neuroprotective. (3) ICV DFX decreased neuroinflammatory markers. (4) Microglial HO-1 is sufficient for DFX neuroprotection in an in vitro model of blood-induced inflammation. (5) ICV DFX neuroprotection and cognitive improvement is dependent on microglial/macrophage HO-1.

The iron-chelating agent, DFX, has been tested for therapeutic use in many animal neurological disease models including Huntington's disease [20], traumatic brain injury [21–23], cerebral ischemia [24–26], and hemorrhagic stroke among others. DFX has been extensively studied in animal models of intraventricular hemorrhage (IVH) and intracerebral hemorrhage (ICH). In IVH animal models,

DFX reduced ventricular enlargement, brain damage, and markers of post-hemorrhagic chronic hydrocephalus [27–31]. In ICH animal models, DFX has been shown to reduce brain damage [32–37], decrease neuroinflammation [34, 38–40], and improve cognitive outcome [38, 41]. Further, DFX was shown to reduce DNA damage [37, 40], oxidative stress [32, 33, 38], neuronal hemoglobin expression [42], and autophagy markers [43], following ICH. Additionally, in a germinal matrix hemorrhage model of neonatal rats, DFX reduced brain damage, ventricular dilation, and improved cognitive outcome [44].

Although DFX treatment has also been studied in SAH animal models, experiments using DFX treatment specifically in a mouse model of SAH are lacking. In rat models of SAH, DFX has been shown to decrease overall mortality, edema, oxidative stress, and neuronal death [15, 16]. Additionally, DFX treatment after SAH has been shown to decrease cortical apoptotic markers [16] and reduce markers of brainstem damage in rats [45], as well as reduce lipid peroxidation markers and improve sodium-potassium ATPase activity in guinea pigs [46]. Our study looked to further elucidate the mechanisms of DFX-induced neuroprotection in a mouse model of SAH.

In our current study, administration of DFX *after* induction of SAH in our mouse model was effective in reducing the cerebral inflammatory response. DFX administered via two different routes, reduced cortical and hippocampal damage after SAH on POD7; the greatest reduction was seen with ICV DFX, followed by IP DFX (Fig. 1b, c). Further, both IP and ICV DFX treatment improved cognitive outcome during a later phase of SAH POD7, but only ICV DFX treated mice showed early improvement on POD4 and 5. Although DFX administration effectively reduced brain damage (Fig. 1b, c) and improved cognitive outcome (Fig. 1d) after SAH, it had no effect on vasospasm (Fig. 1f, g). These results were interesting for two reasons. First, the IP dose of DFX is 25-fold greater than the ICV dose, and yet the ICV dose showed more neuroprotection and earlier cognitive improvement. A potential explanation is that ICV administration allows for proximity to the heme burden, while IP-administered DFX has to effectively cross the blood brain barrier. Second, DFX provided cerebral protection and improved cognition after SAH independent of any effect on vasospasm, similar to previous studies that showed DFX treatment had no effect on vascular response after SAH [47, 48]. Vasospasm-independent cerebral protection provided by DFX is not surprising when one considers recent clinical trials that effectively treated vasospasm but did not improve morbidity or mortality after SAH [7, 8].

DFX has been previously shown to have anti-inflammatory effects in hemorrhagic stroke [14]. We

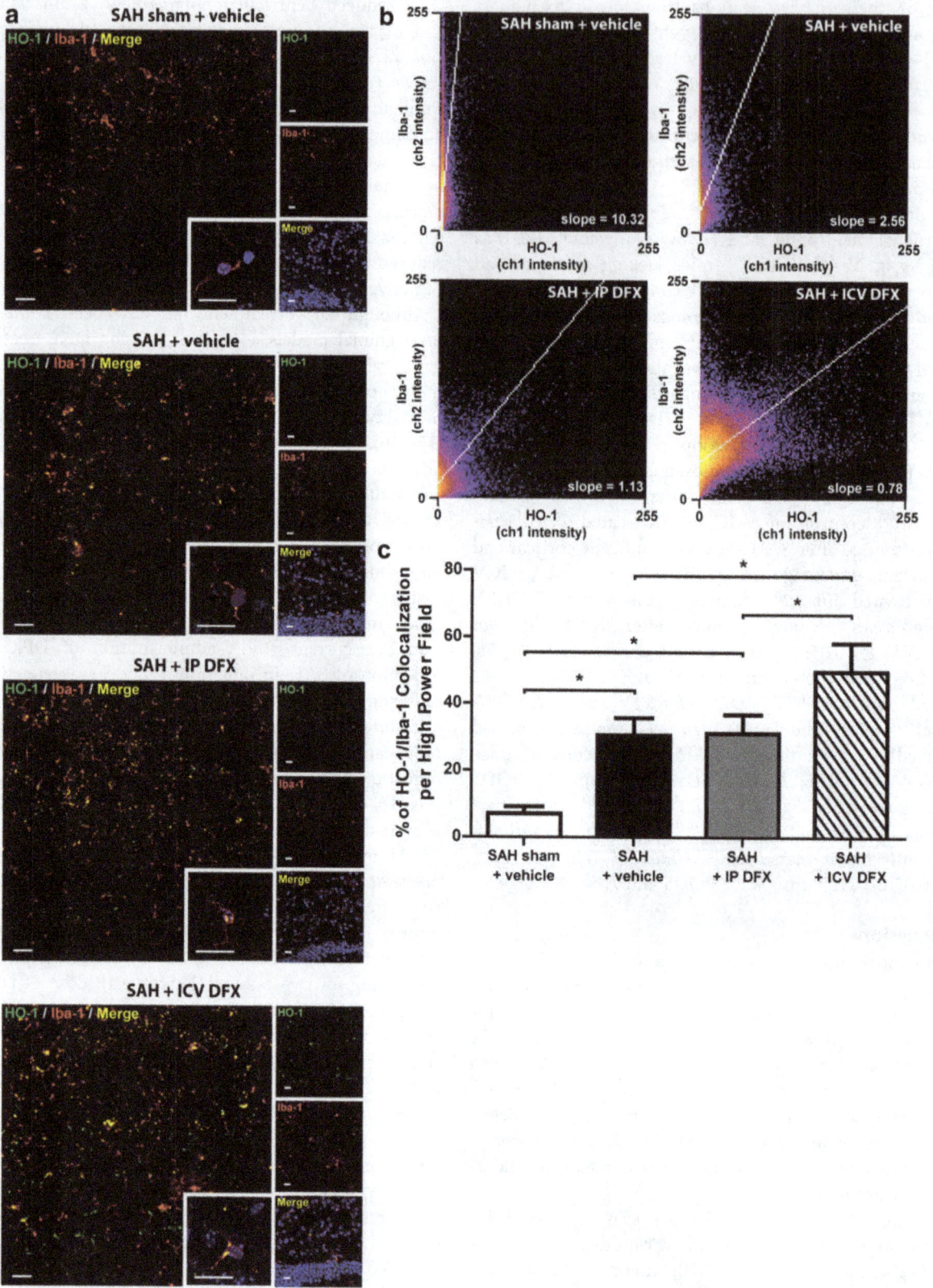

Fig. 4 (See legend on next page.)

Fig. 4 ICV DFX treatment after SAH causes an increase in HO-1/microglia co-localization—Confocal Z-stacked images were taken of the following treatment groups on POD7 in WT mice: SAH sham + vehicle, SAH + vehicle, SAH + IP DFX, and SAH + ICV DFX. **a** Representative confocal images of each experimental group. All images were taken adjacent to the anterior hippocampus, which can be visualized by the DAPI merged image at the bottom right tile. Each color represents the following: *green* = HO-1; *red* = Iba-1/microglia; *yellow* = overlap of green and red/co-localization of HO-1 and microglia; *blue* = DAPI nuclei counterstain. All *scale bars* = 20 μm. **b** Co-localization heat maps for each experimental group. The *x*-axis represents channel-1 (HO-1) pixel intensity, while the *y*-axis represents channel-2 (Iba-1) pixel intensity. *Blue* represents the lowest population frequency possible while *yellow* represents the highest. The lower the slope for each heat map, the more HO-1 staining there is per Iba-1/microglia staining. **c** The percent quantification of co-localization per high-powered field for each experimental group's confocal Z-stacked images. Co-localization percentage was obtained by dividing the total number of yellow-positive cells by the total number of DAPI-positive cells. The highest HO-1/Iba-1 co-localization percentage was seen in the SAH + ICV DFX group, followed by the SAH + IP DFX and SAH + vehicle group (one-way ANOVA $P < 0.05$; *$P < 0.05$; $n = 3$ per group)

investigated whether these anti-inflammatory effects might be partly mediated by changes in immune cell populations, cerebral IL-6 concentration, or mitochondrial superoxide anion production. The SAH + vehicle group showed an upward trend in the cerebral microglial/macrophage cell population as compared to the SAH sham + vehicle group, but DFX did not significantly reduce this increase. Cerebral neutrophils and hematogenous populations of macrophages and neutrophils remained unchanged with DFX administration (Fig. 2a, b). Further, SAH caused a significant increase in both cerebral IL-6 concentrations and mitochondrial superoxide production as compared to sham; in the ICV DFX-treated group, cerebral IL-6 concentrations were reduced and a trend towards decreased reduction in mitochondrial superoxide production was present (Fig. 2c–e). These results indicate that ICV DFX may partially exert protective effects not by changing the total number of microglia/macrophage cells, but instead via modulation of the pro-inflammatory mechanics of these cells, while systemic DFX injection does not.

We investigated whether DFX neuroprotection was dependent on microglia using a microglia-neuron trans-well assay. These assays revealed that DFX offered protection against red blood cell (RBC) induced neuronal damage, even when DFX was added to microglia *after* RBC exposure had already begun (Fig. 3a, b). When we repeated these trans-well assays with HO-1$^{-/-}$ microglia, DFX offered no neuroprotection (Fig. 3c, d). Additionally, we found that DFX treatment increased the protein expression of HO-1 in primary microglial culture (Fig. 3e, f). These results suggest that microglial HO-1 is critical to the mechanism of DFX neuroprotection, possibly, in part, by facilitating the increased expression of microglial HO-1. Our lab has previously shown that administration of carbon monoxide (CO) rescues the neuronal injury seen in co-cultures with HO-1$^{-/-}$ microglia [17]. This indicates that the neuroprotective product of heme breakdown via microglial HO-1 in the context of microglia-neuron co-cultures is CO. Since this current work shows microglial HO-1 to be increased following DFX treatment, it is likely that increased CO production

may be involved. Additionally, DFX would chelate the excess iron from heme breakdown, potentially leading to synergistic benefits produced by DFX administration: increased CO protection and decreased iron toxicity.

When we looked at confocal images of all of our experimental groups, we found that SAH markedly increased the co-localization of microglia and HO-1 compared to sham. Further, we found that ICV DFX treatment affected a significant increase in HO-1 expression within microglia while IP DFX did not (Fig. 4a–c). Because these results demonstrated that ICV DFX most effectively increased microglial HO-1 expression in vivo, we next sought to ascertain the necessity of microglial HO-1 for ICV DFX neuroprotection. Mice lacking myeloid HO-1 (*LyzM^{Cre}:Hmox1$^{fl/fl}$*) and mice lacking neuronal and astrocyte HO-1 (*Nes^{Cre}:Hmox1$^{fl/fl}$*) were exposed to SAH and then treated with ICV DFX. Interestingly, ICV DFX treatment after SAH protected the *Nes^{Cre}:Hmox1$^{fl/fl}$* mice similarly to the *Hmox1$^{fl/fl}$*. Conversely, *LyzM^{Cre}:Hmox1$^{fl/fl}$* mice showed significantly more neuronal damage and cognitive dysfunction compared to *Hmox1$^{fl/fl}$* mice (Fig. 5c–e). This, together with the in vitro data, supported the hypothesis that myeloid HO-1, but not astrocyte or neuronal HO-1, was critical for ICV DFX to reduce brain damage and improve cognition after SAH.

It is still not completely clear why the lack of myeloid HO-1 would suppress DFX neuroprotection in vivo, but we speculate that the DFX mediated increase in myeloid HO-1 cannot occur in the myeloid HO-1 knockout (*LyzM^{Cre}:Hmox1$^{fl/fl}$*) mice. Without the increased myeloid HO-1 expression, the subsequent increase in neuroprotective CO production would be absent. In our previous work, we showed that the neuronal damage and cognitive dysfunction seen in *LyzM^{Cre}:Hmox1$^{fl/fl}$* mice could be saved by administering external CO, showing that CO was the neuroprotective byproduct of myeloid HO-1 heme breakdown [17]. Since our current in vitro data suggests that microglial HO-1 is crucial for DFX neuroprotection, it is possible that increased myeloid HO-1 expression in vivo, due to DFX administration, could

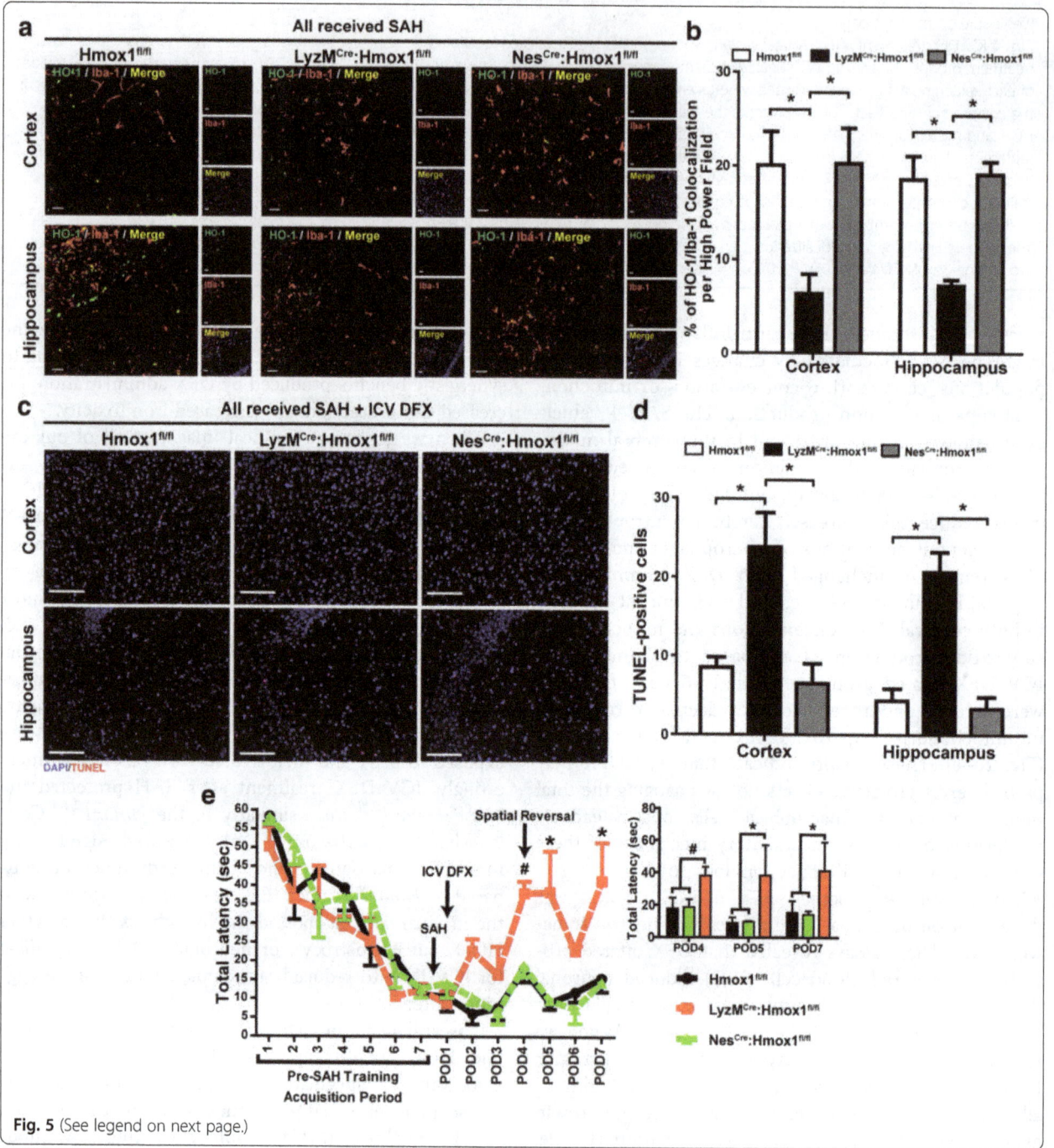

Fig. 5 (See legend on next page.)

(See figure on previous page.)
Fig. 5 Macrophage/microglial HO-1 is critical to ICV DFX neuroprotection and improvement in cognitive outcome after SAH—Cortical and hippocampal damage as well as cognitive outcome were measured after SAH induction and ICV DFX treatment in the following HO-1 conditional knockouts: Hmox1$^{fl/fl}$, LyzM^{Cre}:Hmox1$^{fl/fl}$, and Nes^{Cre}:Hmox1$^{fl/fl}$. **a** Representative confocal images of cortical and hippocampus sections for each genotype after SAH on POD7. Each color represents the following: *green* = HO-1; *red* = Iba-1/microglia; *yellow* = overlap of green and red/co-localization of HO-1 and microglia; *blue* = DAPI nuclei counterstain. All *scale bars* = 20 μm. **b** The percent quantification of co-localization per high-powered field for each genotype's Z-stacked images. Co-localization percentage was obtained by dividing the total number of yellow-positive cells by the total number of DAPI-positive cells. LyzM^{Cre}:Hmox1$^{fl/fl}$ SAH mice showed the least HO-1/Iba-1 co-localization percentage in both the cortex and hippocampus as compared to Hmox1$^{fl/fl}$ and Nes^{Cre}:Hmox1$^{fl/fl}$ SAH mice (two-way ANOVA $P < 0.05$; *$P < 0.05$; $n = 4$ per group). **c** TUNEL (*red*) stained images of cortical and hippocampal sections from each group with DAPI (*blue*) nuclei counterstain on POD7 (*scale bar* = 20 μm). **d** Quantification of TUNEL-positive cells from each treated genotype. Both Hmox1$^{fl/fl}$ and Nes^{Cre}:Hmox1$^{fl/fl}$ SAH mice showed significantly less cortical and hippocampal damage than LyzM^{Cre}:Hmox1$^{fl/fl}$ SAH mice when treated with ICV DFX. (Two-way ANOVA $P < 0.05$; *$P < 0.05$ between groups for cortical damage and **$P < 0.05$ between groups for hippocampal damage; $n = 4$ per group). **e** Morris water maze testing of HO-1 conditional knockout cognition after SAH induction and ICV DFX treatment. *Inset*, bar graph of data for POD4, 5, and 7 shows both Hmox1$^{fl/fl}$ and Nes^{Cre}:Hmox1$^{fl/fl}$ SAH mice performed significantly better than LyzM^{Cre}:Hmox1$^{fl/fl}$ SAH mice on POD5 and 7 when treated with ICV DFX, with a similar trend on POD4. (Two-way ANOVA $P < 0.05$;#$P = 0.07$ between groups on POD4; *$P < 0.05$ between groups on POD5 and 7; $n = 4$ per group)

cause increased CO production and thus result in better protection. Further experimentation would be necessary to test this theory.

We chose the anterior circulation model [18] over the endovascular perforation model and acknowledge that there are limitations; however, we felt that the strengths of the anterior circulation model outweighed the weaknesses. In the anterior circulation model, the increase in intracranial pressure is less severe. Additionally, blood entering the subarachnoid space of a mouse in this method would be that of a donor mouse. On the other hand, the endovascular perforation method better approximates the intracranial pressure crises that can occur in SAH patients.

However, the anterior circulation model has a number of advantages over the endovascular perforation method. First, the amount of blood (60 μl) injected into each mouse, and the resultant increased intracranial pressure is consistent between mice. Because of this, we feel that results obtained using the anterior circulation method are better reproduced. Further, the lower mortality seen with this model is helpful when performing experiments on conditional knockouts, as well as dual injection procedures required for SAH and intracerebroventricular DFX. We have used the anterior circulation method in our past research and believe it to be suitable for our current research interests as well.

In stroke patients, DFX reduced serum markers of oxidative stress and increased antioxidant species [49], while in ICH patients, phase-I testing revealed DFX to be safe and well tolerated [50]. Currently, promising clinical trials investigating the use of DFX for ICH are underway [51]. Our research provides a platform for linear translation of DFX treatment into the human SAH population. Our data show that intracerebroventricular DFX yields the greatest neuroprotection via a mechanism that is dependent on microglial HO-1 and possibly a protective microglial polarization. Given the fact that high-grade SAH patients will have an external

ventriculostomy drain (EVD) placed at admission, a feasibility study for the use of intracerebroventricular DFX in these patients should be explored in the future. Furthermore, monitoring patient HO-1 expression during DFX treatment for hemorrhagic stroke may help clinicians identify patients that are more likely to respond to treatment.

Conclusions

ICV DFX treatment provides superior neuroprotection in a mouse model of SAH. Our results indicate that the mechanisms by which DFX provides neuroprotection after SAH may involve microglial/macrophage HO-1 expression. Monitoring patient HO-1 expression during DFX treatment for hemorrhagic stroke may help clinicians identify patients that are more likely to respond to treatment.

Abbreviations
BIDMC: Beth Israel Deaconess Medical Center; CO: Carbon monoxide; DFX: Deferoxamine; EDTA: Ethylenediaminetetraacetic acid; EVD: External ventriculostomy drain; Fl: Flox; H&E: Hematoxylin and eosin; HO: Heme oxygenase; HO-1/Hmox1: Heme oxygenase-1; IACUC: Institutional Animal Care and Use Committee; ICH: Intracerebral hemorrhage; ICV: Intracerebroventricular; IL-6: Interleukin six; IP: Intraperitoneal; IVH: Intraventricular hemorrhage; LR/WT: Lumen radius/wall thickness; MCA: Middle cerebral artery; M-CSF: Macrophage-colony stimulating factor; NS: Normal saline; PBS: Phosphate-buffered saline; POD: Post-operative day; RBC: Red blood cell; SAH: Subarachnoid hemorrhage; TNF-α: Tumor necrosis factor-alpha; TUNEL: Terminal deoxynucleotidyl transferase dUTP nick end labeling; WT: Wild-type

Acknowledgements
None.

Funding
National Institute of Health Grants K08NS078048 to K.A. Hanafy and U01NS074425 to M.H. Selim. Any unique constructs, techniques, or mice described in this paper will be provided upon request.

Authors' contributions

RHL and RC were all involved in performing the experiments, the data analysis, and the manuscript preparation and editing. MHS was involved in the manuscript editing and the data analysis. KAH was involved in the manuscript preparation, the data analysis, and the project design. All authors read and approved the final manuscript.

Competing interests

The authors declare that they have no competing interests.

Disclosures

M.H. Selim holds an IND for the use of deferoxamine mesylate in hemorrhagic stroke (IND #77306).

References

1. Bederson JB, Connolly ES, Batjer HH, Dacey RG, Dion JE, Diringer MN, et al. Guidelines for the management of aneurysmal subarachnoid hemorrhage: a statement for healthcare professionals from a special writing group of the Stroke Council, American Heart Association. Stroke. 2009;40(3):994–1025.

2. Hop JW, Rinkel GJ, Algra A, van Gijn J. Case-fatality rates and functional outcome after subarachnoid hemorrhage: a systematic review. Stroke. 1997; 28(3):660–4.

3. Suarez JI, Tarr RW, Selman WR. Aneurysmal subarachnoid hemorrhage. N Engl J Med. 2006;354(4):387–96.

4. Suarez JI. Diagnosis and management of subarachnoid hemorrhage. Continuum (Minneap Minn). 2015;21(5 Neurocritical Care):1263–87.

5. Allen GS, Ahn HS, Preziosi TJ, Battye R, Boone SC, Boone SC, et al. Cerebral arterial spasm—a controlled trial of nimodipine in patients with subarachnoid hemorrhage. N Engl J Med. 1983;308(11):619–24.

6. Velat GJ, Kimball MM, Mocco JD, Hoh BL. Vasospasm after aneurysmal subarachnoid hemorrhage: review of randomized controlled trials and meta-analyses in the literature. World Neurosurg. 2011;76(5):446–54.

7. Macdonald RL, Kassell NF, Mayer S, Ruefenacht D, Schmiedek P, Weidauer S, et al. Clazosentan to overcome neurological ischemia and infarction occurring after subarachnoid hemorrhage (CONSCIOUS-1): randomized, double-blind, placebo-controlled phase 2 dose-finding trial. Stroke. 2008; 39(11):3015–21.

8. Macdonald RL, Higashida RT, Keller E, Mayer SA, Molyneux A, Raabe A, et al. Clazosentan, an endothelin receptor antagonist, in patients with aneurysmal subarachnoid haemorrhage undergoing surgical clipping: a randomised, double-blind, placebo-controlled phase 3 trial (CONSCIOUS-2). Lancet Neurol. 2011;10(7):618–25.

9. Etminan N, Vergouwen MDI, Ilodigwe D, Macdonald RL. Effect of pharmaceutical treatment on vasospasm, delayed cerebral ischemia, and clinical outcome in patients with aneurysmal subarachnoid hemorrhage: a systematic review and meta-analysis. J Cereb Blood Flow Metab. 2011;31(6):1443–51.

10. Hanafy KA. The role of microglia and the TLR4 pathway in neuronal apoptosis and vasospasm after subarachnoid hemorrhage. J Neuroinflammation. 2013;10:83.

11. Hanafy KA, Oh J, Otterbein LE. Carbon Monoxide and the brain: time to rethink the dogma. Curr Pharm Des. 2013;19(15):2771–5.

12. Loftspring MC. Iron and early brain injury after subarachnoid hemorrhage. J Cereb Blood Flow Metab. 2010;30(11):1791–2.

13. Gomes JA, Selim M, Cotleur A, Hussain MS, Toth G, Koffman L, et al. Brain iron metabolism and brain injury following subarachnoid hemorrhage: iCeFISH-pilot (CSF iron in SAH). Neurocrit Care. 2014;21(2):285–93.

14. Selim M. Deferoxamine mesylate: a new hope for intracerebral hemorrhage: from bench to clinical trials. Stroke. 2009;40(3 Suppl):S90–1.

15. Lee J-Y, Keep RF, He Y, Sagher O, Hua Y, Xi G. Hemoglobin and iron handling in brain after subarachnoid hemorrhage and the effect of deferoxamine on early brain injury. J Cereb Blood Flow Metab. 2010;30(11):1793–803.

16. Yu Z-Q, Jia Y, Chen G. Possible involvement of cathepsin B/D and caspase-3 in deferoxamine-related neuroprotection of early brain injury after subarachnoid haemorrhage in rats. Neuropathol Appl Neurobiol. 2014;40(3):270–83.

17. Schallner N, Pandit R, LeBlanc R, Thomas AJ, Ogilvy CS, Zuckerbraun BS, et al. Microglia regulate blood clearance in subarachnoid hemorrhage by heme oxygenase-1. J Clin Invest. 2015;125(7):2609–25.

18. Sabri M, Jeon H, Ai J, Tariq A, Shang X, Chen G, et al. Anterior circulation mouse model of subarachnoid hemorrhage. Brain Res. 2009;1295:179–85.

19. Wu H, Wu T, Xu X, Wang J, Wang J. Iron toxicity in mice with collagenase-induced intracerebral hemorrhage. J Cereb Blood Flow Metab. 2011;31(5): 1243–50.

20. Chen J, Marks E, Lai B, Zhang Z, Duce JA, Lam LQ, et al. Iron accumulates in Huntington's disease neurons: protection by deferoxamine. PLoS One. 2013; 8(10):e77023.

21. Zhao J, Chen Z, Xi G, Keep RF, Hua Y. Deferoxamine attenuates acute hydrocephalus after traumatic brain injury in rats. Transl Stroke Res. 2014; 5(5):586–94.

22. Zhao J, Xi G, Wu G, Keep RF, Hua Y. Deferoxamine attenuated the upregulation of lipocalin-2 induced by traumatic brain injury in rats. Acta Neurochir Suppl. 2016;121:291–4.

23. Long DA, Ghosh K, Moore AN, Dixon CE, Dash PK. Deferoxamine improves spatial memory performance following experimental brain injury in rats. Brain Res. 1996;717(1–2):109–17.

24. Mu D, Chang YS, Vexler ZS, Ferriero DM. Hypoxia-inducible factor 1alpha and erythropoietin upregulation with deferoxamine salvage after neonatal stroke. Exp Neurol. 2005;195(2):407–15.

25. Hurn PD, Koehler RC, Blizzard KK, Traystman RJ. Deferoxamine reduces early metabolic failure associated with severe cerebral ischemic acidosis in dogs. Stroke. 1995;26(4):688-694-695.

26. Wilks MQ, Normandin MD, Yuan H, Cho H, Guo Y, Herisson F, et al. Imaging PEG-like nanoprobes in tumor, transient ischemia, and inflammatory disease models. Bioconjug Chem. 2015;26(6):1061–9.

27. Chen Q, Tang J, Tan L, Guo J, Tao Y, Li L, et al. Intracerebral hematoma contributes to hydrocephalus after intraventricular hemorrhage via aggravating iron accumulation. Stroke. 2015;46(10):2902–8.

28. Strahle JM, Garton T, Bazzi AA, Kilaru H, Garton HJL, Maher CO, et al. Role of hemoglobin and iron in hydrocephalus after neonatal intraventricular hemorrhage. Neurosurgery. 2014;75(6):696–705. discussion 706.

29. Chen Z, Gao C, Hua Y, Keep RF, Muraszko K, Xi G. Role of iron in brain injury after intraventricular hemorrhage. Stroke. 2011;42(2):465–70.

30. Gao C, Du H, Hua Y, Keep RF, Strahle J, Xi G. Role of red blood cell lysis and iron in hydrocephalus after intraventricular hemorrhage. J Cereb Blood Flow Metab. 2014;34(6):1070–5.

31. Meng H, Li F, Hu R, Yuan Y, Gong G, Hu S, et al. Deferoxamine alleviates chronic hydrocephalus after intraventricular hemorrhage through iron chelation and Wnt1/Wnt3a inhibition. Brain Res. 2015;1602:44–52.

32. Okauchi M, Hua Y, Keep RF, Morgenstern LB, Schallert T, Xi G. Deferoxamine treatment for intracerebral hemorrhage in aged rats: therapeutic time window and optimal duration. Stroke. 2010;41(2):375–82.

33. Hatakeyama T, Okauchi M, Hua Y, Keep RF, Xi G. Deferoxamine reduces neuronal death and hematoma lysis after intracerebral hemorrhage in aged rats. Transl Stroke Res. 2013;4(5):546–53.

34. Ni W, Okauchi M, Hatakeyama T, Gu Y, Keep RF, Xi G, et al. Deferoxamine reduces intracerebral hemorrhage-induced white matter damage in aged rats. Exp Neurol. 2015;272:128–34.

35. Gu Y, Hua Y, Keep RF, Morgenstern LB, Xi G. Deferoxamine reduces intracerebral hematoma-induced iron accumulation and neuronal death in piglets. Stroke. 2009;40(6):2241–3.

36. Zhao F, Song S, Liu W, Keep RF, Xi G, Hua Y. Red blood cell lysis and brain tissue-type transglutaminase upregulation in a hippocampal model of intracerebral hemorrhage. Acta Neurochir Suppl. 2011;111:101–5.

37. Song S, Hua Y, Keep RF, Hoff JT, Xi G. A new hippocampal model for examining intracerebral hemorrhage-related neuronal death: effects of deferoxamine on hemoglobin-induced neuronal death. Stroke. 2007; 38(10):2861–3.

38. Nakamura T, Keep RF, Hua Y, Schallert T, Hoff JT, Xi G. Deferoxamine-induced attenuation of brain edema and neurological deficits in a rat model of intracerebral hemorrhage. J Neurosurg. 2004;100(4):672–8.

39. Huang F-P, Xi G, Keep RF, Hua Y, Nemoianu A, Hoff JT. Brain edema after experimental intracerebral hemorrhage: role of hemoglobin degradation products. J Neurosurg. 2002;96(2):287–93.

40. Song S, Hua Y, Keep RF, He Y, Wang J, Wu J, et al. Deferoxamine reduces brain swelling in a rat model of hippocampal intracerebral hemorrhage. Acta Neurochir Suppl. 2008;105:13–8.

41. Wan S, Hua Y, Keep RF, Hoff JT, Xi G. Deferoxamine reduces CSF free iron levels following intracerebral hemorrhage. Acta Neurochir Suppl. 2006;96: 199–202.

42. He Y, Hua Y, Lee J-Y, Liu W, Keep RF, Wang MM, et al. Brain alpha- and beta-globin expression after intracerebral hemorrhage. Transl Stroke Res. 2010;1(1):48–56.

43. He Y, Wan S, Hua Y, Keep RF, Xi G. Autophagy after experimental intracerebral hemorrhage. J Cereb Blood Flow Metab. 2008;28(5):897–905.

44. Klebe D, Krafft PR, Hoffmann C, Lekic T, Flores JJ, Rolland W, et al. Acute and delayed deferoxamine treatment attenuates long-term sequelae after germinal matrix hemorrhage in neonatal rats. Stroke. 2014;45(8):2475–9.

45. Hishikawa T, Ono S, Ogawa T, Tokunaga K, Sugiu K, Date I. Effects of deferoxamine-activated hypoxia-inducible factor-1 on the brainstem after subarachnoid hemorrhage in rats. Neurosurgery. 2008;62(1):232-240-241.

46. Bilgihan A, Türközkan N, Aricioğlu A, Aykol S, Cevik C, Göksel M. The effect of deferoxamine on brain lipid peroxide levels and Na-K ATPase activity following experimental subarachnoid hemorrhage. Gen Pharmacol. 1994; 25(3):495–7.

47. Utkan T, Sarioglu Y, Kaya T, Akgün M, Göksel M, Solak O. Effect of deferoxamine and sympathectomy on vasospasm following subarachnoid hemorrhage. Pharmacology. 1996;52(6):353–61.

48. Vollmer DG, Hongo K, Ogawa H, Tsukahara T, Kassell NF. A study of the effectiveness of the iron-chelating agent deferoxamine as vasospasm prophylaxis in a rabbit model of subarachnoid hemorrhage. Neurosurgery. 1991;28(1):27–32.

49. Selim M. Treatment with the iron chelator, deferoxamine mesylate, alters serum markers of oxidative stress in stroke patients. Transl Stroke Res. 2010; 1(1):35–9.

50. Selim M, Yeatts S, Goldstein JN, Gomes J, Greenberg S, Morgenstern LB, et al. Safety and tolerability of deferoxamine mesylate in patients with acute intracerebral hemorrhage. Stroke. 2011;42(11):3067–74.

51. Yeatts SD, Palesch YY, Moy CS, Selim M. High dose deferoxamine in intracerebral hemorrhage (HI-DEF) trial: rationale, design, and methods. Neurocrit Care. 2013; 19(2):257–66.

Toll-like receptor 4 signaling in intracerebral hemorrhage-induced inflammation and injury

Huang Fang, Peng-Fei Wang, Yu Zhou, Yan-Chun Wang and Qing-Wu Yang*

Abstract

Intracerebral hemorrhage (ICH) is a common type of fatal stroke, accounting for about 15% to 20% of all strokes. Hemorrhagic strokes are associated with high mortality and morbidity, and increasing evidence shows that innate immune responses and inflammatory injury play a critical role in ICH-induced neurological deficits. However, the signaling pathways involved in ICH-induced inflammatory responses remain elusive. Toll-like receptor 4 (TLR4) belongs to a large family of pattern recognition receptors that play a key role in innate immunity and inflammatory responses. In this review, we summarize recent findings concerning the involvement of TLR4 signaling in ICH-induced inflammation and brain injury. We discuss the key mechanisms associated with TLR4 signaling in ICH and explore the potential for therapeutic intervention by targeting TLR4 signaling.

Keywords: Toll-like receptor 4, Intracerebral hemorrhage, Inflammation, Hematoma resolution

Introduction

Intracerebral hemorrhage (ICH) is the least treatable type of stroke and has devastating consequences [1]. Hemorrhagic strokes account for 15% to 20% of all strokes and are associated with high mortality and morbidity [2,3]. Primary damage caused by ICH occurs within the first few hours after the onset of bleeding and is mainly due to formation of hematomas, which compress adjacent tissues, thus destroying them [4]. Many patients with ICH deteriorate progressively with no sign of hematoma expansion, suggesting that secondary damage following ICH plays a critical role in neurological deterioration [5,6]. Several lines of evidence show that secondary damage involves inflammation, cerebral edema, and cellular apoptosis, ultimately leading to blood–brain barrier disruption and massive brain cell death [4,7-10]. The molecular mechanisms of secondary damage after ICH have not been well-established, but they may represent novel therapeutic targets to prevent further brain injury.

Secondary damage following ICH is triggered by the presence of intraparenchymal blood, which subsequently activates cytotoxic, oxidative and inflammatory pathways [4,10]. The toxic effects of extravasated blood result mainly from blood components, including red blood cells (RBCs), coagulation factors, complement components and immunoglobulins [4,5,10]. Thrombin, a serine protease produced rapidly after ICH onset, contributes to edema formation and blood–brain barrier damage in early brain injury, and activates the cytotoxic, excitotoxic and inflammatory pathways that are involved in secondary injury following ICH [5,10,11]. Hemoglobin (Hb) released from RBC lysis is a potent cytotoxic chemical that generates free radicals and oxidative damage, causing death of surrounding cells [5,10,12,13]. Hemin, the oxidative form of heme, plays a critical role in Hb-induced brain injury following ICH [5]. Hemin exerts its neurotoxic effects via release of excessive iron, depletion of glutathione and production of free radicals [14]. In addition, an inflammatory response occurs after ICH, which aggravates ICH-induced brain injury, leading to further tissue damage, blood–brain barrier disruption and edema [4,15,16]. The inflammatory mechanisms involved in progression of ICH-induced brain injury include activation of microglial cells, infiltration of inflammatory cells and production of cytokines and chemokines. Neutrophils are believed to contribute to brain injury after ICH [17,18]. Depletion of neutrophils reduced blood–brain barrier disruption, axon injury and inflammation in a rat model of ICH [18] and was found to prevent tissue plasminogen activator (tPA)-induced ICH

* Correspondence: yangqwmlys@hotmail.com
Department of Neurology, Second Affiliated Hospital and Xinqiao Hospital, Third Military Medical University, Xinqiao Zhengjie No.183, Shapingba District, Chongqing 400037, China

in a rat model of cerebral ischemia [17]. Neutrophils may damage brain tissues by producing reactive oxygen species (ROS) and releasing proinflammatory cytokines and matrix metalloproteinases (MMPs) [19,20]. Several lines of evidence show that activation of innate immunity and inflammatory responses contributes to the pathogenesis of secondary injury after ICH [4,5,10,16].

Toll-like receptors (TLRs) belong to a large family of pattern recognition receptors that play a key role in innate immunity and inflammatory responses [21,22]. Thirteen mammalian TLRs have been identified in mice, eleven of which are also found in humans. They recognize distinct pathogen-associated molecular patterns from diverse organisms, including viruses, bacteria, mycobacteria, fungi and parasites [23,24]. In addition, TLRs also recognize damage-associated molecular patterns and mediate host inflammatory responses to injury [22]. TLR1, TLR2, TLR4, TLR5, TLR6 and TLR10 are distributed on the cell surface, and other TLRs (TLR3, TLR7, TLR8, and TLR9) are expressed in the intracellular endosomes [22,25]. TLR consists of leucine-rich repeats in the extracellular ecto-domains that bind various ligands, as well as intracellular Toll-interleukin 1 receptor (TIR) domains that recruit intracellular adaptor proteins, including myeloid differentiation factor 88 (MyD88), TIR domain-containing adaptor-inducing interferons (TRIFs), TIR domain-containing adaptor protein (TIRAP) or TRIF-related adaptor molecule (TRAM). TLR signaling pathways include at least a MyD88-dependent pathway common to all TLRs except TLR3, as well as a MyD88-independent pathway selective to TLR3 and TLR4 [22,26,27]. In the MyD88-dependent pathway, MyD88 activates signal transduction molecules, including interleukin (IL)-1R-associated kinases (IRAKs), tumor necrosis factor (TNF) receptor-associated factor 6 (TRAF6) and transforming growth factor (TGF)-β-activated kinase (TAK1), ultimately leading to activation of nuclear factorκB (NF-κB) and expression of proinflammatory cytokines. In the MyD88-independent pathway, TRIF activates signal transduction molecules including TANK-binding kinase 1 (TBK1) and interferon regulatory factor 3 (IRF3), ultimately leading to expression of interferonβ (IFN-β) [26]. Our recent study shows that both the MyD88 and TRIF signaling pathways are involved in TLR4-mediated inflammatory responses after ICH [28].

It has been reported that TLR4 is upregulated in a rat model of ICH [29,30] and that its signaling pathway contributes to poor outcome after ICH [31]. TLR4 is activated by many endogenous ligands, such as heme and fibrinogen [32,33], which are produced in the brain after ICH. Our recent in vivo study shows that activation of TLR4 by heme causes ICH-induced inflammatory injury via the MyD88/TRIF signaling pathway and that effective blockade of TLR4 by its antibody suppresses ICH-induced inflammation [28]. Thus, the TLR4

signaling pathway could be a promising therapeutic target for ICH treatment.

TLR4 is expressed in microglia, the resident macrophages of the brain. Microglia are activated within minutes after ICH [34,35] and subsequently release chemotactic factors to recruit hematogenous phagocytes to the hemorrhagic areas. Timely clearance of the extravasated RBCs by activated microglia/macrophages can provide protection from local damage resulting from RBC lysis. Successful removal of injured cells can reduce secondary damage by preventing discharge of injurious proinflammatory cell contents. Resolution of hematoma and inhibition of inflammation are considered potential targets for ICH treatment [5,10,36,37]. In this review, we highlight the roles of TLR signaling pathways in ICH and discuss their potential as therapeutic targets.

Innate immunity and inflammation in the pathogenesis of ICH

Microglial cells are activated within minutes after the onset of ICH [34,35]. Activated microglial cells undergo morphological and functional changes that include enlargement and thickening of processes, upregulation of proinflammatory proteins, and behavioral changes, including proliferation, migration and phagocytosis [10,20]. The primary neuroprotective role of activated microglia is to clear the hematoma and damaged cell debris through phagocytosis, providing a nurturing environment for tissue recovery. However, accumulating evidence has shown that microglial activation contributes to ICH-induced secondary brain injury by releasing a variety of cytokines, chemokines, free radicals, nitric oxide and other potentially toxic chemicals [16,34,38,39]. In addition, several studies have shown that inhibition of microglial activation reduces brain damages in animal models of ICH [39-41]. Microglial inhibitors, such as minocycline and microglia/macrophage inhibitory factors (tuftsin fragment 1–3), reduce ICH-induced brain injury and improve neurological function in rodents [40-45]. Clearly, microglial activation mediates ICH-mediated brain injury.

Besides microglia, other blood-derived inflammatory cells, such as leukocytes and macrophages, are also activated after ICH and contribute to ICH-induced brain injury [16]. Neutrophil infiltration occurs less than 1 day after the onset of ICH, and the infiltrating neutrophils die by apoptosis within 2 days [35,46]. Dying leukocytes can cause further brain injury by stimulating microglia/macrophages to release proinflammatory factors [16]. Activated macrophages are indistinguishable from resident microglia in morphology and function [20]. Similar to activated microglia, activated leukocytes and macrophages release a variety of cytokines, chemokines, free radicals and other potentially toxic chemicals [16,20,34].

Cytokines are well-known to be associated with inflammation and immune activation [47]. Although cytokines are released by many cells, including microglia/macrophages, astrocytes and neurons, the major sources of cytokines are activated microglia/macrophages [48]. Many studies have shown that two major proinflammatory cytokines, TNF-α and interleukin1β (IL-1β), exacerbate ICH-induced brain injury. After ICH, TNF-α is significantly increased both *in vivo* and *in vitro* [16,28,34,49], which may contribute to brain edema formation and brain injury in animal models of ICH [49,50]. Consistent with animal studies, clinical studies support the proposition that TNF-α contributes to ICH-induced brain injury. Plasma TNF-α has been shown to correlate with the magnitude of the perihematomal brain edema in patients with ICH [51]. Single-nucleotide polymorphisms in the TNF-α gene promoter are associated with spontaneous deep ICH [52]. Similarly, IL-1β has been found to be upregulated after ICH in an animal model and to produce detrimental effects, including brain edema and blood–brain barrier disruption [28,53,54].

NF-κB, a transcription factor involved in inflammatory responses, is also activated after ICH, leading to upregulation of gene expression that contributes to brain injury [34,55]. Activation of NF-κB occurs within minutes and lasts for at least 1 week after the onset of ICH [56]. NF-κB is a key regulator of many proinflammatory cytokines, such as TNF-α and IL-1β, in various pathological conditions, including ICH [16,28,55,57]. The activity of NF-κB correlates with perilesional cell death after ICH in rats [58]. Activation of NF-κB is positively associated with the progression of apoptotic cell death in patients with ICH [59]. Therefore, understanding the signaling mechanisms underlying ICH-induced NF-κB activation may facilitate identification of therapeutic targets.

Several lines of evidence have shown that NF-κB is activated by RBCs and plasma via signaling pathways involving free radicals, cytokines and glutamate receptors [55]. It is well-known that TLR signaling pathways can lead to NF-κB activation, resulting in production of proinflammatory cytokines [27,60,61]. Increasing evidence has shown that TLR signaling pathways play an essential role in sterile inflammatory diseases in the central nervous system [62-64]. Herein we review recent advances in TLR4 signaling pathways in ICH-induced inflammatory brain injury.

TLR4 signaling in ICH-induced inflammatory brain injury

TLRs, especially TLR4, are involved in the inflammatory responses and neuronal damage associated with cerebral ischemia [22,65]. Expression of TLR4 is upregulated in a mouse model of transient cerebral ischemia [66]. In ischemic brain injury, TLR4-deficient mice show significant suppression of inflammatory cytokine expression, including IRF1, inducible nitric oxide synthase, cyclooxygenase2, MMP9, and IFN-β [67]. TLR4-knockout mice have significantly smaller infarct volumes and better neurological function than wild-type (WT) mice [66,67]. Similar to cerebral ischemia, TLR4 expression is significantly increased after ICH, and TLR4-knockout mice demonstrate improved neurological function after ICH [28-31]. These animal studies agree with recent clinical findings that increased expression of TLR4 is associated with poorer functional outcome and greater residual volume in patients with ICH [68]. However, although TLR4 participates in both cerebral ischemia- and ICH-induced brain injuries, the signaling pathways involved are different. Both the MyD88 and TRIF pathways are involved in TLR4-mediated brain injury in ICH [28], whereas only MyD88 is involved in ischemia [69]. Therefore, the roles of TLR4 in ICH and cerebral ischemia may be different.

The roles of TLR4 in inflammation and neurological impairment following ICH have been studied recently, using TLR4-knockout mice, by our research group and others [28,31]. Compared to WT mice, after ICH, TLR4-knockout mice exhibited significantly decreased brain water content [28] and neurological deficits [28,31]. Furthermore, the perihematomal region in TLR4-knockout mice had lower levels of infiltrating inflammatory cells, including macrophages [28], leukocytes and monocytes [31], as well as lower levels of inflammatory cytokines, such as TNF-α, IL-1β and IL-6, and decreased NF-κB activity [28]. In addition, Sansing *et al.* [31] reported increased gene expression of CD36, CSF2 and CX3CL1 in TLR4-knockout mice compared to WT mice. Taken together, these studies demonstrate that TLR4 activation is involved in ICH-induced neurological deficits and contributes to the detrimental inflammatory response.

TLR4 is expressed in various cell types in the central nervous system, including microglia, neurons and astrocytes, as well as in peripheral blood cells, such as leukocytes, macrophages and platelets [22,28,30,33,70,71]. After ICH, TLR4 mRNA and protein expression is significantly increased by approximately 2 to 6 hours, peaks at day 3, declines somewhat at day 5, but remains elevated relative to baseline even at day 7 [28-30]. Though ICH induces upregulation of TLR4 expression in neurons, astrocytes and microglia, TLR4 is predominantly expressed in CD11b-positive microglial cells in mice [28]. In addition, TLR4 contributes to reduced recruitment of neutrophils and monocytes in the perihematomal area after ICH in TLR4-deficient mice [31]. Therefore, resident microglia in the brain as well as peripheral infiltrating leukocytes and monocytes are likely involved in the roles of TLR4 in ICH-induced brain injury.

Microglial activation in response to ICH contributes to ICH-induced brain injury by releasing cytokines, and inhibition of microglial activation has been shown to improve neurological function in animal models of ICH [38-41]. Recently, we investigated the role of TLR4 in microglial activation following ICH [28]. Exogenous hemin treatment of cultured microglia increases expression of TLR4, as well as proinflammatory cytokines, such as TNF-α, IL-1β and IL-6. This effect is completely abolished by knockout of TLR4 or treatment with anti-TLR4 antibodies, suggesting that TLR4 mediates hemin-stimulated microglial activation [28]. In addition, hemin-induced expression of proinflammatory cytokines TNF-α, IL-1β and IL-6 is completely blocked in TLR4-knockout mice [28]. These data demonstrate that TLR4 signaling mediates heme-induced inflammatory injury, possibly by activating microglial cells and subsequently releasing proinflammatory cytokines. However, Sansing et al. [31] reported that upregulation of IL-1β and IL-6 genes in the perihematomal region did not significantly differ between TLR4-knockout and WT mice, suggesting that TLR4 signaling may not be involved in the transcriptional regulation of proinflammatory cytokines in perihematomal inflammation. Alternately, it may not be possible to detect upregulation of proinflammatory cytokine genes in certain cell types, such as microglia, when the entire perihematomal region is used [31].

Using blood transfer experiments in which TLR4-deficient blood was injected into the brains of WT mice and WT blood into brains of TLR4-deficient mice, Sansing et al. [31] found that TLR4 signaling within the hemorrhage mediated the inflammatory response and contributed to ICH-induced neurological injury. Activation of TLR4 on leukocytes or platelets within the hemorrhage, but not on resident cells, promoted inflammation and resulted in poor functional outcomes. This study clearly demonstrated that TLR4 signaling on peripheral blood cells plays a critical role in ICH-induced brain injury.

Therefore, TLR4 signaling on resident microglia and on blood cells within the hemorrhage is critical for ICH-induced inflammatory injury. Because TLR4 is expressed on resident microglia which are activated within minutes after ICH [34,35], the TLR4 signaling on microglia probably initiates ICH-induced inflammatory injury, causing release of inflammatory cytokines and infiltration of neutrophils. Significant upregulation of TLR4 expression occurs at approximately 2 to 6 hours after ICH [28-30], accompanied by the appearance of infiltrating neutrophils in the hematoma (at approximately 4 hours after ICH) [46]. TLR4 signaling in the neutrophils may further mediate release of proinflammatory cytokines, which contributes to the detrimental inflammatory response [17,18]. There are abundant TLR4 activators in the perihematomal region, including heme [32], fibrinogen [33] and myeloid-related proteins 8 and 14, which are released from degranulating neutrophils [72]. These endogenous activators can stimulate TLR4 on leukocytes, leading to inflammatory injury.

TLR4 signaling pathways in ICH

TLRs are a group of Class I transmembrane proteins that consist of ectodomains, transmembrane domains, and intracellular TIR domains. TLRs recognize and bind various ligands via leucin-rich repeats in the extracellular ectodomains. The receptor-ligand binding results in conformational changes of the receptor, subsequently leading to recruitment of intracellular adaptor proteins, including MyD88, TRIF, TIRAP, or TRAM [22]. Once recruited, these adaptors initiate downstream signaling events, which ultimately lead to activation of transcription factors, such as NF-κB, and subsequent expression of various proinflammatory cytokines, such as IL-6, TNF-α and IL-1 [22,27].

TLR4 interacts with two distinct adaptor proteins (MyD88 and TRIF) and therefore activates two parallel signaling pathways to initiate the activation of transcription factors that regulate expression of proinflammatory cytokine genes [22,26,73]. The MyD88-dependent pathway, common to all TLRs, is essential for activation of NF-κB and production of inflammatory cytokines [26,74]. TRIF is essential for the TLR3- and TLR4-mediated MyD88-independent pathway, which involves the activation of IRF-3, leading to expression of IFN-β [26,27]. Recently, we found that both MyD88 and TRIF signaling pathways are involved in TLR4-mediated inflammatory responses after ICH [28]. Deletion of MyD88 or TRIF in transgenic mice leads to improved neurological function and reduced cytokine release and macrophage infiltration following ICH. After ICH in TLR4-knockout mice, MyD88 and TRIF expression are reduced, further demonstrating the role of these factors in TLR4-mediated ICH sequelae. Furthermore, the ICH-induced increase in NF-κB activity is significantly lower in TLR4-knockout mice than that in WT mice, suggesting that TLR4 mediates ICH-induced inflammation via activation of NF-κB to regulate expression of inflammatory cytokines.

The MyD88 pathway of TLR4 signaling activates not only the NF-κB pathway but also the activating protein1 (AP-1) pathway. AP-1 is a dimeric protein composed of members of the Jun, Fos, and α-fetoprotein families of proteins [75]. AP-1 activation leads to the expression of many proinflammatory mediators, such as MMPs, proteases, and cytokines such as IL-1 and IFN [76,77]. It is well-documented that these proinflammatory mediators are increased after ICH [16,20]. For example, MMPs, including MMP2, MMP3, MMP9, and MMP12, have been reported to be upregulated after ICH as a result of their activation by proteases such as plasmin and tPA [20,78,79]. However, the role of AP-1 in ICH has not been explored yet. AP-1 activation in TLR4 signaling is mainly mediated by mitogen-activated protein kinases (MAPKs), including c-Jun N-terminal kinase (JNK), p38 and ERK [76]. JNK, a stress-activated kinase that mediates apoptosis in neurons and microglia, is activated after ICH, and inhibition of the JNK pathway results in a significant decrease in edema and hematoma volume in mice after ICH [80]. Therefore, proapoptotic signals may play a role in ICH-induced inflammatory injury. However, it remains unknown whether ILR4 can mediate ICH-induced inflammatory injury via AP-1 activation.

Interestingly, lively and Schlichter showed that the expression of inflammatory mediators after ICH is age-dependent [81]. They examined 27 genes, including TLR4, and found that 18 of the 27 genes were different in expression levels or timing between young adult and aged rats [81]. The delayed expression of TLR4 was observed in aged rats, accompanied by a delayed and/or decreased expression of many proinflammatory cytokines such as IL-1β and IL-6 [81]. The TLR4 signaling pathways involved in age-related expression of proinflammatory cytokines is not well-understood. It has been reported that lipopolysaccharide (LPS)-induced production of TLR4-mediated proinflammatory cytokines is age-dependently decreased, accompanied by a decrease in the expression of MAPKs, but not the surface expression of TLR4 [82]. Decreased TLR4/MPAK signaling pathway may be responsible for age-related decrease in the production of inflammatory cytokines.

Because the brain is a sterile organ without any pathogens derived from bacteria or viruses, the endogenous molecules released after ICH become TLR stimulators. Several endogenous molecules have been reported as TLR4 ligands, including heme, fibrinogen, high-mobility group protein B1 (HMGB1), heat shock proteins, hyaluronan, oxidized low-density lipoprotein and amyloid β [32,33,69,83-87]. However, the molecular mechanisms underlying activation of TLR4 signaling pathways by these different ligands are not completely understood. Clearly, different TLR4 ligands can activate distinct signaling pathways. For example, in vivo animal studies show that heme triggers a TLR4 signaling pathway involving both MyD88 and TRIF [28], whereas HMBG1 initiates only the MyD88 pathway [69], and monophosphoryl lipid A, a low-toxicity derivative of LPS, activates only the TRIF pathway [88]. It remains unclear how different TLR4 ligands selectively activate distinct signaling pathways. However, different TLR4 receptor conformations induced by binding of different TLR4 ligands may contribute to the pathway-specific activation [89]. The ligand-biased signaling is well-known for G protein-coupled receptors, such as β-adrenergic receptors [25,90]. Understanding the mechanisms of biased signaling can provide leads for designing more specific drugs.

Many endogenous TLR4 ligands are known to be released during ICH. Some TLR4 ligands are crucial for activating TLR4 to trigger ICH-induced inflammation and inflammatory cytokine expression [28,31,91,92]. Heme,

released from RBC lysis after ICH, is essential for TLR4-mediated inflammation because it potentiates microglial activation and increases cytokine expression [28]. Fibrinogen within the clots after ICH is also critical for activation of TLR4 on platelets or leukocytes within the hemorrhage, which contributes to poor outcome after ICH [31]. HMGB1, known to be essential for ischemic brain injury [65], is reported to be upregulated in the microglia after subarachnoid hemorrhage [91], and the HMGB1 inhibitor glycyrrhizin attenuates ICH-induced brain injury [92]. Additional studies of the roles of endogenous TLR4 ligands in ICH are warranted.

A deeper understanding of TLR4 signaling pathways should enable development of potential therapeutic targets for prevention and treatment of ICH. There are two ways to block TLR signaling: direct blockade by removal of TLR ligands (e.g., heme) and inhibition of TLRs and their downstream signaling pathways. Effective removal of deposited blood and disintegrated cells by promoting hematoma clearance has been demonstrated to reduce ICH-induced neurological deficits in a mouse model of ICH [36,37]. Hematoma resolution could promote clearance of hemin, thus reducing hemin-mediated activation of TLR4 and subsequent inflammatory responses. In addition, effective blockade of TLR4 receptor using an antibody disrupted TLR4 signaling and has neuroprotective effects in a mouse model of ICH [28]. Therefore, effective blockade of TLR4 signaling pathway could be a potential therapeutic strategy for prevention and treatment of ICH.

Blockade of TLR4 signaling as a potential target in the treatment of ICH

As TLR4 signaling plays an important role in ICH-induced inflammatory injury, TLR4 inhibition should be beneficial. TLR antagonists have been developed for a number of inflammatory and autoimmune diseases [93-95] and include anti-TLR antibodies, small-molecule antagonists screened from compound libraries, and antagonists derived from medicinal plants. However, the efficacy of TLR antagonists in ICH has not been well-studied to date.

We have found that a specific antibody (Mts50) blocked TLR4 signaling in a mouse model of ICH [28]. TLR4 antibody treatment significantly reduced cerebral water content and improved neurological function after ICH, similar to effects observed in TLR4-knockout mice, suggesting that blockade of the TLR4 receptor is a potential therapeutic approach in the treatment of ICH. The neuroprotective effects of the TLR4 antibody in ICH may be associated with inhibition of cytokine expression and macrophage infiltration. However, the effectiveness of the antibody on hemin-induced TLR4 activation in macrophages is controversial. We found that the TLR4 antibody effectively suppressed hemin-induced microglial activation in mice [28]. However, Figueiredo et al. reported that this antibody blocked only

LPS-induced, but not hemin-induced, TLR4 activation in macrophages, suggesting that different TLR4 receptor conformations exist in response to different ligands [32]. The discrepancy between the two studies may be due to use of different reagents and animal models, and further studies are needed to evaluate the efficacy of the TLR4 antibody for ICH.

Many TLR4 antagonists have been reported to produce anti-inflammatory effects [93-95]. Some antagonists, such as curumin, 6-shogaol, isoliquiritigenin, and OSL07 (4-oxo-4-(2-oxo-oxazolidin-3-yl)-but-2-enoic acid ethyl ester), block TLR4 signaling by inhibiting homodimerization of TLR4 [96-99]. Other agents, such as sparstolonin B, auranofin, TAK-242, and M62812, have also been reported to block TLR4 signaling pathways selectively [100-103]. However, most of these agents were tested in an animal model of LPS-induced sepsis. The effects of these agents on ICH-induced inflammation have not yet been explored.

In addition to these antagonists, many agents with multiple pharmacological mechanisms have been found to have neuroprotective effects in animal models of ICH via inhibition of TLR4 signaling. For example, oxymatrine, which has anti-inflammatory, antioxidative, and antiapoptotic activities, suppresses TLR4 and NF-κB gene expression and decreases production of proinflammatory cytokines, such as IL-6, TNF-α, and IL-1β [104]. Ginkgolide B, a specific platelet-activating factor receptor antagonist, reduces neuronal cell apoptosis after traumatic brain injury in rats, possibly via inhibition of TLR4 signaling pathways [105]. Progesterone treatment inhibits TLR4 signaling pathways and reduces brain edema and blood–brain barrier impairment after subarachnoid hemorrhage in rats [106]. These agents are not specific TLR4 receptor blockers, but they can inhibit TLR4 signaling to reduce ICH-induced inflammatory injury.

Paradoxically, TLR4 activation with low doses of LPS prior to ischemic brain injury protects against subsequent severe ischemic injury [107-109]. The mechanisms of preconditioning by TLR4 activation in ischemic brain injury are not fully understood. Recent studies have shown that LPS preconditioning redirects TLR4 singling through the TRIF-IRF3 pathway, but not through the MyD88 pathway [109,110]. Enhanced IRF3 activity and increased anti-inflammatory IFN gene expression contribute to the beneficial effects of LPS preconditioning [109]. Though the suppression of NF-κB activity is suppressed in LPS preconditioning mice following ischemic injury, proinflammatory cytokine production does not change, suggesting that besides the TLR4 signaling pathway, other signaling cascades and transcription factors are involved in proinflammatory cytokine production during ischemic injury [109]. However, there have been relatively few studies examining the effects of preconditioning by TLR4 activation on ICH. It remains to be determined whether the TRIF/IRF3 pathway and enhanced anti-inflammatory IFN production are preferentially involved in preconditioning by TLR4 activation in ICH. It has been reported that progesterone inhibits TLR4/NF-κB signaling pathway and decrease proinflammatory cytokine production in rats following subarachnoid hemorrhage [106], suggesting that suppressed proinflammatory signaling may contribute to preconditioning by TLR4 activation in ICH. Therefore, suppressed proinflammatory signaling and/or enhanced anti-inflammatory IFN signaling may be associated with preconditioning by TLR4 activation in ICH. Additional studies of the mechanisms of preconditioning by TLR4 activation in ICH are warranted.

Heme removal and hematoma resolution as potential targets in the treatment of ICH

RBC lysis occurs at approximately 24 hours after the onset of ICH and continues for the next several days, leading to release of cytotoxic hemoglobin [111]. Hemoglobin then degrades to hemin, the oxidative form of heme [14]. Hemin is gradually cleared by hematogenous phagocytes and resident microglia [10]. Once inside these cells, hemin is degraded by heme oxygenase (HO) into biliverdin and carbon monoxide, releasing cytotoxic iron. The toxic effects of hemoglobin/hemin include release of redox-active iron, depletion of glutathione, and production of free radicals [14]. To avoid the toxicity of hemoglobin/hemin, these substances are cleared from the extracellular space via binding to haptoglobin and hemopexin or via phagocytosis by microglia/macrophages.

Haptoglobin, an abundant protein in blood plasma, has the ability to bind hemoglobin. In the brain, it is produced and released by oligodendrocytes, thereby protecting the brain against extravascular hemoglobin toxicity [112]. Expression of haptoglobin is increased around the hematoma in animal models of ICH. Haptoglobin-deficient mice are more vulnerable to ICH-induced brain injury, and mice with haptoglobin overexpression are less susceptible to injury [112]. Sulforaphane, an NF-E2-related factor2 (Nrf2) activator, increases haptoglobin in the brain and reduces brain injury following ICH [112]. In addition, sulforaphane treatment increases expression of Nrf2-mediated antioxidant genes, such as catalase, superoxide dismutase, and glutathioneS-transferase, in the brain after ICH [113]. The antioxidative effects of sulforphane are correlated with reduction of brain damage, measured by brain edema, blood–brain barrier impairment, cortical apoptosis, and motor deficits [114].

Peroxisome proliferator-activated receptorγ (PPARγ) plays an important role in augmenting phagocytosis and promoting hematoma absorption [36,37]. PPARγ is a ligand-dependent transcription factor that regulates the expression of several target genes, such as scavenger receptor CD36 [36,37]. CD36, a class B scavenger receptor, is important for phagocytic activity [115,116]. Treatment with PPARγ agonists, such as rosiglitazone and 15d-PGJ2, increases expression of CD36 and promotes phagocytosis of RBCs by microglia/phagocytes in both *in vitro* and *in vivo* models of ICH [36,37], and anti-CD36 antibodies prevent PPARγ agonist-induced increases in phagocytosis [37]. In addition, in an animal model, treatment of ICH with PPARγ agonists accelerated hematoma resolution and reduced neurological deficits [36,37].

ROS are produced after ICH and contribute to ICH pathogenesis [4,5,13,34]. In addition, phagocytosis generates a large amount of ROS that can damage macrophages and neurons. PPARγ also plays an important role in protecting microglia/macrophages from oxidative damage via upregulation of the antioxidant catalase [36,37]. PPARγ agonists upregulate catalase expression in microglia *in vitro* and *in vivo* after ICH, enhance phagocytosis *in vitro* and increase hematoma absorption *in vivo* [37]. The PPARγ-mediated upregulation of catalase reduces oxidative stress, as demonstrated by a significant reduction of extracellular hydrogen peroxide in cultured microglia [37]. Phagocytosis of RBCs by microglia is also enhanced by upregulation of catalane, as demonstrated by the finding that addition of exogenous catalane to the culture media promotes phagocytosis [37].

PPARγ can also induce neuroprotection after ICH via anti-inflammatory effects. In both *in vitro* and *in vivo* experiments, PPARγ activators reduced expression of proinflammatory genes, including TNF-α, IL-1β, MMP9, and inducible nitric oxide synthase [37]. PPARγ is known to inhibit DNA binding of NF-κB [34,55], which controls expression of proinflammatory cytokines and enzymes, suggesting that the anti-inflammatory effect of PPARγ probably results from inhibition of NF-κB [37,117].

TLR4 signaling in hematoma resolution
Microglia/macrophages express the scavenger receptor CD36, which has been reported to assist in phagocytosis-mediated removal of RBCs after ICH [37]. PPARγ agonists can promote phagocytosis of RBCs by microglia/phagocytes through upregulation of CD36 [36,37]. In addition, PPARγ agonists suppress the subarachnoid hemorrhage-induced inflammatory response by inhibiting TLR4 signaling [118]. Knockout of TLR4 results in upregulation of CD36 in the perihematomal region [31], suggesting that the TLR4 signaling pathway could play a role in hematoma resolution. In agreement with this hypothesis, we found that hematoma resolved significantly faster in TLR4-knockout mice than in WT mice, as shown in Figure 1. Specifically, hematoma started to resolve at 3 days after ICH and almost completely resolved by 5 days. These data demonstrate that the TLR4 signaling pathway is involved in hematoma resolution after ICH, and the underlying mechanisms are currently under investigation.

Conclusions and perspectives
Increasing evidence has shown that TLR4 signaling plays important roles in ICH-induced inflammatory brain injury by stimulating activation of microglial cells, infiltration of leukocytes, and production of cytokines and chemokines [28,31]. The TLR4 signaling pathway involved in ICH-induced inflammatory injury includes ligands (e.g., heme), TLR4 itself, and its downstream pathways, including adaptor proteins (MyD88 and TRIF) and transcription factors, such as NF-κB [28]. Therefore, TLR4 and its signaling pathways are potential targets for developing effective medical treatment of ICH.

There are many challenges to be overcome before inhibition of TLR4 signaling can be used in the prevention and treatment of ICH. Though inhibition of TLR4 signaling by anti-TLR4 antibodies or deletion of TLR4 genes can effectively reduce ICH-induced neurological deficits in mice [28], specific TLR4 antagonists that inhibit TLR4 signaling have not been investigated in models of ICH. In addition, a diverse range of endogenous ligands may activate TLR4 signaling to trigger the inflammatory response that is critical in ICH-induced brain injury. However, it remains unclear how these ligands activate TLR4 signaling, which ligands are the most critical, how TLR4 receptors recruit adaptor proteins and activate transcription factors, and whether TLR4 signaling pathways are similar across cell types (e.g., microglia versus leukocytes). Whether TLR4 interacts with other TLRs in ICH-induced inflammatory injury requires further investigation. Better understanding

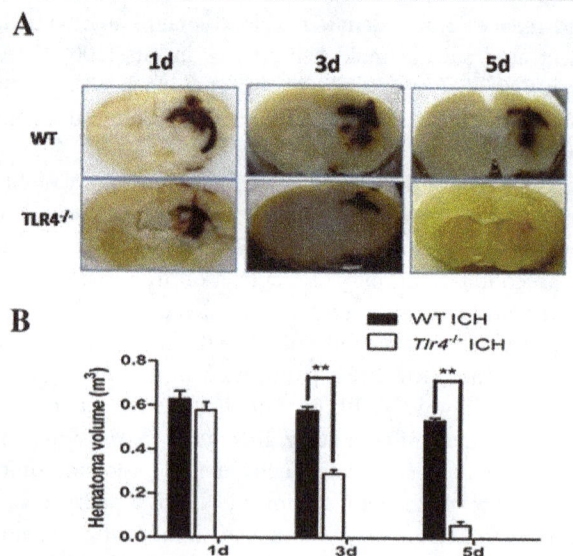

Figure 1 TLR4 knockout results in faster hematoma resolution. (**A**) Representative brain sections from WT and TLR4-knockout mice at 1, 3, and 5 days after intrastriatal injection of blood. (**B**) Compared with WT mice, TLR4-knockout mice had significantly smaller hemotomas at 3 and 5 days after ICH. Hematoma volume was measured on coronal slices (2 mm thick) using image analysis software. Scale bar: 1 mm. **P < 0.05 versus WT mice.

of the roles of TLR4 signaling in ICH will facilitate development of ICH treatments.

Brain injury following ICH is triggered by the presence of intraparenchymal blood. The mechanisms of ICH-induced brain injury are numerous, including cytotoxic, oxidative, and inflammatory pathways. It would be beneficial to develop a medical treatment that promotes hematoma resolution and inhibits cytotoxic, oxidative, and inflammatory insults following ICH. For example, PPARγ activators reduce ICH-induced brain injury by improving hematoma resolution and reducing oxidative injury [36,37]. Another promising intervention is inhibition of TLR4 signaling, which also promotes hematoma resolution (see Figure 1) and inhibits ICH-induced inflammation [28]. However, the molecular mechanisms underlying hematoma resolution and cytotoxic, oxidative, and inflammatory injury following ICH remain elusive. Further research into the complex mechanisms involved in ICH pathogenesis will facilitate identification of novel therapeutic targets.

Abbreviations

Hb: Hemoglobin; HMGB1: High-mobility group box 1 protein; HO: Heme oxygenase; ICH: Intracerebral hemorrhage; IFN-β: Interferon β; IL-1β: Interleukin-1β; LPS: Lipopolysaccharide; MyD88: Myeloid differentiation factor 88; NF-κB: Nuclear factorκB; Nrf2: NF-E2-related factor2; PPARγ: Peroxisome proliferator-activated receptorγ; RBC: Red blood cell; TIR: Intracellular Tollinterleukin 1 receptor; TIRAP: TIR domain-containing adaptor protein; TLR: Toll-like receptor; TNF-α: Tumor necrosis factorα; TRAM: TRIF-related adaptor molecule; TRIF: TIR domain-containing adaptor-inducing interferon; WT: Wild type.

Competing interests

The authors declare that they have no competing interests.

Authors' contributions

All authors read and approved the final manuscript. FH collected literatures and reviewed the literatures. WPF reviewed the literatures. WYC proofreaded and corrected the manuscript. ZY revised the manuscript. YQW wrote the manuscript and approved the final version of the manuscript.

Acknowledgements

This work was supported in part by a grant from the National Natural Science Foundation of China (Nos. 81070932and 81271283).

References

1. Hwang BY, Appelboom G, Ayer A, Kellner CP, Kotchetkov IS, Gigante PR, Haque R, Kellner M, Connolly ES: Advances in neuroprotective strategies: potential therapies for intracerebral hemorrhage. Cerebrovasc Dis 2011, 31(3):211–222.
2. Flower O, Smith M: The acute management of intracerebral hemorrhage. Curr Opin Crit Care 2011, 17(2):106–114.
3. Mayer SA, Rincon F: Treatment of intracerebral haemorrhage. Lancet Neurol 2005, 4(10):662–672.
4. Xi G, Keep RF, Hoff JT: Mechanisms of brain injury after intracerebral haemorrhage. Lancet Neurol 2006, 5(1):53–63.
5. Babu R, Bagley JH, Di C, Friedman AH, Adamson C: Thrombin and hemin as central factors in the mechanisms of intracerebral hemorrhage-induced secondary brain injury and as potential targets for intervention. Neurosurg Focus 2012, 32(4):E8.
6. Elliott J, Smith M: The acute management of intracerebral hemorrhage: a clinical review. Anesth Analg 2010, 110(5):1419–1427.
7. Felberg RA, Grotta JC, Shirzadi AL, Strong R, Narayana P, Hill-Felberg SJ, Aronowski J: Cell death in experimental intracerebral hemorrhage: the "black hole" model of hemorrhagic damage. Ann Neurol 2002, 51(4):517–524.
8. Huang FP, Xi G, Keep RF, Hua Y, Nemoianu A, Hoff JT: Brain edema after experimental intracerebral hemorrhage: role of hemoglobin degradation products. J Neurosurg 2002, 96(2):287–293.
9. Lee KR, Kawai N, Kim S, Sagher O, Hoff JT: Mechanisms of edema formation after intracerebral hemorrhage: effects of thrombin on cerebral blood flow, blood–brain barrier permeability, and cell survival in a rat model. J Neurosurg 1997, 86(2):272–278.
10. Aronowski J, Zhao X: Molecular pathophysiology of cerebral hemorrhage: secondary brain injury. Stroke 2011, 42(6):1781–1786.
11. Sharp F, Liu DZ, Zhan X, Ander BP: Intracerebral hemorrhage injury mechanisms: glutamate neurotoxicity, thrombin, and Src. Acta Neurochir Suppl 2008, 105:43–46.
12. Wagner KR, Packard BA, Hall CL, Smulian AG, Linke MJ, De Courten-Myers GM, Packard LM, Hall NC: Protein oxidation and heme oxygenase-1 induction in porcine white matter following intracerebral infusions of whole blood or plasma. Dev Neurosci 2002, 24(2–3):154–160.
13. Nakamura T, Keep RF, Hua Y, Hoff JT, Xi G: Oxidative DNA injury after experimental intracerebral hemorrhage. Brain Res 2005, 1039(1–2):30–36.
14. Robinson SR, Dang TN, Dringen R, Bishop GM: Hemin toxicity: a preventable source of brain damage following hemorrhagic stroke. Redox Rep 2009, 14(6):228–235.
15. Yenari MA, Xu L, Tang XN, Qiao Y, Giffard RG: Microglia potentiate damage to blood–brain barrier constituents: improvement by minocycline in vivo and in vitro. Stroke 2006, 37(4):1087–1093.
16. Wang J, Dore S: Inflammation after intracerebral hemorrhage. J Cereb Blood Flow Metab 2007, 27(5):894–908.
17. Gautier S, Ouk T, Petrault O, Caron J, Bordet R: Neutrophils contribute to intracerebral haemorrhages after treatment with recombinant tissue plasminogen activator following cerebral ischaemia. Br J Pharmacol 2009, 156(4):673–679.
18. Moxon-Emre I, Schlichter LC: Neutrophil depletion reduces blood–brain barrier breakdown, axon injury, and inflammation after intracerebral hemorrhage. J Neuropathol Exp Neurol 2011, 70(3):218–235.
19. Nguyen HX, O'Barr TJ, Anderson AJ: Polymorphonuclear leukocytes promote neurotoxicity through release of matrix metalloproteinases, reactive oxygen species, and TNF-α. J Neurochem 2007, 102(3):900–912.
20. Wang J: Preclinical and clinical research on inflammation after intracerebral hemorrhage. Prog Neurobiol 2010, 92(4):463–477.
21. Akira S, Uematsu S, Takeuchi O: Pathogen recognition and innate immunity. Cell 2006, 124(4):783–801.
22. Kong Y, Le Y: Toll-like receptors in inflammation of the central nervous system. Int Immunopharmacol 2011, 11(10):1407–1414.
23. Beutler BA: TLRs and innate immunity. Blood 2009, 113(7):1399–1407.
24. Zhu J, Mohan C: Toll-like receptor signaling pathways: therapeutic opportunities. Mediators Inflamm 2010, 2010:781235.
25. Akira S, Takeda K: Toll-like receptor signalling. Nat Rev Immunol 2004, 4(7):499–511.
26. Takeda K, Akira S: TLR signaling pathways. Semin Immunol 2004, 16(1):3–9.
27. Lin Q, Li M, Fang D, Fang J, Su SB: The essential roles of Toll-like receptor signaling pathways in sterile inflammatory diseases. Int Immunopharmacol 2011, 11(10):1422–1432.
28. Lin S, Yin Q, Zhong Q, Lv FL, Zhou Y, Li JQ, Wang JZ, Su BY, Yang QW: Heme activates TLR4-mediated inflammatory injury via MyD88/TRIF signaling pathway in intracerebral hemorrhage. J Neuroinflammation 2012, 9:46.
29. Teng W, Wang L, Xue W, Guan C: Activation of TLR4-mediated NF-κB signaling in hemorrhagic brain in rats. Mediators Inflamm 2009, 2009:473276.
30. Ma CX, Yin WN, Cai BW, Wu J, Wang JY, He M, Sun H, Ding JL, You C: Toll-like receptor 4/nuclear factor-κ B signaling detected in brain after early subarachnoid hemorrhage. Chin Med J (Engl) 2009, 122(13):1575–1581.
31. Sansing LH, Harris TH, Welsh FA, Kasner SE, Hunter CA, Kariko K: Toll-like receptor 4 contributes to poor outcome after intracerebral hemorrhage. Ann Neurol 2011, 70(4):646–656.
32. Figueiredo RT, Fernandez PL, Mourao-Sa DS, Porto BN, Dutra FF, Alves LS, Oliveira MF, Oliveira PL, Graça-Souza AV, Bozza MT: Characterization of

heme as activator of Toll-like receptor 4. *J Biol Chem* 2007, **282**(28):20221–20229.

33. Smiley ST, King JA, Hancock WW: Fibrinogen stimulates macrophage chemokine secretion through Toll-like receptor 4. *J Immunol* 2001, **167**(5):2887–2894.

34. Aronowski J, Hall CE: New horizons for primary intracerebral hemorrhage treatment: experience from preclinical studies. *Neurol Res* 2005, **27**(3):268–279.

35. Xue M, Del Bigio MR: Intracerebral injection of autologous whole blood in rats: time course of inflammation and cell death. *Neurosci Lett* 2000, **283**(3):230–232.

36. Zhao X, Grotta J, Gonzales N, Aronowski J: Hematoma resolution as a therapeutic target: the role of microglia/macrophages. *Stroke* 2009, **40**(3 Suppl):S92–S94.

37. Zhao X, Sun G, Zhang J, Strong R, Song W, Gonzales N, Grotta JC, Aronowski J: Hematoma resolution as a target for intracerebral hemorrhage treatment: role for peroxisome proliferator-activated receptor γ in microglia/macrophages. *Ann Neurol* 2007, **61**(4):352–362.

38. Wang J, Tsirka SE: Contribution of extracellular proteolysis and microglia to intracerebral hemorrhage. *Neurocrit Care* 2005, **3**(1):77–85.

39. Gao Z, Wang J, Thiex R, Rogove AD, Heppner FL, Tsirka SE: Microglial activation and intracerebral hemorrhage. *Acta Neurochir Suppl* 2008, **105**:51–53.

40. Wang J, Rogove AD, Tsirka AE, Tsirka SE: Protective role of tuftsin fragment 1–3 in an animal model of intracerebral hemorrhage. *Ann Neurol* 2003, **54**(5):655–664.

41. Wang J, Tsirka SE: Tuftsin fragment 1–3 is beneficial when delivered after the induction of intracerebral hemorrhage. *Stroke* 2005, **36**(3):613–618.

42. Wu J, Yang S, Xi G, Fu G, Keep RF, Hua Y: Minocycline reduces intracerebral hemorrhage-induced brain injury. *Neurol Res* 2009, **31**(2):183–188.

43. Wu J, Yang S, Hua Y, Liu W, Keep RF, Xi G: Minocycline attenuates brain edema, brain atrophy and neurological deficits after intracerebral hemorrhage. *Acta Neurochir Suppl* 2010, **106**:147–150.

44. Zhao F, Hua Y, He Y, Keep RF, Xi G: Minocycline-induced attenuation of iron overload and brain injury after experimental intracerebral hemorrhage. *Stroke* 2011, **42**(12):3587–3593.

45. Wasserman JK, Schlichter LC: Minocycline protects the blood–brain barrier and reduces edema following intracerebral hemorrhage in the rat. *Exp Neurol* 2007, **207**(2):227–237.

46. Wang J, Dore S: Heme oxygenase-1 exacerbates early brain injury after intracerebral haemorrhage. *Brain* 2007, **130**(Pt 6):1643–1652.

47. Turrin NP, Plata-Salaman CR: Cytokine-cytokine interactions and the brain. *Brain Res Bull* 2000, **51**(1):3–9.

48. Emsley HC, Tyrrell PJ: Inflammation and infection in clinical stroke. *J Cereb Blood Flow Metab* 2002, **22**(12):1399–1419.

49. Hua Y, Wu J, Keep RF, Nakamura T, Hoff JT, Xi G: Tumor necrosis factor-α increases in the brain after intracerebral hemorrhage and thrombin stimulation. *Neurosurgery* 2006, **58**(3):542–550. discussion 542–550.

50. Zhang X, Li H, Hu S, Zhang L, Liu C, Zhu C, Liu R, Li C: Brain edema after intracerebral hemorrhage in rats: the role of inflammation. *Neurol India* 2006, **54**(4):402–407.

51. Castillo J, Dávalos A, Alvarez-Sabín J, Pumar JM, Leira R, Silva Y, Montaner J, Kase CS: Molecular signatures of brain injury after intracerebral hemorrhage. *Neurology* 2002, **58**(4):624–629.

52. Chen YC, Hu FJ, Chen P, Wu YR, Wu HC, Chen ST, Lee-Chen GJ, Chen CM: Association of TNF-α gene with spontaneous deep intracerebral hemorrhage in the Taiwan population: a case control study. *BMC Neurol* 2010, **10**:41.

53. Wu J, Yang S, Xi G, Song S, Fu G, Keep RF, Hua Y: Microglial activation and brain injury after intracerebral hemorrhage. *Acta Neurochir Suppl* 2008, **105**:59–65.

54. Holmin S, Mathiesen T: Intracerebral administration of interleukin-1β and induction of inflammation, apoptosis, and vasogenic edema. *J Neurosurg* 2000, **92**(1):108–120.

55. Wagner KR: Modeling intracerebral hemorrhage: glutamate, nuclear factor-κB signaling and cytokines. *Stroke* 2007, **38**(2 Suppl):753–758.

56. Zhao X, Zhang Y, Strong R, Zhang J, Grotta JC, Aronowski J: Distinct patterns of intracerebral hemorrhage-induced alterations in NF-κB subunit, iNOS, and COX-2 expression. *J Neurochem* 2007, **101**(3):652–663.

57. Allan SM, Rothwell NJ: Inflammation in central nervous system injury. *Philos Trans R Soc Lond B Biol Sci* 2003, **358**(1438):1669–1677.

58. Hickenbottom SL, Grotta JC, Strong R, Denner LA, Aronowski J: Nuclear factor-κB and cell death after experimental intracerebral hemorrhage in rats. *Stroke* 1999, **30**(11):2472–2477. discussion 2477–2478.

59. Wang YX, Yan A, Ma ZH, Wang Z, Zhang B, Ping JL, Zhu JS, Zhou Y, Dai L: Nuclear factor-κB and apoptosis in patients with intracerebral hemorrhage. *J Clin Neurosci* 2011, **18**(10):1392–1395.

60. Barton GM, Medzhitov R: Control of adaptive immune responses by Toll-like receptors. *Curr Opin Immunol* 2002, **14**(3):380–383.

61. Brown J, Wang H, Hajishengallis GN, Martin M: TLR-signaling networks: an integration of adaptor molecules, kinases, and cross-talk. *J Dent Res* 2011, **90**(4):417–427.

62. Shi XQ, Zekki H, Zhang J: The role of TLR2 in nerve injury-induced neuropathic pain is essentially mediated through macrophages in peripheral inflammatory response. *Glia* 2011, **59**(2):231–241.

63. Wu FX, Bian JJ, Miao XR, Huang SD, Xu XW, Gong DJ, Sun YM, Lu ZJ, Yu WF: Intrathecal siRNA against Toll-like receptor 4 reduces nociception in a rat model of neuropathic pain. *Int J Med Sci* 2010, **7**(5):251–259.

64. Hanamsagar R, Hanke ML, Kielian T: Toll-like receptor (TLR) and inflammasome actions in the central nervous system. *Trends Immunol* 2012, **33**(7):333–342.

65. Shichita T, Sakaguchi R, Suzuki M, Yoshimura A: Post-ischemic inflammation in the brain. *Front Immunol* 2012, **3**:132.

66. Hyakkoku K, Hamanaka J, Tsuruma K, Shimazawa M, Tanaka H, Uematsu S, Akira S, Inagaki N, Nagai H, Hara H: Toll-like receptor 4 (TLR4), but not TLR3 or TLR9, knock-out mice have neuroprotective effects against focal cerebral ischemia. *Neuroscience* 2010, **171**(1):258–267.

67. Caso JR, Pradillo JM, Hurtado O, Lorenzo P, Moro MA, Lizasoain I: Toll-like receptor 4 is involved in brain damage and inflammation after experimental stroke. *Circulation* 2007, **115**(12):1599–1608.

68. Rodríguez-Yáñez M, Brea D, Arias S, Blanco M, Pumar JM, Castillo J, Sobrino T: Increased expression of Toll-like receptors 2 and 4 is associated with poor outcome in intracerebral hemorrhage. *J Neuroimmunol* 2012, **247**(1–2):75–80.

69. Yang QW, Lu FL, Zhou Y, Wang L, Zhong Q, Lin S, Xiang J, Li JC, Fang CQ, Wang JZ: HMBG1 mediates ischemia-reperfusion injury by TRIF-adaptor independent Toll-like receptor 4 signaling. *J Cereb Blood Flow Metab* 2011, **31**(2):593–605.

70. Carty M, Bowie AG: Evaluating the role of Toll-like receptors in diseases of the central nervous system. *Biochem Pharmacol* 2011, **81**(7):825–837.

71. Aravalli RN, Peterson PK, Lokensgard JR: Toll-like receptors in defense and damage of the central nervous system. *J Neuroimmune Pharmacol* 2007, **2**(4):297–312.

72. Vogl T, Tenbrock K, Ludwig S, Leukert N, Ehrhardt C, van Zoelen MAD, Nacken W, Foell D, van der Poll T, Sorg C, Roth J: Mrp8 and Mrp14 are endogenous activators of Toll-like receptor 4, promoting lethal, endotoxin-induced shock. *Nat Med* 2007, **13**(9):1042–1049.

73. Buchanan MM, Hutchinson M, Watkins LR, Yin H: Toll-like receptor 4 in CNS pathologies. *J Neurochem* 2010, **114**(1):13–27.

74. O'Neill LA: How Toll-like receptors signal: what we know and what we don't know. *Curr Opin Immunol* 2006, **18**(1):3–9.

75. Jochum W, Passegue E, Wagner EF: AP-1 in mouse development and tumorigenesis. *Oncogene* 2001, **20**(19):2401–2412.

76. Kawai T, Akira S: TLR signaling. *Cell Death Differ* 2006, **13**(5):816–825.

77. Vincenti MP, Brinckerhoff CE: Transcriptional regulation of collagenase (MMP-1, MMP-13) genes in arthritis: integration of complex signaling pathways for the recruitment of gene-specific transcription factors. *Arthritis Res Ther* 2002, **4**(3):157–164.

78. Wasserman JK, Zhu X, Schlichter LC: Evolution of the inflammatory response in the brain following intracerebral hemorrhage and effects of delayed minocycline treatment. *Brain Res* 2007, **1180**:140–154.

79. Xue M, Fan Y, Liu S, Zygun DA, Demchuk A, Yong VW: Contributions of multiple proteases to neurotoxicity in a mouse model of intracerebral haemorrhage. *Brain* 2009, **132**:26–36.

80. Michel-Monigadon D, Bonny C, Hirt L: c-Jun N-terminal kinase pathway inhibition in intracerebral hemorrhage. *Cerebrovasc Dis* 2010, **29**(6):564–570.

81. Lively S, Schlichter LC: Age-related comparisons of evolution of the inflammatory response after intracerebral hemorrhage in rats. *Transl Stroke Res* 2012, **3**(Suppl 1):132–146.

82. Boehmer ED, Goral J, Faunce DE, Kovacs EJ: **Age-dependent decrease in Toll-like receptor 4-mediated proinflammatory cytokine production and mitogen-activated protein kinase expression.** *J Leukoc Biol* 2004, **75**(2):342–349.

83. Stewart CR, Stuart LM, Wilkinson K, van Gils JM, Deng J, Halle A, Rayner KJ, Boyer L, Zhong R, Frazier WA, Lacy-Hulbert A, El Khoury J, Golenbock DT, Moore KJ: **CD36 ligands promote sterile inflammation through assembly of a Toll-like receptor 4 and 6 heterodimer.** *Nat Immunol* 2010, **11**(2):155–161.

84. Ohashi K, Burkart V, Flohe S, Kolb H: **Cutting edge: heat shock protein 60 is a putative endogenous ligand of the toll-like receptor-4 complex.** *J Immunol* 2000, **164**(2):558–561.

85. Vabulas RM, Ahmad-Nejad P, Ghose S, Kirschning CJ, Issels RD, Wagner H: **HSP70 as endogenous stimulus of the Toll/interleukin-1 receptor signal pathway.** *J Biol Chem* 2002, **277**(17):15107–15112.

86. Termeer C, Benedix F, Sleeman J, Fieber C, Voith U, Ahrens T, Miyake K, Freudenberg M, Galanos C, Simon JC: **Oligosaccharides of Hyaluronan activate dendritic cells via toll-like receptor 4.** *J Exp Med* 2002, **195**(1):99–111.

87. Taylor KR, Trowbridge JM, Rudisill JA, Termeer CC, Simon JC, Gallo RL: **Hyaluronan fragments stimulate endothelial recognition of injury through TLR4.** *J Biol Chem* 2004, **279**(17):17079–17084.

88. Mata-Haro V, Cekic C, Martin M, Chilton PM, Casella CR, Mitchell TC: **The vaccine adjuvant monophosphoryl lipid A as a TRIF-biased agonist of TLR4.** *Science* 2007, **316**(5831):1628–1632.

89. Gangloff M: **Different dimerisation mode for TLR4 upon endosomal acidification?** *Trends Biochem Sci* 2012, **37**(3):92–98.

90. Schmidt P, Krook H, Goto M, Korsgren O: **MyD88-dependent toll-like receptor signalling is not a requirement for fetal islet xenograft rejection in mice.** *Xenotransplantation* 2004, **11**(4):347–352.

91. Murakami K, Koide M, Dumont TM, Russell SR, Tranmer BI, Wellman GC: **Subarachnoid hemorrhage induces gliosis and increased expression of the pro-inflammatory cytokine high mobility group box 1 protein.** *Transl Stroke Res* 2011, **2**(1):72–79.

92. Ohnishi M, Katsuki H, Fukutomi C, Takahashi M, Motomura M, Fukunaga M, Matsuoka Y, Isohama Y, Izumi Y, Kume T, Inoue A, Akaike A: **HMGB1 inhibitor glycyrrhizin attenuates intracerebral hemorrhage-induced injury in rats.** *Neuropharmacology* 2011, **61**(5–6):975–980.

93. Kanzler H, Barrat FJ, Hessel EM, Coffman RL: **Therapeutic targeting of innate immunity with Toll-like receptor agonists and antagonists.** *Nat Med* 2007, **13**(5):552–559.

94. Liu X, Zheng J, Zhou H: **TLRs as pharmacological targets for plant-derived compounds in infectious and inflammatory diseases.** *Int Immunopharmacol* 2011, **11**(10):1451–1456.

95. Gearing AJ: **Targeting toll-like receptors for drug development: a summary of commercial approaches.** *Immunol Cell Biol* 2007, **85**(6):490–494.

96. Park SJ, Kang SH, Kang YK, Eom YB, Koh KO, Kim DY, Youn HS: **Inhibition of homodimerization of Toll-like receptor 4 by 4-oxo-4-(2-oxo-oxazolidin-3-yl)-but-2-enoic acid ethyl ester.** *Int Immunopharmacol* 2011, **11**(1):19–22.

97. Youn HS, Saitoh SI, Miyake K, Hwang DH: **Inhibition of homodimerization of Toll-like receptor 4 by curcumin.** *Biochem Pharmacol* 2006, **72**(1):62–69.

98. Ahn SI, Lee JK, Youn HS: **Inhibition of homodimerization of toll-like receptor 4 by 6-shogaol.** *Mol Cells* 2009, **27**(2):211–215.

99. Park SJ, Youn HS: **Suppression of homodimerization of Toll-like receptor 4 by isoliquiritigenin.** *Phytochemistry* 2010, **71**(14–15):1736–1740.

100. Liang Q, Wu Q, Jiang J, Duan J, Wang C, Smith MD, Lu H, Wang Q, Nagarkatti P, Fan D: **Characterization of sparstolonin B, a Chinese herb-derived compound, as a selective Toll-like receptor antagonist with potent anti-inflammatory properties.** *J Biol Chem* 2011, **286**(30):26470–26479.

101. Park SJ, Lee AN, Youn HS: **TBK1-targeted suppression of TRIF-dependent signaling pathway of toll-like receptor 3 by auranofin.** *Arch Pharm Res* 2010, **33**(6):939–945.

102. Kuno M, Nemoto K, Ninomiya N, Inagaki E, Kubota M, Matsumoto T, Yokota H: **The novel selective toll-like receptor 4 signal transduction inhibitor tak-242 prevents endotoxaemia in conscious guinea-pigs.** *Clin Exp Pharmacol Physiol* 2009, **36**(5–6):589–593.

103. Nakamura M, Shimizu Y, Sato Y, Miyazaki Y, Satoh T, Mizuno M, Kato Y, Hosaka Y, Furusako S: **Toll-like receptor 4 signal transduction inhibitor, M62812, suppresses endothelial cell and leukocyte activation and prevents lethal septic shock in mice.** *Eur J Pharmacol* 2007, **569**(3):237–243.

104. Huang M, Hu YY, Dong XQ, Xu QP, Yu WH, Zhang ZY: **The protective role of oxymatrine on neuronal cell apoptosis in the hemorrhagic rat brain.** *J Ethnopharmacol* 2012, **143**(1):228–235.

105. Yu WH, Dong XQ, Hu YY, Huang M, Zhang ZY: **Ginkgolide B reduces neuronal cell apoptosis in the traumatic rat brain: possible involvement of Toll-like receptor 4 and nuclear factor κB pathway.** *Phytother Res* 2012, **26**(12):1838–1844.

106. Wang Z, Zuo G, Shi XY, Zhang J, Fang Q, Chen G: **Progesterone administration modulates cortical TLR4/NF-κB signaling pathway after subarachnoid hemorrhage in male rats.** *Mediators Inflamm* 2011, 2011:848309.

107. Tasaki K, Ruetzler CA, Ohtsuki T, Martin D, Nawashiro H, Hallenbeck JM: **Lipopolysaccharide pre-treatment induces resistance against subsequent focal cerebral ischemic damage in spontaneously hypertensive rats.** *Brain Res* 1997, **748**(1–2):267–270.

108. Rosenzweig HL, Lessov NS, Henshall DC, Minami M, Simon RP, Stenzel-Poore MP: **Endotoxin preconditioning prevents cellular inflammatory response during ischemic neuroprotection in mice.** *Stroke* 2004, **35**(11):2576–2581.

109. Vartanian KB, Stevens SL, Marsh BJ, Williams-Karnesky R, Lessov NS, Stenzel-Poore MP: **LPS preconditioning redirects TLR signaling following stroke: TRIF-IRF3 plays a seminal role in mediating tolerance to ischemic injury.** *J Neuroinflammation* 2011, **8**:140.

110. Stevens SL, Leung PY, Vartanian KB, Gopalan B, Yang T, Simon RP, Stenzel-Poore MP: **Multiple preconditioning paradigms converge on interferon regulatory factor-dependent signaling to promote tolerance to ischemic brain injury.** *J Neurosci* 2011, **31**(23):8456–8463.

111. Wagner KR, Sharp FR, Ardizzone TD, Lu A, Clark JF: **Heme and iron metabolism: role in cerebral hemorrhage.** *J Cereb Blood Flow Metab* 2003, **23**(6):629–652.

112. Zhao X, Song S, Sun G, Strong R, Zhang J, Grotta JC, Aronowski J: **Neuroprotective role of haptoglobin after intracerebral hemorrhage.** *J Neurosci* 2009, **29**(50):15819–15827.

113. Zhao X, Sun G, Zhang J, Strong R, Dash PK, Kan YW, Grotta JC, Aronowski J: **Transcription factor Nrf2 protects the brain from damage produced by intracerebral hemorrhage.** *Stroke* 2007, **38**(12):3280–3286.

114. Chen G, Fang Q, Zhang J, Zhou D, Wang Z: **Role of the Nrf2-ARE pathway in early brain injury after experimental subarachnoid hemorrhage.** *J Neurosci Res* 2011, **89**(4):515–523.

115. Fadok VA, Warner ML, Bratton DL, Henson PM: **CD36 is required for phagocytosis of apoptotic cells by human macrophages that use either a phosphatidylserine receptor or the vitronectin receptor ($\alpha_v\beta_3$).** *J Immunol* 1998, **161**(11):6250–6257.

116. Ren Y, Silverstein RL, Allen J, Savill J: **CD36 gene transfer confers capacity for phagocytosis of cells undergoing apoptosis.** *J Exp Med* 1995, **181**(5):1857–1862.

117. Zhao X, Zhang Y, Strong R, Grotta JC, Aronowski J: **15d-prostaglandin J2 activates peroxisome proliferator-activated receptor-γ, promotes expression of catalase, and reduces inflammation, behavioral dysfunction, and neuronal loss after intracerebral hemorrhage in rats.** *J Cereb Blood Flow Metab* 2006, **26**(6):811–820.

118. Beutler B: **Inferences, questions and possibilities in Toll-like receptor signalling.** *Nature* 2004, **430**(6996):257–263.

Permissions

The contributors of this book come from diverse backgrounds, making this book a truly international effort. This book will bring forth new frontiers with its revolutionizing research information and detailed analysis of the nascent developments around the world.

We would like to thank all the contributing authors for lending their expertise to make the book truly unique. They have played a crucial role in the development of this book. Without their invaluable contributions this book wouldn't have been possible. They have made vital efforts to compile up to date information on the varied aspects of this subject to make this book a valuable addition to the collection of many professionals and students.

This book was conceptualized with the vision of imparting up-to-date information and advanced data in this field. To ensure the same, a matchless editorial board was set up. Every individual on the board went through rigorous rounds of assessment to prove their worth. After which they invested a large part of their time researching and compiling the most relevant data for our readers.

The editorial board has been involved in producing this book since its inception. They have spent rigorous hours researching and exploring the diverse topics which have resulted in the successful publishing of this book. They have passed on their knowledge of decades through this book. To expedite this challenging task, the publisher supported the team at every step. A small team of assistant editors was also appointed to further simplify the editing procedure and attain best results for the readers.

Apart from the editorial board, the designing team has also invested a significant amount of their time in understanding the subject and creating the most relevant covers. They scrutinized every image to scout for the most suitable representation of the subject and create an appropriate cover for the book.

The publishing team has been an ardent support to the editorial, designing and production team. Their endless efforts to recruit the best for this project, has resulted in the accomplishment of this book. They are a veteran in the field of academics and their pool of knowledge is as vast as their experience in printing. Their expertise and guidance has proved useful at every step. Their uncompromising quality standards have made this book an exceptional effort. Their encouragement from time to time has been an inspiration for everyone.

The publisher and the editorial board hope that this book will prove to be a valuable piece of knowledge for researchers, students, practitioners and scholars across the globe.

List of Contributors

Xiang-Dong Zhu, Jing-Sen Chen, Feng Zhou, Qi-Chang Liu, Gao Chen and Jian-Min Zhang
Department of Neurosurgery, The Second Affiliated Hospital, School of Medicine, Zhejiang University, 88 Jiefang Road, Hangzhou 310000, PR China

Frederick Bonsack IV, Cargill H. Alleyne Jr and Sangeetha Sukumari-Ramesh
Department of Neurosurgery, Medical College of Georgia, Augusta University, 1120 15th Street, CA1010, Augusta, GA 30912, USA

Ze-Li Zhang and Qi-Bing Huang
Department of Emergency Surgery, Qilu Hospital of Shandong University, No. 107 Wenhuaxi Road, 250012 Jinan, Shandong Province, People's Republic of China

Yu-Guang Liu, Hong-Wei Wang, Yan Song, Zhen-Kuan Xu and Feng Li
Department of Neurosurgery, Qilu Hospital of Shandong University and Brain Science Research Institute of Shandong University, No. 107 Wenhuaxi Road, 250012 Jinan, Shandong Province, People's Republic of China

Khalid A Hanafy
Division of NeuroCritical Care, Department of Neurology, Harvard Medical School, Beth Israel Deaconess Medical Center, The Center for Life Science, 3 Blackfan Circle, Boston, MA 02215, USA

Min Chen, Xifeng Li, Xin Zhang, Xuying He, Lingfeng Lai, Guohui Zhu, Wei Li, Hui Li, Qinrui Fang, Zequn Wang and Chuanzhi Duan
The National Key Clinic Specialty, The Neurosurgery Institute of Guangdong Province, Guangdong Provincial Key Laboratory on Brain Function Repair and Regeneration, Department of Neurosurgery, Zhujiang Hospital, Southern Medical University, Guangzhou 510282, China

Yanchao Liu
Department of Neurosurgery, The First People's Hospital of Foshan and Foshan Hospital of Sun Yat Sen University, Foshan, Guangdong 528000, China

Jie Wu, Liang Sun, Haiying Li, Haitao Shen, Weiwei Zhai, Zhengquan Yu and Gang Chen
Department of Neurosurgery & Brain and Nerve Research Laboratory, The First Affiliated Hospital of Soochow University, 188 Shizi Street, Suzhou, Jiangsu Province 215006, China

Hans Worthmann, Meike Dirks, Ramona Schuppner and Karin Weissenborn
Department of Neurology, Hannover Medical School, 30623 Hannover, Germany

Na Li
Department of Neurology, Hannover Medical School, 30623 Hannover, Germany
Department of Neurology, Beijing Tiantan Hospital, Capital Medical University, Beijing, China

Jens Martens-Lobenhoffer and Stefanie M. Bode-Böger
Department of Clinical Pharmacology, Otto-von-Guericke-University of Magdeburg, University Hospital, Magdeburg, Germany

Ralf Lichtinghagen
Department of Clinical Chemistry, Hannover Medical School, Hannover, Germany.

Jan T. Kielstein
Department of Nephrology and Hypertension, Hannover Medical School, Hannover, Germany
Medical Clinic V, Academic Teaching Hospital Braunschweig, Braunschweig, Germany

Peter Raab and Heinrich Lanfermann
Institute of Diagnostic and Interventional Neuroradiology, Hannover Medical School, Hannover, Germany

Jun Zeng, Yizhao Chen, Zhichong Xie and Shizhong Zheng
Department of Neurosurgery, Zhujiang Hospital, The National Key Clinical Specialty, The Neurosurgery Institute of Guangdong Province, Guangdong Provincial Key Laboratory on Brain Function Repair and Regeneration, The Engineering Technology Research Center of Education Ministry of China, Southern Medical University, Guangzhou 510282, China

Rui Ding
Department of Neurosurgery, Jingmen No. 1 People's Hospital, Jingmen 448000, Hubei, China

Liang Feng
Department of Neurosurgery, Affiliated Hospital of Xiangnan University, Chenzhou 423000, Hunan, China

Zhenghao Fu
Department of Neurosurgery, The Fifth Affiliated Hospital of Southern Medical University, Guangzhou 510900, Guangdong, China

Shuo Yang
Department of Neurosurgery, Gaoqing Campus of Central Hospital of Zibo, Gaoqing People's Hospital, Gaoqing, Zibo 256300, Shandong, China

Xinqing Deng
Department of Neurosurgery, 999 Brain Hospital, Jinan University, Guangzhou 510510, Guangdong, China

Liang Feng, Yizhao Chen and Jun Zeng
The National Key Clinical Specialty, The Engineering Technology Research Center of Education Ministry of China, Guangdong Provincial Key Laboratory on Brain Function Repair and Regeneration, Department of Neurosurgery, Zhujiang Hospital, Southern Medical University, Guangzhou 510282, China

Rui Ding
Department of Neurosurgery, Jingmen No. 1 People's Hospital, Jingmen 448000Hubei, China

Zhenghao Fu
Department of Neurosurgery, The Fifth Affiliated Hospital of Southern Medical University, Guangzhou 510900, China

Shuo Yang
Department of Neurosurgery, Gaoqing Campus of Central Hospital of Zibo, Gaoqing People's Hospital, Gaoqing, Zibo 256300 Shandong, China

Xinqing Deng
Department of Neurosurgery, 999 Brain Hospital, Jinan University, Guangzhou 510510 Guangdong, China

Hengli Zhao, Pengyu Pan, Yang Yang, Hongfei Ge, Weixiang Chen, Jie Qu, Jiantao Shi, Gaoyu Cui, Xin Liu, Hua Feng and Yujie Chen
Department of Neurosurgery, Southwest Hospital, Third Military Medical University, 29 Gaotanyan Street, Shapingba District, Chongqing 400038, China

Bo Ma, Jason Patrick Day, Harrison Phillips and Bryan Slootsky
Department of Anesthesiology, Center for Translational Research in Neurodegenerative Disease, University of Florida College of Medicine, Gainesville, FL 32610, USA

Sylvain Doré
Department of Anesthesiology, Center for Translational Research in Neurodegenerative Disease, University of Florida College of Medicine, Gainesville, FL 32610, USA
Departments of Neuroscience, Neurology, Psychiatry, Psychology and Pharmaceutics, University of Florida College of Medicine, Gainesville, FL 32610, USA

Emanuela Tolosano
Departments of Molecular Biotechnology and Health Sciences, University of Torino, Torino, Italy

Slaven Pikija, Constantin Hecker and Christian Ramesmayer
Department of Neurology, Christian Doppler Medical Center, Paracelsus Medical University, Ignaz-Harrer-Straße 79, 5020 Salzburg, Austria

Johann Sellner
Department of Neurology, Christian Doppler Medical Center, Paracelsus Medical University, Ignaz-Harrer-Straße 79, 5020 Salzburg, Austria
Department of Neurology, Klinikum rechts der Isar, Technische Universität München, Munich, Germany

Laszlo K. Sztriha
Department of Neurology, King's College Hospital, Denmark Hill, London, UK

Monika Killer-Oberpfalzer
Research Institute for Neurointervention, Christian Doppler Medical Center, Paracelsus Medical University, Salzburg, Austria

Friedrich Weymayr
Division of Neuroradiology, Christian Doppler Medical Center, Paracelsus Medical University, Salzburg, Austria

Larissa Hauer
Department of Psychiatry, Psychotherapy and Psychosomatics, Christian Doppler Medical Center, Paracelsus Medical University, Salzburg, Austria

Chun-Hu Wu and Chai-You Lai
Department of Physiology and Biophysics, National Defense Medical Center, Taipei, Taiwan, Republic of China
Graduate Institute of Life Sciences, National Defense Medical Center, Taipei, Taiwan, Republic of China

Chien-Cheng Chen and Chao-Chang Lin
Department of Physical Medicine and Rehabilitation, Cheng Hsin General Hospital, Taipei, Taiwan, Republic of China

Szu-Fu Chen
Department of Physiology and Biophysics, National Defense Medical Center, Taipei, Taiwan, Republic of China
Department of Physical Medicine and Rehabilitation, Cheng Hsin General Hospital, Taipei, Taiwan, Republic of China

Tai-Ho Hung
Department of Obstetrics and Gynecology, Chang Gung Memorial Hospital at Taipei and College of Medicine, Chang Gung University, Taipei, Taiwan, Republic of China

Min Chao
School of Medicine, National Defense Medical Center, Taipei, Taiwan, Republic of China

Robert H. LeBlanc III, Ruiya Chen and Magdy H. Selim
Department of Neurology, Beth Israel Deaconess Medical Center, Harvard Medical School, 3 Blackfan Circle, Boston, MA 02140, USA

Khalid A. Hanafy
Department of Neurology, Beth Israel Deaconess Medical Center, Harvard Medical School, 3 Blackfan Circle, Boston, MA 02140, USA
Division of Neurointensive Care Medicine, Beth Israel Deaconess Medical Center, Harvard Medical School, 3 Blackfan Circle, Boston, MA 02140, USA

Huang Fang, Peng-Fei Wang, Yu Zhou, Yan-Chun Wang and Qing-Wu Yang
Department of Neurology, Second Affiliated Hospital and Xinqiao Hospital, Third Military Medical University, Xinqiao Zhengjie No.183, Shapingba District, Chongqing 400037, China

Index

A

Alzheimer's Disease, 2, 24, 59, 70, 113, 116, 134, 143-144, 167-168

Aneurysmal Subarachnoid Hemorrhage, 1, 11-12, 34, 42-43, 78, 182

Anti-inflammatory Phenotype, 58, 64

Antioxidant Pathway, 79-80, 91

Asymmetric Dimethylarginine, 71, 77-78

B

Basal Ganglia Hemorrhage, 27-28

Blood-brain Barrier, 10, 32, 44-46, 50, 55-57, 77, 79-80, 95, 97, 113, 128, 130-132, 134, 143, 152-153, 155, 168, 184, 186, 189, 191-192

Body Mass Index (BMI), 147

Brain Injury, 9, 11, 13-14, 17, 20-21, 26, 33, 45, 56, 58-59, 61, 68-71, 74, 77, 79-81, 87, 91, 94-99, 106, 109-116, 128, 133, 137, 140, 144, 163, 168, 177, 182, 184-193

Brain Oedema, 96, 115, 127-128, 130

C

Cellular Apoptosis, 184

Central Nervous System, 11, 13, 20, 24, 45, 59, 69-70, 94-95, 115-116, 128, 131, 134, 143, 165, 168, 191-192

Cerebrospinal Fluid, 2, 9, 11, 72, 77-78

Cerebrovasospasm, 1-8, 10

Cytokine, 1-2, 9, 11, 15, 17, 39, 41, 46, 49, 56-57, 64, 84, 88, 96, 166, 186-189, 192-193

Cytoplasm, 28, 31, 54-55, 86

Cytotoxic Edema, 71-75, 78

D

Deferoxamine, 169-174, 176-177, 181-183

Dimethylarginine, 71-72, 75, 77-78

Drug Delivery, 81, 101

E

Edema, 25, 28-33, 44-45, 51-54, 56, 71-78, 80, 85, 91, 95, 99, 101, 103, 106, 113-114, 118, 122, 130, 132, 153, 155, 158-160, 165, 168, 170, 177, 184, 186, 189, 192

Endovascular Thrombectomy, 145, 150

F

Fluorescence Intensity, 14-16, 18-20, 62, 66-67, 82

Functional Outcome, 1, 4, 6, 10, 24, 27, 29, 32, 70, 75, 77, 145, 151, 167, 186

G

Glycyrrhiza Uralensis, 95-97

H

Hematoma Enlargement, 71-77

Hematoma Resolution, 42, 184, 188-192

Heme Oxygenase, 34, 80, 95, 97, 133-134, 143-144, 169-170, 181-182, 189, 191-192

Hemoglobin, 21, 24, 34, 56, 72, 94-97, 99, 113, 133-135, 137-144, 153, 155, 157, 159, 177, 182-184, 189, 191

Hemopexin, 133-134, 143-144, 189

Hemorrhagic Lesion, 50-51, 98, 103, 107

Hemorrhagic Stroke, 3, 33, 42, 76, 133, 153, 159, 169, 177, 181-182, 191

High-mobility Group Box 1 (HMGB1), 1-2, 11

Hydrogen Sulfide, 115, 132

I

Immunohistochemistry, 14, 22, 27-28, 32, 36, 38-39, 41, 46, 49, 51, 79, 81, 95, 133, 135, 154, 156, 162

Inducible Nitric Oxide Synthase, 44, 52, 77, 98-99, 107, 146, 186, 190

Inflammasome Activation, 79-80, 89, 94, 96-100, 102, 105, 110-113, 115-118, 120, 123-125, 128, 130-132

Inflammation, 1-2, 9-11, 13, 19-20, 26, 28, 31, 35, 41, 44-45, 54, 56-59, 64, 66, 70, 77, 90, 97, 113, 125, 132, 143-147, 152-153, 166-168, 177, 184-189, 191-193

Interleukin, 11, 15, 24-25, 32-33, 57, 70, 77, 80, 95, 98-99, 102, 105, 110, 112, 124, 128, 130, 157, 161, 167, 173, 181, 185, 191-193

Intracerebral Hemorrhage, 3, 5, 7, 9, 13, 19, 28, 32-34, 41, 44, 55-59, 69-72, 77-81, 95-100, 102, 113, 132-134, 143-145, 151-154, 159, 168, 181-184, 191-193

Intracerebroventricular Injection, 34, 37, 60, 65-66, 82, 101, 117, 144, 170

Ischaemic Stroke, 25, 116, 144

Isoliquiritigenin, 79-80, 95-97, 189, 193

L

Leukocytes, 111, 156, 161, 185-188, 190-191

Lymphocyte Ratio, 76, 78, 145-146, 148-151

M

Macrophage, 13, 15, 17-24, 34-35, 42, 70, 88, 94, 97, 144, 155-157, 161, 167-170, 172, 175, 177, 179, 181, 185, 187-188, 192

Mesenchymal Stem Cell, 44-45, 55-56, 167

Methylene Blue Assay, 116, 118

Microglia, 9, 13, 17-26, 34-35, 39, 42, 45, 49, 51, 54, 61, 64, 66-70, 72, 77, 88, 97, 100, 108, 111, 115, 117-118, 121, 128, 134, 144, 153, 155-158, 177, 179, 182, 185-192

Microglia Polarization, 58-59, 61, 64, 66, 68-69

Microglial Activation, 13, 19, 23-24, 26, 113, 132, 134, 138-139, 142, 152-153, 161-163, 165-166, 168, 185-188, 192

Microglial Cell, 39, 126-128, 136, 172

Monocytes, 72, 76-78, 100, 111, 113, 161, 186

Mortality, 1-10, 13, 28, 34, 45, 72, 80, 96, 98, 116, 134, 136, 145-147, 149, 151, 153, 170, 177, 181, 184

Msc Transplantation, 48, 50

Myeloperoxidase, 49, 83, 95, 98, 104, 112, 119, 121, 123, 130, 156, 167

N

Neurobehavioral Deterioration, 80

Neurobehavioural Function, 118

Neuroinflammation, 2, 11, 13, 20, 23-26, 33, 42-43, 56, 70, 78, 96-97, 99, 111, 113, 115-116, 130, 132, 151-152, 166-168, 170, 177, 182, 191, 193

Neuronal Apoptosis, 34, 37-43, 104, 107, 127, 170, 182

Neuroprotection, 23-25, 57, 96, 113, 127, 144, 150, 153, 165-167, 169-170, 173-174, 177, 179, 181-182, 190, 193

Neutrophil, 44, 57, 76-78, 98, 106, 108, 111, 120, 123, 127, 131-132, 145-146, 148-152, 161-162, 165-166, 168, 177, 185, 191

Nitric Oxide Synthase, 32, 44, 52, 72, 77-78, 97-99, 107, 113, 146, 186, 190

O

Oligodendrocyte, 144

Oxidative Damage, 153, 184

Oxidative Stress Injury, 144

Oxyhemoglobin, 34, 42, 58

P

Perihematomal Brain Tissue, 27-28, 85, 92, 95

Peroxynitrite, 44, 55-57, 76-77, 96-99, 109, 111-113, 132

Phagocytosis, 25, 133-134, 136, 138, 140, 142, 144, 185, 189-190, 193

Pro-inflammatory Cytokine, 11, 193

Programmed Death Protein, 58, 69

Protein Level, 3, 7, 63-64, 66, 86, 159

S

Stroma-free Hemoglobin, 133, 143

Subarachnoid Hemorrhage, 1-2, 11-12, 34-37, 39-43, 72, 77-78, 96, 132, 146, 169-170, 173-174, 182-183, 188-191, 193

Synthetic Liver, 152, 167

T

Thrombectomy, 145, 150-151

Tlr4 Pathway, 34-35, 37, 39, 41, 182

Trypsinization, 60

V

Vasospasm, 3, 5-7, 9-12, 34-43, 78, 169-170, 173-174, 177, 182-183

www.ingramcontent.com/pod-product-compliance
Lightning Source LLC
Chambersburg PA
CBHW082014190326
41458CB00010B/3190